Praise for *Reversing A*

"It is the dawn of the era of treatable Alzheimer's and pre-Alzheimer's—after more than a century of failure, reports are appearing documenting success after success. *Reversing Alzheimer's* by Dr. Timothy Smith provides clear explanations of the disease mechanisms and a practical, useful approach to combat this scourge. I recommend this book wholeheartedly."

> —Dale Bredesen, MD, author of the *New York Times* bestseller *The End of Alzheimer's*

"Alzheimer's is a dreaded and increasingly common diagnosis for millions of people and their families every year. Drawing on the most recent research and clinical applications, Dr. Smith provides an evidence-based, practical, and effective guide for individuals to prevent and even reverse early-stage neuropsychological disorders. His book is an optimistic blend of science and hope."

> —Kenneth R. Pelletier, PhD, MD, Clinical Professor of Medicine, UC San Francisco School of Medicine, and author of *Change Your Genes, Change Your Life*

"Alzheimer's and dementia are often optional! About half the people diagnosed with Alzheimer's don't even have it. They have other treatable conditions that are being missed. Meanwhile, research shows that metabolic factors have a profound impact on cognitive function, as well as Alzheimer's risk and severity. Sadly, physicians are simply not taught about this research. This book will empower *you* to help you and your loved ones recover!"

> —Jacob Teitelbaum MD, author of *From Fatigued to Fantastic!*

"As someone working daily with cognitively impaired individuals and seeing great results, I can vouch for Dr. Timothy Smith's approach! He provides a powerful, practical, easy-to-follow road map to both prevention and reversal of Alzheimer's disease! Highly recommended!"

—Ann Hathaway, MD, functional medicine physician, Bredesen Protocol researcher, and Director, Orthomolecular Health Medicine Board

"The best health book I have read in years. Dr. Smith describes the neurodegenerative process in an easy-to-understand way. Dementia is not inevitable, and *Reversing Alzheimer's* proves that."

—Stephen Langer, MD, author of *Solved: The Riddle of Illness*

"Utilizing the latest research, Dr. Smith reveals the real causes of Alzheimer's and helps each of us create a personalized, comprehensive treatment program to ensure that our own central nervous system—including our brain—achieves and stays in optimal condition."

—Kani Comstock, author of *Journey into Love*

REVERSING ALZHEIMER'S

REVERSING ALZHEIMER'S

How to Prevent Dementia and Revitalize Your Brain

Timothy J. Smith, MD

HIDDEN PATH PUBLISHERS

Hidden Path Publishers
www.hiddenpathpublishers.com

Disclaimer: This book is not intended for use in the treatment or prevention of disease or as a substitute for medical treatment or as an alternative to medical advice. All matters regarding your health require medical supervision. Please consult your physician or health professional before beginning any diet or fitness program as well as about any condition that may require diagnosis or medical attention.

Every attempt has been made to present accurate and timely information. This field is constantly changing, which will account for many of the changes in references, resources, information, statistics, technology, approaches, or techniques that no doubt will occur by the time this book is purchased or read.

The author and publisher assume neither liability nor responsibility to any person or entity with respect to any direct or indirect loss or damage caused, or alleged to be caused, by the information contained herein, or for errors, omissions, inaccuracies, or any other inconsistency within these pages, or for unintentional slights against people or organizations.

ORDERING INFORMATION

Quantity sales. Special discounts are available on quantity purchases by corporations, associations, and others. For details, contact the "Special Sales Department" at the address above.

Orders by US trade bookstores and wholesalers. Please contact BCH: (800) 431-1579 or visit www.bookch.com for details.

Printed in the United States.

First Edition

Cataloging-in-Publication Data

Names: Smith, Timothy J., author.
Title: Reversing Alzheimer's : how to prevent dementia and revitalize your brain / Timothy J. Smith, MD
Description: Includes bibliographical references and index. | Graton, CA: Hidden Path Publishers, 2020.
Identifiers: LCCN: 2020910412 | ISBN: 978-1-7350480-2-4
Subjects: LCSH Alzheimer's disease--Prevention. | Alzheimer's disease--Treatment. | Alzheimer's disease--Research. | Alzheimer's disease--Nutritional aspects. | Alzheimer's disease--Physiological aspects. | Integrative medicine. | BISAC HEALTH & FITNESS / Diseases / Alzheimer's & Dementia | MEDICAL / Holistic Medicine.
Classification: LCC RC523.2 .S625 2020 | DDC 616.8/311--dc23

26 25 24 23 22 21   10 9 8 7 6 5 4 3 2 1

Text designer: Marin Bookworks
Editor: PeopleSpeak

This book is dedicated to Elizabeth Foote-Smith, my amazing mother—
and to each and every Alzheimer's patient the world over,
their families, and their caregivers.

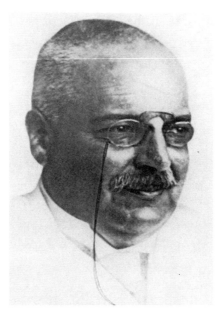

Alois Alzheimer (1864–1915).
The original of this portrait is kept in the historical library of the
Max Planck Institute of Neurobiology, Martinsried, Germany.

Contents

Preface..ix

Introduction: A Dramatic Breakthrough...1

Part 1. The Problem and the Solution...5

Chapter 1.   What Is Alzheimer's Disease?...9

Chapter 2.   How to Prevent and Reverse Alzheimer's.........................21

Chapter 3.   How We Would Treat Mom's Alzheimer's Today..............26

Chapter 4.   Alois Alzheimer and the Discovery of
             Alzheimer's Disease..38

Chapter 5.   Two Exceptionally Long Droughts and the Discovery
             of the Multiple Modality Model.......................................45

Chapter 6.   The Search for a Cure..50

Chapter 7.   Vascular Dementia and My Stroke of Luck.......................55

Chapter 8.   Neuroplasticity, Neurogenesis, Neuroregeneration,
             and the Power of Exercise..62

Part 2. Biomarker Testing: Identifying the Causes of Alzheimer's.....73

Chapter 9.   Testing Your Alzheimer's Biomarkers—Why and How.....75

Chapter 10. High Blood Pressure Causes Vascular Dementia................84

Chapter 11. High Blood Sugar Shrinks Your Memory Centers.............90

Chapter 12. High Cholesterol Promotes Alzheimer's Disease.............104

Chapter 13. B-Complex Vitamins Reverse Cognitive Decline.............109

Chapter 14. Vitamin D Defeats Dementia...115

Chapter 15. Sleep Apnea Increases Dementia Risk.............................121

Chapter 16. The Human Microbiome and the Gut-Brain Connection...131

Chapter 17. A Healthy Thyroid Prevents Cognitive Decline...145

Chapter 18. Neurotoxic Metals Can Ravage Your Brain...161

Chapter 19. Bioidentical Estradiol Prevents Neurodegeneration
in Women...175

Part 3. Your Anti-Alzheimer's Diet...183

Chapter 20. Eating to Reverse Cognitive Decline...185

Chapter 21. The Very Low-Carb Ketogenic Diet...197

Chapter 22. Autophagy: A Powerful Anti-Alzheimer's Weapon...205

Chapter 23. Coconut Oil and MCTs: Brain Food...213

Chapter 24. Polyphenols: Miracle-Gro for Your Brain...218

Chapter 25. Blueberries: Brain-Boosting Bonanza...224

Chapter 26. Cocoa and Chocolate: Memory-Boosting Superfoods...233

Part 4. Nutritional Supplements That Reverse Alzheimer's...243

Chapter 27. Low-Dose Lithium Reverses Dementia...247

Chapter 28. DHA and Flaxseed Oil: The Omega-3 Brain Power Oils...254

Chapter 29. Curcumin: The Secret to India's Low Alzheimer's Rate?...263

Chapter 30. Green Tea: Jack-of-All-Trades...270

Chapter 31. Citicoline: Potent Stroke Protection...272

Chapter 32. Bacopa: Botanical Brain Booster...279

Chapter 33. Phosphatidylserine: Guarding against Cognitive Decline...283

Chapter 34. Berberine: Protection against Vascular Dementia...288

Conclusion: Epigenetics and the Future of Alzheimer's Research...295

Appendix 1. Laboratory Test Order...301

Appendix 2. High-Polyphenol Foods...303

Notes...307

Acknowledgments...333

Index...335

About the Author...353

Preface

As a physician, I have witnessed the horrors of Alzheimer's countless times. The disease killed my mother and three of her four siblings. Watching my patients and loved ones slip into confusion and forgetfulness is dreadful—the mental memory slates of their minds gradually and systematically wiped clean, including even their own identities. Perhaps more frightening is their inability to care for themselves and protect themselves from danger.

My mother, Elizabeth Foote-Smith, was an intelligent and accomplished woman—a college professor, author, researcher, musician, and artist. But despite her exceptional brain, Mom ended up completely demented—slumped in a wheelchair in a nursing home, her brain riddled with damage—incapable of understanding who or where she was. No words can express how sad this is. I believe that if we knew twenty years ago what we know today, her Alzheimer's probably could have been prevented.

Mom maintained an enviable level of physical and cognitive health through her seventies and early eighties, writing books and research papers, maintaining an active social life, managing a household with two dogs, and exercising every day. Mom was always feisty, but as she moved into her mideighties, she became withdrawn, irritable, paranoid, cantankerous, and argumentative; she'd quibble over trivialities. She started misplacing things and forgetting names.

Searching for answers, I turned to the dementia literature. After all, about a hundred years had passed since Alois Alzheimer, MD, published the first accounts of the disease named after him, billions of research dollars had been spent, and thousands of researchers had generated tens of thousands of papers—so I figured I'd find some ideas that might help. I figured wrong. To my astonishment and disappointment, the literature pointed to no medication, no treatment of any kind, that could favorably impact the course of my mother's disease or even relieve her symptoms, and she slowly declined.

In the last few months of her life, Mom did not know who or where she was. She couldn't identify people or objects. One day I took her for a ride out to the beach at Bodega Bay, and when we got back, I asked her if she knew where we had been. She shook her head.

I once rolled her wheelchair over to the piano. Four years earlier she had done performances of Rachmaninoff and Beethoven for family and friends and could discuss the deeper meaning of classical music; now she stared blankly at the keyboard, unable to play a single note, unable to even remember what the piano was for.

One morning, a nurse's aide got Mom out of bed and into her wheelchair and pushed her down the hall, dropping her off in front of the nurses' station so they could keep an eye on her. The aide neglected to fasten Mom's seatbelt, but no one noticed this seemingly innocuous error. Unable to remember that she couldn't stand or walk, Mom tried to get out of the wheelchair. She fell and fractured her femur (thigh bone). She was writhing on the floor in agonizing pain. Fortunately, a nurse saw her fall, knew the femur was fractured, and quickly gave Mom a morphine shot.

Mom was moved to a nearby hospital. She never regained consciousness. She died ten days later.

That was seventeen years ago. If Mom went into cognitive decline today, we would deploy the wealth of tools I discuss in this book. We'd diagnose the causes of her brain disease and reverse them. Her prognosis would be exceptionally good.

In the last seventeen years, our scientific understanding of how the brain works has seen exponential growth. We discovered that our brains possess the fantastic ability to grow new neurons from stem cells as needed and can rapidly change their structure and function in response to environment and experience. We also now realize that Alzheimer's disease is caused by multiple metabolic disruptions. Although this new understanding of Alzheimer's came too late for my mother, it has catapulted us into a dramatically different mind-set. It has become compellingly clear that in each patient we must identify and repair the unique biochemical malfunctions that are causing the disease.

I hope you find this book useful. If it helps you and your loved ones, I am certain that this would have made my mother very happy.

A Dramatic Breakthrough

Over one hundred years ago, in 1915, Alois Alzheimer, MD, died in obscurity in Europe after having described the disease that carries his name. The century since his death has brought remarkable research developments, but one thing hasn't changed: we still have no effective medicines for this deadly disease—nothing that relieves its symptoms or arrests its relentless progression—and definitely no cure.

The toll continues to mount. According to the Alzheimer's Association, one in three of us alive today will die with dementia.

In the past hundred years we've progressed from horses and trains to jet planes and rocket ships. We've transcended scribbled notes and typewriters, moving to word processors and computers that can think, remember, and do Google searches for anything we can imagine. We've gone from telegraphs and single-wire party-line telephones to an incredible global communications network where we can talk with just about anybody, anywhere, anytime.

In science and medicine, we've got magnetic resonance imaging (MRI), robotic surgery, and now CRISPR, the ability to edit and reprogram our own genome and thus alter our evolutionary destiny. We have explored the fantastic, miniature, extremely busy world of molecular biologic metabolic activity inside our cells, whose richness and organizational complexity defy the human imagination. Yet despite all these astonishing accomplishments, we have no effective treatment for dementia. Time is running out, and an Alzheimer's epidemic is upon us.

That is all about to change. Finally, after a century of abject failures, we have a dramatic breakthrough. Thanks to the thousands of dedicated clinicians and researchers who built a scientific framework for understanding metabolic disease in the context of alternative, functional, and molecular medicine, we now understand what causes Alzheimer's and what we need to do to reverse it. This book describes these exciting discoveries, shows you how and why they work, and provides a road map for applying this information to prevent—and even reverse—this horrific disease.

We owe profound thanks to Dale Bredesen, MD, a brilliant and insightful neuroscientist. He took the foundational work done by clinicians and researchers to the next level, showing that Alzheimer's is caused by a broken metabolism and can be reversed by applying a multicausal, molecular medicine approach. For this, he deserves a Nobel Prize.

Our new understanding of Alzheimer's disease as *multiple systemic disruptions of normal metabolism* radically alters how we address the disease. Functional medicine provides the theoretical platform for a new multiple-modality approach. FM physicians like me rely on the peer-reviewed mainstream scientific understanding of the molecular biology and genetics of disease causation. We focus on finding the root causes of disease that undermine optimum function: nutritional deficiencies, improper food choices, insufficient exercise, stress, hormonal imbalances, infection, and toxic chemical exposures.

FM doctors view health as a state of vitality rather than just the absence of disease. We assume that the body wants to be healthy, has the power to heal itself, and will do so if supported properly and left to its own devices. FM doctors apply the principles outlined in this book to reverse dementia by prescribing nutritional medicines that alter gene expression in the direction of improved brain biochemistry.

The process is pretty straightforward. First, biomarker testing is done to identify the unique combination of biochemical malfunctions that are causing memory loss in you or your loved ones. (These are standard tests that can be done at any medical laboratory.) Based on that information, a treatment program can be designed and implemented—an individualized protocol that addresses each dysfunction to restore metabolic harmony, reverse the abnormal markers, repair the damaged neurons, and get the entire central nervous system up and running properly again.

Learning how to do this is what this book is about.

HOW THIS BOOK IS STRUCTURED

Part 1 presents the fascinating history of Alzheimer's disease. I explain what the disease is, why it took so long to find treatments that work. I describe our new systems-based functional medicine understanding of the disease and our tools for diagnosing it. I show why, in each patient, identifying and addressing each of the multiple causes is necessary. I introduce the topics of neurogenesis (the growth of new nerve cells) and neuroplasticity (the brain's ability to respond to change) and explain how the loss of neuroplasticity is the underlying cause of all dementia. The principal cause of this loss of neuroplasticity is damage to brain cells in the hippocampus, the part of the brain that stores and retrieves our memories.

Part 2 describes biomarker testing to identify the molecular imbalances that cause Alzheimer's. I reveal which lab tests to do, how they work, and why they are important. I explain what the results mean and provide detailed instructions for correcting the values that are out of range.

Part 3 is a comprehensive guide to the anti-Alzheimer's diet—eating practices and food choices that have been shown in research studies to prevent and reverse the disease. Certain foods (blueberries, curry dishes, coconut oil) enhance neurogenesis and neuroplasticity and repair a damaged hippocampus. Other foods (grains, sugars, common cooking oils) cause cognitive decline, encourage brain disease, and must be avoided.

Part 4 is about several amazing nutritional medicines that have been shown to prevent and reverse dementia, such as low-dose lithium,

Bacopa monnieri, omega-3 essential fatty acids (EFAs), curcumin (turmeric), berberine, phosphatidylserine, and citicoline. I explain what they are, how they work in the body, and how to use them.

The conclusion discusses epigenetics and the future of Alzheimer's research. We have long known how the genes in our DNA express themselves, but until the past few years we could not explain what controls that expression. Epigenetics finally explains the when and why of gene and DNA expression. We now know that personal lifestyle choices—what we eat, whether we exercise, which supplements we take—determine which genes are expressed and when. This breakthrough information transforms the playing field for anti-aging medicine and dementia. Thanks to epigenetics, we can finally make enlightened choices that control our genetic destiny and reverse Alzheimer's.

Let's get started.

PART 1

The Problem and the Solution

In chapter 1 you'll learn the medical definition and diagnostic criteria for Alzheimer's disease, the reason Alzheimer's is the third most likely cause of mortality, and additional mind-boggling statistics. I explain why our current approach to Alzheimer's is not working and outline a new way to diagnose and treat the disease. I also show how multiple metabolic and biochemical imbalances cause the disease, what to do if you suspect dementia, and when to get tested.

In chapter 2, we move on to a description of our new theoretical framework for understanding the disease. It's the first ever to successfully reverse the disease and is based on the most up-to-date peer-reviewed published scientific research using mainstream, alternative, complementary, functional, and naturopathic medical models.

Then, in chapter 3, you'll meet my mother, Elizabeth, and see how we would have treated her if she had Alzheimer's today (rather than twenty years ago).

Chapter 4 presents the fascinating history of the discovery of the disease. You'll learn about Dr. Alzheimer's first patient, his disastrous (and forgotten-for-a-century) lecture to the medical establishment, and the modern reanalysis of DNA from Professor Alzheimer's 1905 brain slides (rediscovered in 1992).

Chapter 5 is about the remarkable research by Dale Bredesen, MD, proving that identifying and correcting multicausal, multisystem metabolic disruptions using functional medicine therapies reverses Alzheimer's.

Chapter 6 is a history of how discoveries in molecular biology and genetics paved the way for the breakthroughs described in this book. The discovery that our brains can grow new nerve cells (neurogenesis) has led to the concepts of neuroplasticity and synaptoplasticity (neuronal restructuring in response to environment and experience). More recently, we have discovered how to apply new epigenetic information to choices of diet, exercise, and supplements to tweak our DNA so that it delivers better cellular structural material to bolster healthy neuronal metabolism.

Chapter 7 is about vascular dementia and the lessons a small stroke taught me.

In chapter 8, you'll learn about BDNF (brain-derived neurotrophic factor)—the powerful neurohormone that stimulates the growth of new brain cells, enhances memory, improves IQ, and reverses cognitive impairment—and I'll show you how to increase your levels.

CHAPTER 1

What Is Alzheimer's Disease?

Alzheimer's disease is memory loss, but it's not just the inability to recall a phone number or a name. It is forgetting on a more profound level; it's losing access to the memories necessary to live a normal life.

All of us occasionally lose keys or forget names, dates, and places. We usually remember them later. Alzheimer's patients forget more often and don't remember later.

Alzheimer's patients often have language problems. They may not be able to find the correct word, or they may forget simple words and replace them with inappropriate or even incomprehensible words.

They may become disoriented. Even on a short trip in a familiar town they may ask, "Where are we going. What are we doing?"

Personality change is common in Alzheimer's patients, and it's often tinged with suspicion, confusion, or fearfulness.

Judgment is often compromised. For example, Alzheimer's patients may dress inappropriately or forget to complete necessary tasks.

Loss of initiative is common. We all get tired of the daily grind of work and social obligations, but we get over it and carry on. Alzheimer's patients become passive and detached, requiring prompting or cues to get involved.

They have problems with abstract thinking, which can translate into trouble keeping track of a checking account or dialing the wrong sequence of numbers on a phone.

We all have mood swings, but people with Alzheimer's can have rapid or wide mood swings for little or no reason. They may react inappropriately emotionally, such as suddenly becoming extremely sad over a long-lost relative.

They will misplace things. Putting away groceries properly can be a great test for this. (The ice cream should not end up on the back porch.)

In a very real sense, our memories are who we are. With Alzheimer's, these fade or disappear altogether, and with them, a sense of self—not knowing who, what, or where you are or not knowing what to do because the continuity of doing things requires lots of memory.

CONFUSING TERMS

Alzheimer's disease (AD) is used two different ways. To neurologists and neuroscience researchers, the term refers to a specific diagnosis of a type of dementia characterized by amyloid beta plaques and neurofibrillary tangles.

The term is also used by laypeople in everyday conversation as a synonym for dementia to describe any type of memory loss. This colloquial, though technically inaccurate, usage could refer to mild cognitive decline, Alzheimer's disease, or other types of dementia.

In this book, I'll try to keep things simple by using the term *Alzheimer's disease* in the common, broader sense to refer to any and all dementias.

ABOUT DEMENTIA

Dementia is not a specific disease. The term describes a wide range of symptoms associated with a decline in memory or other thinking skills, severe enough to compromise one's ability to perform everyday activities.

Dementia always starts with mild cognitive impairment (MCI) and is usually, but not always, accompanied by memory loss. MCI might or might not progress to dementia and might or might not become Alzheimer's. Either way, detected and treated early, it is reversible.

No single test can determine whether someone has Alzheimer's or dementia. Doctors diagnose dementia based on a careful medical history, a physical examination, laboratory tests, imaging, and a mental status exam focused on changes in thinking, day-to-day function, and behavior.

The problem of diagnosis is compounded by the fact that definitively diagnosing Alzheimer's disease in a living person is impossible. That requires an autopsy and a microscopic examination of brain tissue. When referring to living patients, only specialists can authoritatively diagnose Alzheimer's disease, and even specialists will be wrong some of the time. Though advanced imaging techniques have improved diagnostic accuracy, autopsy remains the gold standard for diagnosis.

A diagnosis of dementia, on the other hand, can be made on the basis of symptoms alone (in a living patient, without an autopsy). If someone has significant memory problems, most likely that person is demented.

SOME SOBERING STATISTICS

The Alzheimer's Association estimates that one in three persons alive today in the United States will die with dementia.[1] Every 67 seconds, someone in the United States develops Alzheimer's disease. Fourteen percent of Americans over the age of seventy-one have some form of dementia, and over 5 million Americans now have Alzheimer's disease. The estimated proportion of the general population aged sixty and over with dementia at a given time is 5 to 8 percent. More than one hundred thousand Americans die of Alzheimer's each year.[2]

The economic impact is huge: $818 billion a year in the United States alone.[3] Nearly 16 million unpaid caregivers provide some 18.4 billion hours of care, worth an estimated $238 billion, according to the Alzheimer's Association.[4]

Dementia is a worldwide public health disaster: nearly 44 million people are living with Alzheimer's disease or dementia. Every three seconds, someone in the world is diagnosed with dementia, and every year, there are nearly 10 million new cases. The World Health Organization estimates that the total number of people with dementia will reach 82 million in 2030 and 152 million in 2050.

Until recently, Alzheimer's had been considered the sixth most common cause of death, but Alzheimer's deaths have been underreported. Some people with the disease never receive a diagnosis. Many others have dementia-related conditions, such as aspiration pneumonia, listed as the primary cause of death, while the underlying cause, Alzheimer's, is not reported. Studies funded by the National Institute on Aging have shown that the number of deaths due to Alzheimer's disease in people seventy-five and older could be six times higher than the official count. This would make it the *third leading cause of death*, behind heart disease and cancer.[5] A related study by Jennifer Weuve and colleagues at Rush University Medical Center in Chicago found that 32 percent of deaths in persons sixty-five years or older were due to AD and projected that by 2050, this number will rise to 43 percent, or 1.6 million deaths.[6]

What's more, the brain changes that lead to Alzheimer's may begin twenty years or more before symptoms appear.[7]

The human toll of AD is not reflected in these mind-boggling numbers. For example, caregivers experience overwhelming stress and require support from medical, social, financial, and legal systems. People with dementia and their families are frequently discriminated against and denied basic rights and freedoms available to others. Often physical and chemical restraints are used in age care facilities and acute care settings. Increased awareness will reduce discrimination and improve the quality of life for people with dementia, as well as their families.

Addressing dementia is a public health necessity. Interventions aimed at improving the quality of life for people with dementia by reducing the modifiable risk factors outlined in this book should be instituted at a local level in clinics and healthcare settings.

This book will show you how to determine the causes of dementia and apply effective treatments to modifiable risk factors. Addressing them works.

A NEW WAY TO DIAGNOSE AND TREAT ALZHEIMER'S DISEASE AND A NEW LANGUAGE EMPHASIZING CAUSALITY

The remainder of this chapter outlines current mainstream concepts used to describe and diagnose Alzheimer's disease and dementia. A major goal of this book, however, is to present a new and very different way of defining Alzheimer's disease. Breakthroughs in understanding the causes of dementia—the molecular biological underpinnings—are shifting our attention away from the *effects* of the disease (symptoms, signs, plaques and tangles, and atrophy) and redirecting the spotlight onto *causality*. Each individual case of Alzheimer's disease, we now know, represents a combination of several possible causes. Patient A might have low vitamin D, elevated homocysteine, high blood sugar, and sleep apnea. Patient B might have a disrupted gut microbiome, high blood pressure, lacunar strokes, mercury exposure, and hypothyroidism. Patient C might have a different biochemical landscape with similarities and differences. Figuring out each patient's unique combination of causes is achieved through molecular biomarker testing, which we use to generate an individual biochemical profile.

Defining the biochemical changes that cause the disease empowers corrective action in the form of treatments that alter the course of the disease. We can lower homocysteine and blood pressure, fix hypothyroidism, lower high blood sugar, supplement vitamin D, and remove sources of cadmium, lead, and mercury. The earlier we make this causative diagnosis and implement corrective therapies, the greater the chance of reversal.

The odds of any healthy person getting Alzheimer's is one in three. If your brain is working fine and you want to keep it that way, do the testing to determine your areas of vulnerability, and then treat them preventively. By adopting a preventive lifestyle, you can dramatically reduce the probability of developing the disease.

Now that we can identify and correct the multiple metabolic factors that cause Alzheimer's, clinicians will need to integrate this new information into clinical practice. For many, this will be akin to learning a new language. I hope that doctors and patients alike will find this book useful in easing that transition.

DIAGNOSING DEMENTIA

Dementia is a symptom complex (again, it's *not* a specific disease) characterized by cognitive dysfunction, memory loss, personality changes, and impaired reasoning. Dementia is commonly seen across a wide spectrum of neurodegenerative diseases of which Alzheimer's disease and vascular dementia are by far the most common.

The Handbook of Alzheimer's Disease and Other Dementias—an encyclopedic reference work written by specialists for physicians and other health professionals—defines dementia as a "syndrome of acquired persistent intellectual impairments characterized by deterioration in at least three of the following domains: memory, language, visuospatial skills, personality or behavior, and manipulation of acquired knowledge (including executive function)."[8]

The symptoms of dementia can be grouped into four main categories:

- *Cognitive symptoms* include memory loss, mental decline, confusion, disorientation, language problems, inability to speak or understand, making things up, and inability to recognize common objects.
- *Behavioral symptoms* include irritability, restlessness, lack of restraint, wandering and getting lost, and falling.
- *Psychological changes* include personality changes, anxiety, depression, mood swings, loneliness, hallucinations, and paranoia.
- *Musculoskeletal symptoms* include inability to coordinate muscle movements, unsteady walking, and jumbled speech.

Assessing Levels of Cognitive Functioning

Cognitive testing determines the presence and extent of cognitive decline. If you suspect cognitive decline, performing baseline testing is helpful as it will (1) determine whether your cognition is compromised and (2) provide a basis for comparison down the road to determine whether your program is working.

(Don't confuse cognitive/mental status testing with metabolic marker testing. Cognitive testing is a way to determine whether a loss in brain function has occurred; it in no way identifies or addresses possible causes. Metabolic marker testing, on the other hand, identifies the causes of the damage and provides the road map to treatment.)

Mental status testing evaluates memory, ability to solve simple problems, and other thinking skills. Such tests give an overall sense of whether a person is aware of his or her symptoms; knows the date, time, and where he or she is; and can remember a short list of words, follow instructions, and do simple calculations.

The Mini-Mental State Examination (MMSE) and the Mini-Cog test are two commonly used assessments.

The MMSE (also known as the Folstein test) is a thirty-point questionnaire designed to test a range of everyday mental skills. It is used extensively in clinical and research settings to evaluate the severity and progression of cognitive impairment and to follow cognitive changes over time.[9]

The Mini-Cog is an assessment in which a health professional asks the patient to complete two tasks: (1) remember and a few minutes later repeat the names of three common objects and (2) draw a face of a clock showing all twelve numbers in the right places and a time specified by the examiner.[10]

Types of Dementia

Alzheimer's disease, a specific type of dementia, is defined as a progressive neurodegenerative disorder displaying two classical hallmark pathologies: extracellular (outside the neurons) amyloid beta plaques and intraneuronal (inside nerve cells) neurofibrillary tangles. Again, a corpse, biopsy, and microscope are required.

Vascular dementia (VaD) is loss of cognitive function due to atherosclerotic damage to brain blood vessels that blocks the flow of blood. This obstruction may develop gradually or suddenly. Uncontrolled hypertension is *by far* the single leading cause of blood vessel damage, stroke, and dementia.

A lacunar stroke is a specific type of stroke that occurs when blood flow is blocked to one of the small arterial vessels that lie just beneath the outer cerebral cortex. Lacunar strokes are the most common cause of vascular dementia, and about one-fifth of all strokes are this type. The most common cause of lacunar strokes is chronic high blood pressure. (Read the story of my lacunar strokes in chapters 7 and 10.) The cumulative damage caused by repeated lacunar strokes leads to dementia. (For an in-depth discussion of VaD, see chapter 7.)

Mixed dementia is the simultaneous coexistence of more than one type of dementia. Though mixed dementia may include any combination of types, over 90 percent of patients have the mixed AD/VaD type.

Because both AD and VaD cause the same symptoms, it is usually impossible to differentiate between the two in living patients. Nor is it possible, in any given patient, to determine how much of his or her dementia is caused by Alzheimer's and how much is caused by vascular dementia. A definitive diagnosis is possible only on autopsy. Pure AD (AD without the vascular component) is rare.

Less common dementias include the following:

- Dementia from Parkinson's disease and similar disorders
- Lewy body dementia
- Frontotemporal dementia (Pick's disease)
- Creutzfeldt-Jakob disease
- Dementia caused by
  - Drug interactions

- Infection
- Brain tumors
- Depression

Advanced Disease

Though it selectively attacks specific memory areas in the hippocampus, Alzheimer's also changes the entire brain, causing nerve cell death and tissue loss throughout. Over time, the brain dramatically shrinks, and nearly all its functions are compromised.

As dementia gradually progresses, memory loss is increasingly accompanied by impaired judgment, personality changes, loss of concentration, confusion, disorientation, restlessness, irritability, inability to communicate, forgetfulness, and inattention to personal hygiene. These conditions worsen until patients are no longer able to read, write, speak, take care of themselves, recognize loved ones, or even swallow and walk. Survival after onset of symptoms is usually five to ten years but can be as long as twenty years.

In advanced Alzheimer's disease, massive cell loss shrivels the outer cortex, damaging areas involved in thinking, planning, and remembering. Shrinkage (atrophy) is especially severe in the hippocampus, the area of the cortex that plays a key role in formation of new memories (fig. 1.1).

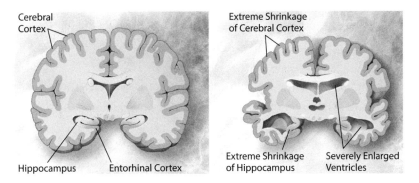

Figure 1.1. Brains with and without Alzheimer's disease

Under a microscope, tissue from an Alzheimer's patient's brain reveals devastating changes. It has many fewer nerve cells and synapses than tissue from a healthy brain. Clumps of amyloid beta plaque have accumulated in the tissue between nerve cells. These disrupt normal nerve cell functioning by blocking cell-to-cell synaptic signaling. These amyloid clumps also cause a local inflammatory reaction and activation of immune system cells that gobble up disabled nerve cells. When we focus our microscope on the insides of the sick, dying, and dead nerve cells, we also spot neurofibrillary tangles—twisted strands of tau protein.

IF MILD COGNITIVE IMPAIRMENT APPEARS, IT IS TIME TO TEST

Forgetfulness and memory delays are often part of the normal aging process. We all slow down as we get older, and we sometimes need more time to learn a new fact or remember an old one.

Between "normal," age-related memory loss and true dementia lies a condition called mild cognitive impairment. Individuals with MCI have persistent memory problems—for example, difficulty remembering names and following conversations or marked forgetfulness. Symptoms of MCI may also include depression, irritability, anxiety, and even aggressive or apathetic behavior. MCI patients generally have normal reasoning skills, judgment, and perception. Many individuals who develop MCI will never progress to dementia, but some will—and in the early stages it is not possible to determine who will go on to develop full-blown dementia.

Until very recently, we could not determine whether those earliest signs of a failing memory were a part of normal aging or the first symptoms of a dread disease. We could not treat the memory loss, so we could do nothing in the mild cognitive impairment stage but wait and see whether it was the beginning of dementia.

That has all changed. Now that cognitive decline and AD have been linked to abnormalities of specific biomarkers that can be identified and reversed, we are no longer at the mercy of fate—or even of our DNA. We can protect our brains from the ravages of both MCI and AD by getting tested and addressing those abnormal markers. Lowering our elevated blood sugar or cholesterol, getting our sleep apnea and hypertension under control, making sure we get daily exercise, taking vitamin D if needed, avoiding neurotoxic exposures, eating dementia-preventive foods, and taking nutritional medicine supplements that reverse dementia will prevent and reverse these causative disease processes.

WHAT TO DO IF YOU SUSPECT DEMENTIA

If friends and family have told you that they notice increasing memory loss that interferes with your daily activities, work productivity, and social interactions, it's time to seek professional help. The first step would be to consult your family doctor or healthcare provider for an evaluation—and, if necessary, a referral to a neurologist for diagnostic assistance and to rule out causes of dementia best treated via conventional medicine, such as stroke, drug interactions, infection, brain tumor, depression, and Parkinson's disease.

If the diagnosis is AD, VaD, or MCI, however, a conventional neurologist might be a poor choice for *treatment* because the mainstream approach to dementia is therapeutically bankrupt. To put it bluntly: no conventional treatment works.

What's more, the current mainstream medicine neurology system will fail to appreciate and diagnose—or even understand—the true causative elements. Neurologists are typically not trained in the metabolic approach and will prescribe only conventional drug therapy, which is ineffective because it fails to address the multiple causative metabolic imbalances that are the driving force behind the disease. Drugs merely suppress the symptoms and are only marginally effective at that. You want to stop and reverse the course of the disease, if possible, and no pharmaceutical agent can do that. Dementia is a progressive disease, so don't waste valuable time trying drugs when you could have been addressing causes. The proactive multimodality approach, which identifies and addresses causative factors, makes a lot more sense.

MCI is reversible using the methods outlined in this book, but as the disease progresses, it becomes more entrenched and increasingly resistant to treatment. To increase the probability of successful reversal, the best approach is to assume that all significant memory problems are early signs of dementia and begin the diagnostic and treatment process as soon as possible. Find a physician who understands that symptom suppression does not work and wants to focus on reversal by addressing the underlying causes, using the program outlined in this book.

CHAPTER 2

How to Prevent and Reverse Alzheimer's

This book describes a new theoretical framework for understanding Alzheimer's disease. The therapeutic system based on this framework is the first ever to successfully reverse the disease. It is based on the most up-to-date peer-reviewed published scientific research. It applies mainstream, alternative, complementary, functional, and naturopathic medical models.

Alternative means finding biocompatible treatments that bypass the drugs and surgery of mainstream medicine. *Complementary* means integrating mainstream and alternative approaches, using the best of both. *Functional* means identifying and addressing known biochemical and metabolic causes of disease rather than treating the symptoms. *Naturopathic* means encouraging the body's ability to heal, using foods and nondrug medicines whenever possible.

Nontoxic, nondrug, bioidentical, biocompatible therapies restore metabolic harmony and gently nourish the brain back to health. These include dietary changes, brain-nourishing foods, a daily exercise program, toxin avoidance, and nutritional medicines, including vitamins, minerals, herbs, essential fatty acids, phytonutrients, and bioidentical hormones.

Although drugs have their place in medicine, they should be used not as a first choice but as a last resort.

A NEW WAY TO DIAGNOSE DEMENTIA

I am a big fan of the microscope. As a medical student I spent hundreds of hours peering into a magical world of untold complexity. But a microscope can take you down to the cellular level only; it is unable to reveal the molecular world of activity unfolding inside each cell. Every human cell has a biochemical complexity rivaling that of a large city, almost none of which can be seen by looking through a microscope. Viewing a cell through a microscope is like looking at New York City from the moon: you know a lot is happening down there, but almost none of it is visible.

The metabolic dysfunctions that cause dementia transpire at the molecular level. Solving the riddle of dementia requires that we shift our focus to the deeper, submicroscopic realms of molecular biology where the changes that lead to neurodegenerative disease occur. To be able to see what is happening (and what is going wrong) at that level, we need to blow it up, and we do that by examining the kinds of chemical molecules that are present. This is a challenging task because hundreds of thousands of different kinds of molecules exist, and they are constantly moving and changing. Biomarker testing, however, provides a powerful tool that allows us to sort through the possibilities and identify the abnormalities that are causing neurodegeneration.

MULTIPLE SYSTEMS, MULTIPLE CAUSES

The symptoms we see in dementia patients—diminished cognition, memory defects, emotional changes, and behavioral problems—are classic signs of central nervous system (CNS) malfunction, so we could easily assume that the pathology that causes dementia originates in the CNS. That would be a mistake.

Even though the CNS is the window through which we view the symptoms, the actual causes of dementia usually originate outside the CNS—most commonly in the vascular, immune, endocrine, and gastrointestinal (GI) systems. Those causes include nutritional deficiencies, hormonal disruptions, blood sugar regulating abnormalities, athero-sclerotic changes, hypertension, toxic exposures, inflammatory reactions, sleep disturbances, gut microbiome disruption, gut wall (intestinal mucosal) inflammatory damage, intestinal absorption issues, autoimmune reactions, inappropriate diet, and insufficient exercise (fig. 2.1). Though they originate elsewhere, these metabolic disruptions undermine the harmonious functioning of nerve cells, causing neurodegenerative disease.

What Causes Alzheimer's?

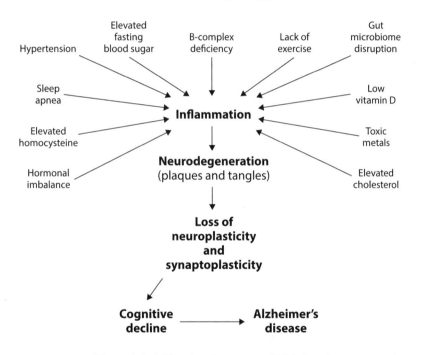

Figure 2.1. Addressing the causes of Alzheimer's

To initiate reversal of Alzheimer's, we must first identify these derangements using Alzheimer's metabolic biomarker testing, which provides a unique profile—a biochemical landscape that serves as a guide to the deep causes of neurodegeneration. An abnormal result on an AD biomarker test reveals that the changes leading to AD are underway and pinpoints exactly where, in the amazingly complex metabolic network of bodily systems, the malfunction is located. Abnormal results also guide us directly to specific and effective treatment options.

Testing reveals which molecular systems are malfunctioning and allows us to identify the changes that are leading toward dementia. Using this information, we can easily generate a treatment program that addresses each causative factor (i.e., each abnormal lab value). For example, if your vitamin D is low, you'll know you need to take a D supplement. If your thyroid hormone level is low, that needs to be balanced. If your homocysteine is high, you will need to supplement your diet with B-complex vitamins. If a polysomnogram reveals sleep apnea, you'll need to use a CPAP (continuous positive air pressure) machine. If hair analysis shows a high mercury level, you'll know to stop eating fish and have amalgam fillings removed. If your blood pressure, blood sugar, or cholesterol are elevated, those need to be fixed.

For each marker, I have written a chapter explaining why it is important, how the testing works, what the results mean, and how to fix them if they're out of balance (see chapters 10–19). Once your treatment program has been in place for a few months, retesting is necessary to determine whether the program is working to reverse the neurodegenerative metabolic disruptions.

Metabolic testing provides a comprehensive picture that is useful whether a person already has symptoms of cognitive decline or simply wants to learn which areas are vulnerable.

THE AD BIOMARKERS

Here are the tests that identify the specific causes of Alzheimer's and neurodegenerative disease:

- Blood pressure
- Fasting blood sugar
- Cholesterol

- Homocysteine, vitamin B12, and folic acid
- Vitamin D
- Polysomnogram (to diagnose sleep apnea)
- Gut microbiome assessment
- Thyroid
- Hair analysis for toxic metals (mercury, lead, aluminum, and cadmium)
- Ferritin (to detect excess iron)
- Sex steroid hormones (estrogen, progesterone, testosterone, and DHEA-S [dehydroepiandrosterone sulfate])

Once testing has identified the "broken" metabolic systems, the next step is implementation of your treatment program to restore metabolic harmony, reverse the abnormal markers, repair the damaged neurons, and get them up and running again. Then you can take it to the next level by learning how to reprogram your brain for neurogenesis: a surge in the growth of new healthy brain cells (see chapter 8).

START NOW!

It is impossible to overemphasize the importance of early preventive action. The early changes that lead to dementia begin decades before overt symptoms appear. The earlier these are addressed, the greater your protection from eventual cognitive decline. These changes can be easily identified using biomarker testing, and—once again, if detected early—the disease can be reversed with simple diet and supplement changes. Know your markers! Manage them.

CHAPTER 3

How We Would Treat Mom's Alzheimer's Today

My mom epitomizes the kind of person this book would have helped, had this information been available twenty years ago when she began showing signs of cognitive decline. This chapter looks at how we would have treated Elizabeth if we had known then what we know today.

ADDRESSING AD *AND* VaD

Vascular dementia and Alzheimer's disease are the two most common types of dementia. In AD, the dementia is caused by a breakdown of *nerve cells* and brain tissue. VaD, on the other hand, usually results from high blood pressure that damages the *blood vessels* that supply the brain. This, in turn, damages downstream nerve cells.

Brain blood vessel disease is rampant in older adults, and with it comes the risk of Alzheimer's disease. MRI studies reveal that 63 percent of people over sixty have multiple white matter hyperintensities—evidence of a previous lacunar stroke. That number goes up to 96 percent in people over eighty.[1]

In any given patient, vascular dementia and Alzheimer's almost always coexist. Over 90 percent of people diagnosed with Alzheimer's suffer from both VaD and AD. Since VaD and AD cause more or less the same symptoms, they are clinically indistinguishable in living patients.[2] Mom, like most people, had both.

We now know that the vascular portion of the dementia damage equation virtually always involves abnormalities in one or more of the four vascular markers: blood pressure, blood sugar, cholesterol, and homocysteine. This is important information because these abnormalities are all treatable and reversible, and spotting them early tells us what needs to be fixed to prevent brain damage. With proper attention to the vascular markers, we can alter how genes are expressed and alter the course of the disease. In Mom—as in all dementia patients—the VaD component would have been eminently treatable.

First, I'll focus on the four main vascular markers. Then I'll go on to discuss each of the other markers.

BLOOD PRESSURE

Twenty years ago, doctors had not yet connected the dots between high blood pressure and dementia. Now we know that any elevation of blood pressure increases the risk of dementia, so I would have made certain that Elizabeth's elevated blood pressure was aggressively tracked and treated. (Normal blood pressure is 120/80 or less; pressures above 130/85 are cause for concern and must be lowered.)

The importance of blood pressure control cannot be overemphasized. Even slight blood pressure elevations can damage the brain, causing VaD. Also known as multi-infarct dementia, vascular dementia can be stopped and reversed only if the high blood pressure that causes it is caught early, treated aggressively, and normalized.

The pounding from Elizabeth's long-term elevated blood pressure damaged the blood vessels in her brain. The cumulative damage from untreated hypertension coupled with multiple small strokes played a major role in Elizabeth's death. (See chapter 10 for more about blood pressure and dementia.)

BLOOD SUGAR

Fasting blood sugar (FBS) had been tested in Elizabeth, but twenty years ago, we didn't know that even minimal increases over normal (anything over 90 milligrams per deciliter [mg/dL]) indicated damage to her blood-sugar-regulating systems. This damage posed a danger to her brain. Elizabeth's FBS ran in the mid- to high 90s (numbers routinely dismissed as normal back then). We didn't know it, but she was at significant risk of diminished cognition, stroke, memory problems, hippocampal (memory center) damage, brain atrophy, and dementia. (See chapter 11 for more details.)

Today, we would bring down Elizabeth's blood sugar by putting her on a very low-carbohydrate ketogenic diet, eliminating all grains and sugars, and having her do as much exercise as possible given her age and health.

We would include lots of high-polyphenol foods. These compounds help the body regulate blood sugar—for example, blueberries, cherries, raspberries, blackberries, pomegranate, grapes, green tea, nuts, curcumin, cabbage, eggplant, greens, onions, garlic, and olives. (See chapters 20, 24, 25, 26, 29, and 30 and appendix 2 for other choices.)

CHOLESTEROL

We would make sure Elizabeth's cholesterol and lipids were normal. Mom's cholesterol ran around 220–230 mg/dL. Back then, we thought this was a little high, but since her diet was excellent and her heart was fine, we didn't worry much about it. The research is now very clear, however: a cholesterol number over 200 increases the risk of strokes and dementia.[3] With the wisdom of hindsight—and more definitive research—it is easy to see that her high cholesterol, coupled with her modestly elevated blood pressure and blood sugar, played a significant role in accelerating the progression of her Alzheimer's. We should have gotten her numbers down.

We'd treat her cholesterol naturally with red yeast rice extract, plant sterols, bergamot, and berberine, and if that didn't get it under 200, we would add the smallest possible (effective) dose of a statin. (See chapter 12.)

HOMOCYSTEINE

In 1998, researchers found that individuals low in B-complex vitamins are more likely to have elevated homocysteine levels and are more likely to develop Alzheimer's disease.[4] We didn't test homocysteine routinely back then, but it is safe to assume Mom's level was high, indicating a B-complex deficiency, which is extremely common in people over fifty.

In 2010, researchers discovered that (regardless of homocysteine level), people who supplement their diet with B-complex vitamins were less likely to develop cognitive impairment.[5] Researchers also showed that supplementing with B-complex vitamins not only lowers homocysteine levels but reverses brain atrophy and prevents Alzheimer's. However, this research came out in 2013, ten years after Elizabeth died. Now we know that all eight of the B-complex vitamins play crucial roles in supporting healthy brain metabolism and that they work together as a team. A deficiency of any of them can cause cognitive erosion and cerebral atrophy and dramatically heighten the probability of dementia.[6] At the earliest sign of memory problems, we'd have put Elizabeth on both the active form of B-complex and regular B-complex vitamins plus a multivitamin. (See chapter 13 for details.)

VITAMIN D

Twenty years ago, we knew vitamin D was important for strong bones, but we had no idea how important it is for brain health and a raft of other chronic diseases. Optimum levels of vitamin D are also necessary to prevent cancer, autoimmune disease, and blood sugar imbalances.

Nowadays, we know that a low level of D causes dementia risk to skyrocket.[7] Most people with cognitive impairment have a vitamin D deficiency (levels less than 50 nanograms per milliliter [ng/mL]), and studies have shown that the greater the deficiency, the higher the risk.[8] Individuals with the lowest vitamin D levels are twenty-five times more likely to develop mild cognitive impairment when compared to those with the highest vitamin D levels.

Why is D so important for the brain? Perhaps it's because vitamin D is not a vitamin; it is a neurohormone that exerts a broad and powerful spectrum of effects that control the health of our nervous systems. It suppresses inflammation, stimulates removal of amyloid beta plaque deposits from the cerebral cortex, prevents oxidative nerve damage, regulates blood sugar and blood pressure, optimizes the effectiveness of glial cells (supporting cells of the nervous system), and regulates calcium balance inside and outside of cells. A complete list would be very much longer because D controls the expression of about 25 percent of our genes.

To reverse the disease process, we would get Mom's levels of 25-hydroxy vitamin D up into the 70–100 ng/mL optimum range. (For more about D, see chapter 14.)

GUT MICROBIOME

The bacteria in our gut microbiome (GM) outnumber the body's cells by a factor of one hundred and provide over 95 percent of our genetic material.[9] This powerful force helps us break down food and extract nutrients from it, generate energy, produce certain vitamins, stave off infections, bolster our immunity, and—perhaps most important of all—enhance brain health and vitality. Your GM controls the destiny of your brain by exerting powerful control over nerve impulse transmission, neuroinflammatory reactions, and neuroimmunity.[10]

We would take a close look at Mom's bowel health to determine whether her gut microbiome population had been damaged and whether healthy probiotic bacterial microbes had been replaced by pathogenic species. If Elizabeth had food intolerances, indigestion, gastric acid reflux, bloating, gas, loose stools, cramps, irritable bowel syndrome (IBS), leaky gut, any autoimmune disease, or other signs of microbiome distress, we would prescribe digestive enzymes, acidophilus to repopulate her GI tract with healthy microbes, prebiotics to nourish and support the probiotics, natural antibiotics that kill pathogenic bugs while leaving the good guys alone, and biofilm disrupters

that break down the walls bacteria build around their colonies to protect them from the immune cells and antibiotics that would otherwise
kill them. (See chapter 16.)

SLEEP APNEA

Obstructive sleep apnea (OSA) involves an involuntary cessation of
breathing in which the walls of the pharynx collapse. As inhaled air
flows past the partially collapsed walls, they flap in the wind, so to
speak, causing the snoring sound.

Such episodes of airway occlusion reduce the oxygen supply to the
brain and blood vessels. Recurring oxygen deficit causes body-wide
inflammatory damage to the vascular endothelium (the inner lining
of blood vessels) and central nervous system, causing high blood pressure and stroke and setting the stage for dementia.

Apnea episodes may occur thirty times or more per hour and often
hundreds of times during a night. The sleeper is unaware of these stoppages, but they chisel away at the quality of sleep without triggering
full awakening. OSA victims may experience daytime fatigue but often
have no clear symptoms to warn them that brain damage is accumulating. OSA is associated with a high risk of hypertension, stroke, other
cardiovascular disease, and Alzheimer's.

Experts publishing their data in a 2018 article in the *American
Journal of Respiratory and Critical Care Medicine* estimate the worldwide prevalence of obstructive sleep apnea at 1 billion people.[11] OSA
affects an estimated 30 million Americans. About 24 percent of women
and 9 percent of men have it.[12] Over 90 percent of these people remain
undiagnosed and untreated. A study of 15,699 sleep-disordered
patients participating in the Sleep Heart Health Study revealed that
only 0.6 percent of sleep apnea patients were actively receiving physician treatment for their sleep apnea. Most of them were unaware they
had the disease.[13]

According to American Academy of Sleep Medicine president
Dr. Timothy Morgenthaler, "Obstructive sleep apnea is destroying

the health of millions of Americans, and the problem has only gotten worse over the last two decades."[14]

Most people who snore have sleep apnea. Mom didn't snore and probably didn't have sleep apnea, but we never even considered that possibility because twenty years ago, when she developed cognitive decline, we didn't know that sleep apnea caused dementia.

Snoring is the most common symptom of sleep apnea, so all snorers should be tested. Sleep apnea can cause high blood pressure, so a polysomnogram should be done on all hypertensives.

LOW THYROID

The thyroid gland controls metabolism everywhere in the body, including the brain and CNS. Low thyroid (hypothyroidism), also known as subclinical hypothyroidism, is a very common condition that can impair brain function and cause cognitive decline.

According to the American Thyroid Association, an estimated 20 million Americans have some form of thyroid disease, and up to 60 percent of those with thyroid disease are unaware of their condition. Women are five to eight times more likely than men to have thyroid problems. Undiagnosed thyroid disease may put patients at risk for numerous serious conditions.[15]

Hypothyroidism has been dubbed the "unsuspected illness" because it usually presents with vague symptoms that impersonate other ailments and physicians often miss the diagnosis. The epidemic of undiagnosed hypothyroidism causes a great deal of human suffering and disability, including dementia.[16]

Mom had three classic symptoms of low thyroid: fatigue, constipation, and depression. From these, plus lab testing, I had diagnosed her hypothyroidism many years earlier, and her treatment program had reversed the disease.

Untreated hypothyroidism serves as a launchpad for dementia— so if Mom hadn't already been diagnosed, we would have taken a close look at her thyroid numbers. Her dementia would likely have begun sooner and progressed more rapidly if her hypothyroidism hadn't been treated. (See chapter 17.)

TOXIC METALS

Mom's dementia may have been caused or accelerated by her exposure to toxic heavy metals. To explore this possibility, we would do a hair toxic mineral analysis—a simple, easy, reliable, inexpensive, and revealing test that is done from home. (See chapter 18 for more details.)

The following toxic metals are most likely to cause neurodegeneration:

- *Mercury*—from fish (this includes *all* seafood, including farm-raised) and amalgam dental fillings. People who consume a serving of fish more than once a week usually have dangerously high levels.
- *Lead*—from old paint, imported dishes, water contamination, lead pipes and fittings, brass or bronze faucets and valves, and many national brands of chocolate.
- *Cadmium*—from almost all brands of chocolate and cocoa.
- *Aluminum*—from deodorants and cookware.
- *Arsenic*—from building materials, pressure-treated wood, and pesticides.
- *Iron*—Iron is an essential mineral, but high levels are neurotoxic. Causes include too many iron supplements, cooking with an iron skillet, liver disease, and repeated blood transfusions.

EXERCISE AND BDNF

Everyone knows about the vital importance of exercise. But you might not be aware that exercise is the single most effective way to improve brain function—including both cognitive power and memory.

Mom jogged—and later walked—several miles every day. She also used hand weights. Mom knew exercise was good for her, but she had no idea how good it was. Exercise, we now know, stimulates the production and release of brain-derived neurotrophic factor, a hormone-like molecule that enables the four most important features necessary to prevent and reverse dementia: neurogenesis (growing new nerve cells), neuroregeneration (healing damaged nerve cells), and neuroplasticity and synaptoplasticity (having a nervous system with synapses responsive to change). (See chapter 8 for more on this subject.) I am certain Mom's daily exercise slowed or stalled the progression of her dementia for several years.

Although nothing comes close to exercise in terms of power to release BDNF, certain foods, nutritional supplements, and practices also trigger its production:

- Intermittent fasting
- Lithium
- Omega-3 fatty acids such as DHA (docosahexaenoic acid) and flaxseed oil
- Blueberries
- B-complex vitamins (including B12)
- Folic acid (methylfolate)
- Curcumin
- Zinc
- Caffeine
- Resveratrol
- Flavonoids (green tea, cocoa, chocolate)
- Other flavone-rich foods such as strawberries, raspberries, blackberries, cherries, peaches, apples, pear, oranges, romaine lettuce, celery, tomatoes, garbanzo beans, almonds (and much more, see chapter 24)

The following have been shown to inhibit BDNF production:

- Ethanol (all alcoholic beverages)
- Vitamin A deficiency
- Vitamin E deficiency
- High saturated-fat diet
- Sugar

DIET

Mom's diet would be limited to foods shown to prevent or reverse dementia. She'd be on a ketogenic diet, which eliminates all grains, sugars, and other high-carbohydrate foods while emphasizing healthy fats and modest amounts of high-quality protein.

We'd make sure she got large doses of antidementia oils: medium chain triglycerides (MCTs) from coconut, omega-3s from flaxseed, and DHA derived from algae. Other brain-beneficial fats include avocado, walnut, and olive oils. (See chapters 21, 23, and 28.)

We'd also remove sources of pro-inflammatory omega-6 oils such as soy, sunflower, safflower, corn, cottonseed, and canola. A little saturated fat (from clean, humanely raised lean meat and eggs) is okay, but we'd keep her intake on the low side because too much saturated fat blocks the availability of the all-important omega-3 oils.

We'd take advantage of the incredible neuroregenerative powers of polyphenols by loading Mom's diet with fruits such as blueberries, raspberries, strawberries, cherries, blackberries, pomegranate, and grapes and polyphenol-rich vegetables such as artichokes, broccoli, red cabbage, celery, eggplant, garlic, dark leafy greens, kohlrabi, leeks, onions (red, white, and yellow), scallions, peppers, peas, spinach, sweet potatoes, tomatoes, nuts, and green tea.

I'd make sure that most days she ate two eggs cooked in coconut oil. Absolutely no fish or other seafood and no processed foods would be allowed.

You will learn a lot more about antidementia dieting in chapter 20.

Autophagy

Autophagy is the practice of fasting twelve to sixteen hours every day to activate cellular housekeeping systems that remove the waste material that would otherwise cause metabolic dysfunction and neurodegenerative disease. It is relatively easy to do. (See chapter 22.)

Autophagy is how our cells eject or recycle all kinds of used-up or broken biomolecules—an enormous hodgepodge of cellular debris, including proteins, nucleic acids, carbohydrates, lipids, viruses, bacteria, and toxins.

It also plays a dramatic role in slowing and reversing cognitive decline. Optimizing autophagy in nerve cells is essential for repair, renewal, and regeneration—for both maintaining a cognitive edge in a healthy brain and restoring it in a brain with cognitive decline.

Nutritional Supplements

Research studies have shown that specific nutritional medicines prevent and reverse cognitive decline. In this book I have included only those with the strongest research support.

I would have prescribed several nutritional supplements for Mom. At the top of the list would be lithium, a "magical mineral" that not only prevents Alzheimer's but has been shown to increase BDNF, stimulate neurogenesis, and reverse cerebral atrophy. Lithium has been shown to halt the progression of—and even reverse—Alzheimer's disease. Anyone who wants to prevent dementia and keep the sharpest possible mental edge should include this mineral in his or her supplement program. (See chapter 27.)

Since Mom had a significant vascular component to her dementia, the herb berberine would also have been an excellent choice.

Several other nutritional medicine supplements have been shown to provide basic brain support, enhance cognition, and block or reverse the Alzheimer's disease process. Examples include B-complex vitamins, curcumin, Bacopa, DHA, flaxseed oil, phosphatidylserine, green tea extract, citicoline, and probiotics.

I would also prescribe specific supplements to correct specific metabolic defects—for example, berberine for high blood sugar, B-complex for high homocysteine, red rice yeast extract for elevated cholesterol, curcumin for inflammation, and vitamin D3 for low vitamin D.

To assure purity and effectiveness, I'd make sure Mom's supplements were professional-level quality and didn't come from any drugstore chain or big box store. Trying to save money on vitamins is a really bad idea. Substandard quality, offshore unregulated products, and toxic source materials are common in the cheaper products. Purity and efficacy go hand in hand. Professionally produced, pharmaceutical quality nutritional medicines are highly recommended.

It saddens me that Mom couldn't benefit from these new treatment approaches.

CHAPTER 4

Alois Alzheimer and the Discovery of Alzheimer's Disease

Let's take a brief trip back in time to 2:30 p.m. on November 3, 1906—a Saturday afternoon—in southern Germany. We're attending a lecture remembered for its profound influence on the history of medicine, all the more remarkable because its importance went unnoticed for over half a century. At the time, not a single soul—not even the presenter himself, neuropathologist and psychiatrist Alois Alzheimer—suspected the revolutionary impact this brief case presentation would make.[1]

We are sitting with about eighty psychiatrists and neurologists at the 37th Meeting of Southwest German Psychiatrists in Tübingen, a quaint and picturesque university town on the Neckar River about 230 kilometers west of Munich. In the audience with us sit neuropsychiatric heavyweights such as neuropathologist Franz Nissl (a name familiar to all medical students for the neuronal stain he discovered)—and Carl Jung.

Notes in hand, Alois Alzheimer, MD, a forty-two-year-old lecturer at the Munich University Hospital, sits in the front row, awaiting his turn in a succession of speakers.

In Munich, Alzheimer was thriving under the tutelage of Emil Kraepelin, the preeminent psychiatrist of that era, who is remembered today as the father of scientific psychiatry. Early in Alzheimer's career, Kraepelin had encouraged Alzheimer to focus on histopathology (the study of brain tissue on slides under a microscope) as a way to make clinicopathological connections in which microscopic findings are correlated with clinical data to better understand the disease process.

Though we take this approach for granted now, at the turn of the twentieth century it was a novel concept. Psychiatrists of that era were still wedded to Freudian thinking to understand and explain neuropsychiatric pathology. Even though infectious diseases causing psychiatric symptoms had been spotted under a microscope (the most common of which was syphilis), the consensus was that these were odd exceptions to the rule and that most psychiatric symptoms were invisible and due to psychological factors, such as poor parenting and psychic trauma, rather than damaged tissue. Kraepelin and his understudy believed that mental symptoms could often be explained by damage visible under a microscope, and Alzheimer's presentation in Tübingen was an attempt to advance this idea.[2]

Alzheimer's early attempts at clinicopathological connections (linking symptoms with pathology) were severely hampered by a lack of scientific understanding of what was going on inside cells. Researchers of that era did not understand DNA, RNA, mitochondria, liposomes, and cell membranes. The fields of molecular biology and genetics, the basis for our current understanding of disease, did not exist, so Alzheimer's remarkably precise descriptions of what he saw under a microscope explained very little about the disease process.

Alzheimer's case today focused on a dementia patient named Auguste Deter. Alzheimer had admitted this German housewife to the hospital and followed her closely for six years until her death. On autopsy, which was a few months earlier, he had spotted significant pathological changes in her diseased brain—and these, coupled with his clinical observations during her hospitalization, generated what he believed to be groundbreaking revelations about dementia.

Alzheimer had been going through an extremely difficult period in his life. Eleven years earlier, at age thirty-one, he had fallen deeply in love with and married the very wealthy Cecilia Geisenheimer (née

Wallerstein), whose wealthy banker husband had recently died. His wife's extensive inheritance instantly catapulted Alzheimer into a level of prosperity that allowed him to fund his own psychiatric research.[3]

But then tragedy struck. In 1901, his beloved wife died shortly after giving birth to their third child, leaving Alzheimer a thirty-seven-year-old widower with three young children.

Perhaps to overcome his grief, Alzheimer rededicated himself to research and poured himself into his hospital work. One of the mental patients he admitted to the hospital in this period was Auguste Deter, who was destined to become one of the most famous neuropsychiatric patients in medical history because she was the first to be diagnosed with what would come to be called Alzheimer's disease.

AUGUSTE DETER AND THE "DISCOVERY" OF ALZHEIMER'S DISEASE

Deter was a fifty-one-year-old woman with an eight-month history of short-term memory loss, disorientation, and hallucinations. Over the previous eight months, Deter's memory had been failing. She was having difficulty organizing the household and preparing food. Her personality had been changing—and not for the better. Her illness had initially been managed at home, but her husband, Karl, a railroad worker, was unable to both work and take care of her, so he took her to the hospital.

By the time she was admitted, Auguste Deter could not find her way around her own home, she dragged objects to and fro, and she hid herself. She got easily lost in familiar situations and developed a fear of people—even those she knew well. Periodically she became delirious, dragged her bedding around, and seemed to have auditory hallucinations. She imagined that someone wanted to kill her, and at times she shouted wildly.

Alzheimer first examined Auguste Deter on November 25, 1901, at the Municipal Asylum of Frankfurt. Not for one moment did he suspect that his clinical investigation of this patient would make him world famous for generations to come, nor was there reason to suspect that her name—and his—would grace neurology textbooks for centuries.

Alzheimer found that Deter was severely disoriented; she had lost her connection to time and place. She was anxious and confused. Although she spoke clearly, she often stopped midsentence before continuing. She could read, but she pronounced words in a flat, meaningless fashion or spelled them out letter by letter, which suggested to Alzheimer that she was having difficulty attaching meaning to words.

Alzheimer's notes indicate that Deter had impaired memory, aphasia, disorientation, and psychosocial incompetence (which at that time fit the legal definition of dementia). Over and over again during the initial interview, when stumped by one of Alzheimer's questions, Deter would repeatedly say, "Ich hab mich verloren" (I have lost myself)—an apt metaphor for the tragic changes in mental capacity suffered by all dementia patients.

Auguste Deter's condition gradually worsened. She became more distant, her activities became increasingly random and meaningless, and her speech became unintelligible. Eventually, she stopped talking altogether, and her vocalizations were limited to humming or shouting wildly, often for hours on end. In her fifth and final year of hospitalization, she became completely withdrawn, most of the time lying apathetically hunched in her bed.

THE DEATH OF AUGUSTE DETER

In 1903, after fourteen years at the Frankfurt hospital, Alzheimer was invited to join Emil Kraepelin at the Royal Psychiatric Clinic in Munich. There, Alzheimer became famous for his inspired teaching. Students and scientists flocked to Munich from around Europe for the privilege of studying under him. Several of his students went on to neurologic fame, including Friedrich H. Lewy, known today for the eponymic Lewy bodies seen in Parkinson's disease, and Hans-Gerhard Creutzfeld and Alfons Maria Jakob, the neurologists who first described the prion disease known as mad cow disease.

Despite his exciting new tasks in Munich, Alzheimer never lost interest in the special case of Auguste Deter. On April 9, 1906, he received a call from Frankfurt that Deter had died the previous day, just five weeks short of her fifty-sixth birthday.

He requested that Deter's brain and medical records be sent to him in Munich, and there he conducted an autopsy. Alzheimer gained revolutionary insights into the nature of the dementia that had ravaged the last five years of Deter's life. He was able, for the first time ever in a case of dementia, to correlate clinical psychiatric findings with documentable microscopic evidence.[4]

ALZHEIMER PRESENTS DETER'S CASE

Alzheimer's talk was entitled *Eine eigenartige Erkrankung der Hirnrinde* (A peculiar disease of the cerebral cortex). After recounting Deter's clinical symptoms and his physical examination, Alzheimer displayed his own drawings of Deter's brain cells and the abnormalities he spotted there. (He labeled them "very strange changes in the neurofibrils.")

Normal neurons contain long, thin, microscopic fibers that provide support and shape. In normal healthy cells, the neurofibrils run together in bundles of parallel fibers, much like a cable or a lock of hair made up of many small parallel strands. When these strands are damaged, they curl up, forming neurofibrillary tangles—clearly visible on the images Alzheimer presented (see fig. 4.1).

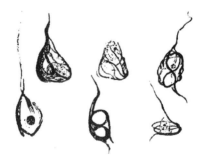

Figure 4.1. Neurofibrillary tangles from Auguste Deter,
drawn by Alois Alzheimer

Alzheimer described abundant senile amyloid plaques, which could be found throughout Deter's entire cerebral cortex. Unlike tangles, which occur inside nerve cells, plaques are distributed in the matrix between nerve cells. Alzheimer noted that these could be discerned without any staining and speculated that they had formed by the "deposition of a peculiar substance." We now know that this substance was amyloid beta.

He closed his presentation with a powerful prediction: microscopic histological analysis, coupled with clinical correlations, could—as he had just demonstrated—reveal discrete pathologies, and this was the path of the future. His esteemed (but misguided) audience was unimpressed by Alzheimer's assertion that physical lesions could cause psychiatric symptoms.

A TEPID RESPONSE

When Alzheimer concluded his talk, none of the attendees cared to discuss the case; in fact, no one even asked a question! There was no appreciation of the monumental significance of this presentation. The next speaker stepped up.

To add insult to injury, the organizers of the medical gathering considered his talk unsuitable for publication in the meeting proceedings. The local newspaper, the *Tübinger Chronik*, which covered the meeting in its November 5, 1906, issue, briefly mentioned his talk but limited its coverage to a single sentence: "Dr. Alzheimer from Munich reported of a peculiar, severe disease process which in a period of four and a half years causes a substantial loss of neurons." No other publications, scientific or otherwise, bothered to mention it.

Alzheimer's train trip back to Munich must have been sorrowful indeed. He had invested so much in this project, hoping the world (or at least a neurological corner of it) would value his observations. His peers clearly didn't share his desire to shine a bright microscopic light into dark and inaccessible regions of the brain. He had found the exact location of Deter's brain damage, correlated it with the clinical signs of malfunction, and proved the connection between the patient's lesions and her disease—an understanding that later changed the world.

REDISCOVERY OF ALZHEIMER'S SLIDES AND MODERN REANALYSIS

Fortunately, after a lengthy search, Alzheimer's original histopathology slides and clinical notes were rediscovered almost a century later (in 1992 and 1995, respectively) in a basement at the Institute of Neuropathology of the University of Munich. In a remarkable feat of science, a smidgen of Auguste Deter's one hundred-year-old DNA was extracted from the slides and in 1998 underwent state-of-the-art neuropathological and molecular genetic analysis. The researchers state "As described by Alzheimer in his original report (*Allg Zeitschr Psychiatr* 1907; 64:146–148)[5], there were numerous neurofibrillary tangles and many amyloid plaques, especially in the upper cortical layers of this patient."[6]

That might have gotten his peers' attention!

Two Exceptionally Long Droughts and the Discovery of the Multiple Modality Model

In high school, in the 1950s, my buddies and I would take an occasional afternoon off. Our principal might've called this hooky, but we looked at it as more of a well-deserved minivacation. We'd hop an elevated train, zip down to the north side of Chicago, and enjoy a Cubs game. At Wrigley Field, we'd fork over fifty cents each for a bleacher seat. The Cubbies would usually lose, but we didn't care; it was just a fun way to spend the afternoon—way better than algebra. We had no idea, as we sipped our Cokes and taunted the rival outfielders, that our beloved team was about halfway through an epic, century-plus losing streak and on the way to setting one of the most remarkable records in modern baseball: between 1908 and 2016, the Cubs failed to win a World Series, thus setting the record for longest title drought (not just in baseball but in North American professional sports history): 108 years.

During almost exactly the same time frame, the Alzheimer's researchers chalked up an equally remarkable record: not a single effective treatment for 108 years.

Alois Alzheimer first presented his dementia discoveries in 1906, just two years before the Cubs' drought began. Starting then, and for over a century, researchers struggled to find a cure but without success. Thousands of medical scientists toiled, billions of research dollars were spent, and hundreds of promising drugs were tested, but this effort generated not a single effective treatment for the disease. Then, finally, in 2014, Dale Bredesen hit the ball out of the park by publishing a pilot research study showing not only that Alzheimer's could be reversed but how to do it—thus ending one of the longest treatment droughts in medical history.

Bredesen is the brilliant and perspicacious founding president and CEO of the Buck Institute for Research on Aging in Marin County, California, and director of the Mary S. Easton Center for Alzheimer's Disease Research at the University of California, Los Angeles. His study entitled "Reversal of Cognitive Decline: A Novel Therapeutic Program," addressed Alzheimer's, for the first time, as a disease caused by a broken metabolism—a dramatic departure from the way scientists had traditionally thought about the disease. In the study, he identified the key causative metabolic imbalances in each study patient. Then he designed individualized treatment programs that addressed these causative metabolic factors.[1]

The outcome was astonishing. Nine out of the ten patients showed definite improvement. (The tenth had advanced disease.) While blazing a new research trail, Dr. Bredesen accomplished something equally splendid: he gave these patients their lives back.

WHY IT TOOK SO LONG

Why did it take over a century to come up with a treatment that worked? We didn't know enough. Several major scientific discoveries were necessary before all the pieces of a very complex puzzle could be assembled.

Until the 1990s, we knew almost nothing about the inner workings of nerve cells. When we finally began to figure out what transpires inside nerve cells, the process turned out to be far more complex than anyone had imagined.

The human brain contains about 100 billion nerve cells that make trillions of synaptic connections.[2] Each cell is an elaborate biochemical factory able to manufacture hundreds of thousands of compounds.

Each neuron talks to itself and to other nerve cells using a chemical language whose lexicon contains tens of thousands of chemical "words." Figuring all that out slowed the research process.

We had to discover and learn about genes, DNA, messenger RNA, genetic translation and expression, enzymes, proteins, hormones, cell signaling, membranes, membrane receptors, neurotransmitters, epigenetics, 3D protein chemistry, genetic sequencing, the microbiome, and much more. We had to learn about how nerve cells are nourished, how they grow, what goes wrong when they get sick and damaged, and how they recover and regenerate. We needed to learn that essential nutrients (especially B-complex, vitamins C and D, certain essential fatty acids, and some minerals such as lithium and zinc) are absolutely necessary for nerve cell health and cognitive functioning. We had to learn that toxins in food, water, and air could exert powerful adverse effects on nerve cells.

Not only did the microbiome have to be discovered, but we then had to deal with the startling consequences of learning that 98 percent of the genes controlling our brain were not in our brain or body at all but in the quadrillion or so bacteria residing in our gut.[3] And just in the past couple of decades, neuroscience breakthroughs have shown us how we grow new nerve cells, how damaged nerve cells heal, how the nervous system adapts to changing environments, and how hormone-like nerve growth factors such as BDNF mediate and control these processes.

I don't mean to imply we have arrived in terms of completely understanding dementia. We're still just scratching the surface. But we have reached a point where enlightened treatment is possible.

Each of these breakthroughs in molecular biology and genetics, in its own way, guided scientists to the central idea that metabolic disruption must be the driving force behind Alzheimer's disease.

Soon came a second realization. Since many different phenomena can disrupt nervous system metabolism, Alzheimer's disease must be multicausal.

And then scientists had a third insight. Any useful therapy would have to address multiple causes, and this would require a multiple modality approach.

THE METABOLIC DYSFUNCTION, MULTIPLE-CAUSALITY, MULTIPLE-MODALITY MODEL

The earliest seeds of the multiple-causality/multiple-modality, metabolic approach employed by Dr. Bredesen date back to the birth of nutritional medicine in 1967. In that year, one of my first teachers, two-time Nobel Prize winner Linus Pauling, PhD, coined the term *orthomolecular* to describe treatments aimed at curing disease by identifying and correcting metabolic imbalances and repairing biochemical deficiencies. The field burgeoned over the next few decades as researchers shed ever brighter light on the intimate connections between nutrition, biochemistry, and disease, filling a vital gap in the medical scene, which was, up to then, dominated by the drugs and surgery of mainstream medicine. An increasing number of doctors realized that nutrition and biochemistry are powerful, nontoxic tools that can be used to reverse disease by addressing the underlying causes.

Momentum grew for the orthomolecular approach. Today thousands of doctors practice various mixtures of alternative, nutritional, complementary, and functional medicine, integrating these with mainstream practices. In recent years, the functional medicine movement has taken the leadership role in this process.

Functional medicine is the school of medicine most closely aligned with the multiple-causality/multiple-modality concept. Functional medicine provides the roots for the ideas expressed in this book.

The term *functional medicine* was coined by—and is intimately associated with the work of—another of my teachers, Jeffrey Bland, PhD, a great biochemist who is known for his insight, sense of humor, and ability to bring complex molecular biology to life in his lectures. FM views health as a state of vitality rather than just the absence of disease and is based on a peer-reviewed mainstream scientific understanding of the molecular biology and genetics of disease causation. Its focus is on finding the root causes of disease that undermine optimum function. Causes might include improper food choices, nutritional deficiencies, hormonal imbalances, insufficient exercise, stress, and environmental toxic chemical exposures.

Physicians who subscribe to—and think in terms of—FM principles will find it much easier to adopt and apply the metabolic dysfunction, multiple-causality, multiple-modality model described in this book. Physicians who have worked only within the mainstream conventional model of medicine will be at a distinct disadvantage.

Functional medicine doctors hold a deep appreciation for genetic and biochemical differences. In diagnosis and treatment, they take environmental and ecosystem influences into account.

FM doctors assume the body wants to be healthy, has the power to heal itself, and will do so if properly supported and otherwise left to its own devices. Rather than finding a diagnostic label for a disease and then prescribing from a matching list of drugs, FM doctors try to identify and address causative mechanisms by asking these kinds of questions:

- What organ and system malfunctions would cause this symptom picture?
- What biochemical and metabolic imbalances could lead to this disorder?
- How can we assist the body's efforts to restore healthy function and homeostatic balance?

Treatment methods are natural whenever possible. The idea is to restore balance to the patient's network of metabolic systems—and to accomplish this by only using molecules that nourish systems. Avoiding toxic agents that disturb systems is especially important.

CHAPTER 6

The Search for a Cure

In terms of finding a cure, or even a treatment that helps control symptoms, our one hundred-year Alzheimer's progress report is pretty dismal. To date, every candidate drug tested in large-scale clinical trials in patients with Alzheimer's dementia has failed to show a significant effect in slowing the usual five to ten-year course of this fatal illness. More than two hundred Alzheimer's drugs have been tested, and a few can temporarily relieve a few of the symptoms, but none stops the inexorable progression of the disease.

As biochemistry, neuroscience, cell biology, and neurochemistry marched forward throughout the twentieth century, thousands of researchers struggled to understand cognitive decline, memory impairment, and Alzheimer's disease. Great strides were made in explaining brain structure and function, but no effective treatment emerged. Let's trace a little of that history.

During the first half of the twentieth century, virtually no research specifically addressed Alzheimer's disease, and public awareness was very low. In the 1950s, a fledgling drug industry spotted an Alzheimer's epidemic in the making and set its sights on a cure. "If we can just identify the *cause* of Alzheimer's," the logic went, "we'll be able to develop a drug for it." This "one cause, one treatment" (so-called monotherapy) idea made sense back then, but doubts began to surface when the search morphed into a fifty-year wild goose chase that burned through billions of research dollars without delivering a single useful drug.

Again and again, researchers came up with promising new drugs that could cure Alzheimer's in mice but always flopped in humans.

These researchers are very smart people, so one has to wonder why one of them didn't stand up and say—along about failure 198 or 199—"Hey, folks, this is not working. We are not making progress here. Might we be barking up the wrong tree?" Or maybe those voices *did* exist but were squelched by profit-motivated Big Pharma executives who thought they knew better. One in three people alive today are expected to die with dementia, which creates an enormous market. Coming up with something—anything—that worked could spawn the biggest blockbuster of all time.

Through the latter half of the twentieth century, under increasing pressure to fashion an effective drug, researchers repeatedly jumped the gun. Eager for a breakthrough and hungry for funding, when they found a hot new pharmaceutical that looked like it might work, they'd boast widely that an effective new drug therapy was "just around the corner" or "just over the horizon," but it would always fizzle. Despite failure after failure, the pharmaceutical industry persists, pumping billions upon billions into the fruitless search for the magic drug that good science tells us can't possibly exist.

The new, deeply scientific approach described in this book involves relatively inexpensive lab testing and treatments that can be purchased without a prescription. There is no pot of gold at the end of this rainbow, however, so the drug companies are not interested.

DISCOVERIES THAT PAVED THE WAY FOR AN EFFECTIVE TREATMENT

While the dementia drug fiasco plays itself out, molecular biologists, neuroscientists, and alternative-minded physicians have begun, just in the past few years, to distance themselves from the pharmaceutical approach and address Alzheimer's not as a pathology per se, but as a *multicausal molecular imbalance*.[1] This has been an especially fruitful paradigm shift—one that has led, for the first time, to successful reversal.

In Alzheimer's day—and for the next fifty years—very little was known about the complicated chemistry going on inside cells, especially nerve cells. The term molecular biology would not be coined until 1938. To understand the pathogenesis of Alzheimer's, we needed to know about genetics, but DNA wasn't discovered until the '50s. We needed cell biology, which came of age in the '80s, and molecular biology, which has blossomed in the past twenty years. An appreciation for the importance of free radicals and antioxidants materialized in the '90s, and only in the past ten years or so have we come to appreciate the importance of inflammation as a key player in neurodegenerative disease.

The most exciting discovery of all was saved for last, however. Everyone—researchers, clinicians, and laypeople alike—had accepted the dogma that humans were bestowed with a certain number of brain cells at birth, and we had better protect them because that was all we were ever going to get. Then, in the 1960s, Joseph Altman and Gopal Das published the first studies demonstrating that rodents exhibited neurogenesis.[2]

This work was ignored by the medical community, and for the next forty years, debates raged as research evidence mounted, but not until the early 2000s did the idea of neuroregeneration become fully accepted. Now everybody agrees that our brain's memory centers regenerate throughout our lives.[3] The related concepts of neuroplasticity and synaptoplasticity emerged just a few years ago.

Why is all of this important? Because it is empowering. This research means that the choices you make will determine whether or not you get dementia. Now we know the brain is not stagnant and its number of neurons is not fixed; as long as you are alive, your brain is constantly adapting and changing in response to your level of activity, your exposures, the food you eat, your stress level, your emotions, and the medicines you take. Regardless of your age, you are always capable of growing new brain cells from stem cells.

Perhaps most astonishing of all is the realization—and proof—that whether or not neuroregeneration and synaptoplasticity actually happen inside *your* brain is under your control. Whether you have a healthy, cognitively crisp, dementia-resistant brain is up to you. By making the right choices, you have the power to literally change your genetic destiny!

THE CAUSE OF ALZHEIMER'S DISEASE

As these neuroregeneration revelations unfolded, several other parallel lines of research were converging on the idea that dementia is not a simple breakdown in one molecular biological pathway, nor is it a deficiency of a neurotransmitter or a buildup of plaque or a broken circuit that, once identified, could be fixed with a single magical drug. Seeing dementia in this new natural, nutritional, biochemical, alternative, integrative, and functional context underscores the absurdity of the single-drug idea.

The newer studies all tell us that dementia is a multisystem disorder caused by a multiplicity of disrupted biochemical pathways—a cacophony caused by multiple simultaneous malfunctions in the body's vast and complex network of molecular interactions. These disruptions cause inflammation, which, if it persists, results in neurodegeneration, and neurodegeneration is accompanied by an abrupt cessation of those crucial functions that keep our brains crisp and healthy: neurogenesis, neuroregeneration, synaptoplasticity, and neuroplasticity.

These biochemical errors—*the causes of dementia*—vary greatly from one person to the next. They can be detected and then treated and normalized long before actual symptoms appear. By testing and treating your own personal risk factors for dementia, you can alter the course of the disease. This is true whether your brain is young and healthy or you have already moved into MCI.

What goes wrong in Alzheimer's has everything to do with how cells are nourished. Accordingly, nutritional, metabolic, and endocrine factors that have gone out of kilter are in a very real sense broken but amenable to repair, especially if treatment is initiated in the early stages of the disease. Not only is Alzheimer's reversible, but the medicines that work to reverse it are for the most part nontoxic and natural: diet, food-derived medicines, natural bioidentical hormones, and exercise.

Recent research has dramatically altered our understanding of neurodegenerative disease. The discovery that cognitive decline, dementia, and Alzheimer's disease are caused by simultaneous impairments in multiple metabolic systems and the realization that these broken systems can be repaired are incredible breakthroughs. They have been enhanced by the discovery of epigenetic control over DNA expression, which has further elevated our ability to determine whether or not we get dementia. For more about these remarkable epigenetic breakthroughs, see the conclusion of this book. Compromised cognition no longer needs to be a death sentence.

CHAPTER 7

Vascular Dementia and My Stroke of Luck

It was December 17, 2012. My wife was rushing me to Memorial Hospital in Santa Rosa. My entire lower left lower body was numb. I figured I must be having a stroke.

The excitement began about twenty minutes earlier. Our daughters were both in town, and the family ritual is dinner at our favorite restaurant. We had just ordered when I started feeling a little light-headed. As we waited for our food, that feeling intensified, so I stepped outside for a walk around the block to try to clear my head.

The fresh air didn't help, so I began thinking, "Hmm, could this be a stroke?" I decided probably not. I walked back into the restaurant and sat down, still not feeling right. The food hadn't arrived yet.

My younger daughter, Emma, looked intently at me. "Dad, are you okay?" she asked. The concern showed in her voice.

"Yeah, I just needed a little fresh air. But I do still feel a bit spacey."

As I sat back down, I noticed that my left leg had begun to feel numb, starting just to the left of my bellybutton and spreading all the way down to my foot. With that, I could narrow down my self-diagnosis to a TIA (transient ischemic attack) or a stroke. I figured we'd better hightail it to the hospital.

At the ER I was fast-tracked because of the stroke possibility. An MRI of my brain confirmed a 0.8 millimeter blockage of a blood vessel in my brain. As strokes go, this was a very small one, a temporary blockage of a tiny arteriole that supplies the nerves that convey feeling sensations from my left abdomen and leg to the brain.

I was admitted for overnight observation. In the morning, Dr. Peters, a thoughtful and gracious neurologist with a big smile and a neatly trimmed mustache, appeared and we sat down together at a computer screen to go over my MRI. He pointed to a tiny bright white dot in my right parietal lobe.

"There's your stroke," he said.

"Okay." I was still getting used to the idea that I was a stroke patient. "Looks pretty small."

"Yes, but you've had quite a few of these already." He directed my attention to several small fluffy-looking white spots scattered around in the same general area of my parietal lobe. There were perhaps sixteen of them.

"These small puffs of white are what we call white matter intensities and they indicate the presence of cerebral small vessel disease. Each is a tiny bit of scar tissue, a permanent piece of evidence left behind by a previous small lacunar stroke. Radiologists have several different names for them—white matter hyperintensities, white matter disease, small vessel ischemic disease, periventricular white matter changes, perivascular chronic ischemic white matter disease of aging, age-related white matter changes, and leukoaraiosis—but they are all the same thing, and all are caused by lacunar strokes."

"I've never had any symptoms."

"That's why we call them silent, Tim. You already knew that. You just didn't know you'd been having them. Most strokes are silent. Yours are the lacunar type commonly seen in aging brains—virtually always the result of improperly controlled blood pressure, cholesterol, and blood sugar—and as you know, Tim, the cumulative effect of these is Alzheimer's disease."[1]

"Yes. And clearly I haven't been working on my numbers as hard as I should have been. So I have had quite a few strokes already. I guess I'm fortunate to become aware of this problem while the damage is still minimal."

"Absolutely. Many are not so lucky. You could have had a big one last night."

Whoa. Suddenly I got it. That was the moment when I started referring to this as my "stroke of luck."

This memory is as permanently etched on my brain as are those sixteen white spots, telling me—no, screaming at me—"If you want to avoid Alzheimer's and all the misery that accompanies it, you are going to have to make some big lifestyle changes." I could no longer deny I had to work a lot harder to get my blood pressure, cholesterol, and blood sugar back on track. These white spots were not just harbingers of more strokes—I had to view them as the first baby steps down a nasty road that leads straight to vascular dementia, the road that my mother and three of her siblings had gone down.

A VERY COMMON PROBLEM

I started wondering how many millions of people are on the same hapless trajectory but aren't fortunate enough to get a shot across the bow like I did. Some online searching revealed flabbergasting numbers. About a third of seniors over seventy have had silent strokes. Even more eye-popping, 95 percent of people over sixty-five have small vessel disease (also known as white matter disease, or WMD) of the brain.[2]

I am not alone. I say that with considerable sadness.

Vascular dementia, the kind that is caused by many small strokes, is clinically indistinguishable from the purely neuronal form known as Alzheimer's disease. AD and VaD usually appear together, coexisting in varying proportions. Almost all dementia patients have some degree of both. The degree to which VaD is mistaken for AD is not known but must be very high.

The cognitive decline of VaD begins with the cumulative effects of multiple minor strokes (a.k.a. lacunar strokes or silent strokes), like mine. The earliest stage of this process includes the ministrokes that show up on an MRI as white matter hyperintensities. These cause minimal damage and usually no symptoms, so they are casually dismissed by the reading radiologist but are clear evidence that small strokes have occurred and that the small blood vessels that feed the brain are being damaged and blocked. In the short run, the price of these silent strokes is minor neurodegeneration, loss of neuroplasticity, and perhaps MCI. As damage piles up, however, symptoms of compromised thinking and memory gradually appear. This is the road to dementia.

Each white matter intensity is a stroke that happened, and though those strokes may have been small, the cumulative cognitive decline caused by them is routinely misdiagnosed as MCI or senility rather than vascular blockages. This diagnostic distinction is clinically important. While senility or MCI may be considered untreatable, the metabolic vascular changes that cause these silent strokes can (and must) be addressed and reversed. These WMD strokes are the earliest sign of developing dementia and should always be considered a wake-up call that strokes are happening and that abnormal metabolic markers need to be addressed. Virtually all of them can be molecularly traced back to untreated elevations of blood pressure, high fasting blood sugar, excess cholesterol, sleep apnea, low vitamin D, insufficient B-complex vitamins, and high homocysteine. We'll go into much more detail about each of these metabolic problems in subsequent chapters, but it is important to be aware that the presence of WMDs on an MRI is an important early warning sign of brain damage and progression toward dementia. It is a powerful call to action that is routinely disregarded.[3]

The early changes leading to dementia begin decades before the symptoms appear. It is impossible to overemphasize the importance of prevention. Know your markers. Manage them. Stop the progression of this disease in the early stages while you are still symptom-free and your cognitive decline is easily reversible.

When stroke-driven small-vessel damage has become more extensive, unequivocal symptoms will appear:

- Impaired planning and judgment
- Confusion or problems with short-term memory

- Declining ability to pay attention or follow instructions
- Laughing or crying inappropriately
- Impaired function in social situations
- Difficulty finding the right words
- Wandering or getting lost in familiar places
- Walking with rapid, shuffling steps
- Losing bladder or bowel control
- Difficulty counting money and making monetary transactions

We are all vulnerable to VaD. Unfortunately, doctors who see MCI in a patient rarely consider—and even more rarely address—the causal connection that traces back to their patient's metabolic issues. They usually assume the patient has early Alzheimer's and that nothing can be done. This is a huge error because stroke doubles the risk of dementia,[4] and at this stage, the disease is totally reversible.

IF YOU HAVE A STROKE

I was lucky. My stroke was a minor one, and clot-busting drugs were not necessary. However, with a major stroke, time is of the essence. If clot-busting drugs are administered within three hours, they will dissolve the clot, restoring blood flow and protecting the brain from major damage. The only treatment for ischemic strokes that is approved by the US Food and Drug Administration (FDA) is intravenous tPA (tissue plasminogen activator).

People who develop stroke symptoms, such as arm weakness, speech problems, or facial droop, should call for help immediately and hurry to a nearby emergency room. Call ahead to make sure it has tPA on hand; if it doesn't, locate the nearest hospital that does.

When your brain is starved of oxygen, every second counts; speedy restoration of blood flow to the brain is crucial for brain cell survival. The earlier tPA is administered, the better the outcome.

Research studies published in *Stroke* and *Neurology* found that getting to the hospital faster and administering tPA sooner—even by just a few minutes—nets big gains.[5] Data from over two thousand stroke patients showed that for every minute earlier that they received tPA, patients gained an average of one extra week of healthy life.[6]

CITICOLINE IMPROVES COGNITIVE FUNCTIONING, PREVENTS STROKES, AND REVERSES STROKE DAMAGE

All strokes—regardless of type or size—kill brain cells and move the person toward VaD. The only meaningful treatment strategy is prevention: identify and manage one's risk factors (see part 2) to speed healing and prevent recurrences. Ideally, one would identify and correct the hypertension, elevated blood sugar, elevated cholesterol and other vascular markers before a stroke appears. However, if prevention fails and a stroke has occurred, tPA is the first and most important treatment. The next step is to begin citicoline.

As soon as possible after the acute impact of the stroke is under control, one should start taking citicoline (cytidine 5'-diphosphocholine, or CDP-choline), a natural, bioidentical cognition-enhancing medicine that protects against ischemic stroke, prevents additional strokes, and reverses stroke damage.[7] Taking citicoline immediately after a stroke decreases the degree of damage and dementia caused by stroke and brain trauma. Doses of 2,000 mg/day have been found effective in research studies. Citicoline helps at every stage, but for the best outcomes in reversing the damage of an acute stroke, dosing should begin in less than forty-eight hours.

Citicoline protects against the ravages of dementia because it is the precursor to acetylcholine, our main brain neurotransmitter. In healthy individuals, citicoline improves memory, cognition, and general brain health. It also enhances neurogenesis and neurorepair.[8]

In acute ischemic stroke, citicoline has therapeutic effects. If you have had strokes in the past, or are at risk of stroke, or you have had silent strokes detected only on imaging, citicoline offers protection from future episodes. For this purpose, I recommend 1,000 mg a day.

Extensive research and clinical experience have demonstrated that long-term treatment with citicoline is a safe and effective way to improve poststroke cognitive decline and enhance functional recovery. Citicoline is free of side effects and toxicity at all doses.

Citicoline, considered a food by the FDA, is widely used in Europe and Asia to speed healing from stroke, treat and reverse the effects of stroke, and reduce the risk of subsequent dementia. Researchers have documented positive responses in stroke, MCI, and AD patients. Sadly, citicoline is almost never recommended by US physicians, who are generally unaware of its tremendous potential to reduce damage and accelerate recovery in the aftermath of a stroke—and perhaps even prevent the next one. (See chapter 31.)

CHAPTER 8

Neuroplasticity, Neurogenesis, Neuroregeneration, and the Power of Exercise

You're feeling pretty chipper. Just back from a three-mile brisk walk, you worked up a light sweat and cleared out the brain fog. You figure you got a good workout.

As you walked along, your thoughts may have drifted to the weather, your sore back, road conditions, and the daily hassles that drive us all a little nuts. But you probably weren't thinking about brain growth factors. You probably weren't thinking, "I feel smarter now" or "I just generated a bunch of BDNF—a powerful neurohormone that stimulates the growth of new neurons in my cerebral cortex." But you did! Physical activity generates BDNF, which grows new brain cells, enhances memory, improves IQ, and reverses cognitive impairment.[1]

EXERCISE: THE KEY TO NEUROPROTECTION

BDNF invigorates nerve cells in three ways. First, it stimulates neurogenesis, the growth of new nerve cells from your own stem cells. Second, it enhances neuroplasticity—your nervous system's ability to reorganize your nerve pathways. Last, but definitely not least, it amplifies synaptoplasticity—making new synaptic interconnections between neurons by encouraging them to grow new tendrils that reach out and make new connections with nearby nerve cells. So BDNF gives you new brain cells that are more open and flexible and more communicative.

The BDNF generated during your exercise also increased the size of your brain. Each brisk walk or run adds just a bit of gray matter, but researchers have shown that the cumulative effect of regular jogging generates an annual 2 percent gain in brain size and cell count. Couch potatoes are headed in the other direction.[2]

BDNF PROTECTS AGAINST ALZHEIMER'S

Given the above information, it should come as no surprise that the brains of AD patients have been found to contain significantly lower levels of BDNF than the brains of healthy patients[3] and that restoring BDNF reverses neurodegenerative conditions. Your program for cognitive decline prevention and reversal should therefore be aimed at upgrading your body's production of BDNF. This book points out numerous ways to do just that.

Although exercise is the most effective method to increase your BDNF, levels can be raised many other ways: following a ketogenic diet, applying caloric restriction, and consuming some delicious foods, such as blueberries, walnuts, coconut oil, almonds, green tea, chocolate and cocoa, and (believe it or not) coffee. Supplemental low-dose lithium and DHA also do it. You'll find a more complete list later in this chapter. For now, I want to shift the conversation to your hippocampus because that is the place in your brain where most of your BDNF is made.

THE HIPPOCAMPUS: YOUR BRAIN'S MEMORY CENTER

The hippocampus is a funny-named, funny-shaped area located deep in the brain's temporal lobe, near the center of the brain (fig. 8.1). Though the hippocampus accounts for only about 1 percent of the brain's total volume, it is the reservoir for all past knowledge and experience. It controls virtually all aspects of memory: storage, retrieval, and processing. Memories of everything that ever happened to you are stored there, ready to be accessed and used on a moment's notice. Every place you have been, every trip you have taken, every person you have met, every interpersonal interaction—a lifetime of information has been salted away in this relatively small and specialized area of the brain.

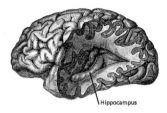

Figure 8.1. The hippocampus

The hippocampus is also your brain's center for coordinating learning, concentration, time management, goalsetting, clear thinking, and long-term planning. It stores and manages every word you have learned, searches for the right one from tens of thousands, and helps you organize words into meaningful sequences. Walking, jogging, playing sports, traveling, running errands, working, and just plain "doing stuff" are all forms of navigation that depend on memories processed by the hippocampus. Navigational memory in the hippocampus is crucial for finding our way around and keeping track of events that occur, like those that enabled you to get through this morning's walk.

How did the hippocampus get its name? *Hippocampus* is the Greek word for seahorse (hippos, "horse," and kampos, "sea monster"). The term was originally used to describe an ancient Greek and Phoenician mythological sea creature with a horse's head and the body of a fish. Some mythologically savvy neuroanatomist noticed that the brain's memory area was shaped like a seahorse (fig. 8.2), and the word resonated.

The hippocampus is where physical activity exerts its most potent BDNF-producing effect and is where almost all our BDNF is made. Not surprisingly, it is also the central location for most neurogenesis,

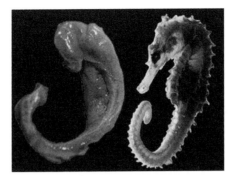

Figure 8.2. The hippocampus (left) named after the seahorse (right)
(Photo by Laszlo Seress, 1980; modified by Anthonyhcole, 2010, CC BY-SA 8.0)

neuroplasticity, and synaptoplasticity. The breakdown of these processes in the hippocampus in the earliest stages of cognitive decline can be spotted on an MRI.

NEUROGENESIS, NEUROREGENERATION, AND NEUROPLASTICITY FOR LIFE

Neurologists (and pretty much everybody else) used to think that the adult brain was static. They believed we were born with a finite number of brain cells, and any that died would not be replaced.

They were wrong. Scientific research disproving the fixed-brain idea began in the 1960s and '70s, but it took over two decades for the idea to gain traction in the scientific community. Now no one doubts that our brains continue to regenerate, continuously making new cells and circuits throughout our lives.[4]

Our brains remain malleable until death—continually changing in response to our lifestyle, environment, exposures, diet, and exercise. Even the elderly can generate new nerve cells for life and can create measurable changes in brain size and capacity. This is especially true in the hippocampus, where neurogenesis has been shown to persist throughout life.[5]

The synapse (the gap between nerve cells that relays nerve impulses to the next nerve cell in the circuit) has also received a major upgrade from recent research. We used to think that the synapse's only job was to transfer information between one neuron and the next. It was thought that these connections were relatively fixed, like the solder between two electric wires. But new research has shown that the gap between neurons—and even the neurotransmitter chemicals that nerve cells secrete into the synapse—are also plastic. The term for this is *synaptoplasticity*, the ability of synapses to strengthen or weaken over time in response to increases or decreases in their activity. Since memories are generated by vast networks of synapses in the brain, many experts think that synaptoplasticity is central to understanding the mechanisms of learning and memory.

INCREASING YOUR BDNF LEVELS

BDNF, neurogenesis, neuroplasticity, and synaptoplasticity are under your control, and you can choose to enhance them with diet, supplements, and exercise to prevent and reverse dementia. An overwhelming number of research studies tell us that high-level brain fitness is associated with increased production of BDNF and its ability to unleash neurogenesis, neuroplasticity, and synaptoplasticity. These, in turn, are virtually always associated with increased hippocampal volume, better memory, across-the-board cognitive enhancement, and improved overall brain function.[6]

Exercise, in particular, turbocharges BDNF production. A modest amount of moderate intensity physical activity is necessary to take advantage of the brain's natural capacity for plasticity, resulting in improved cognitive performance, better academic achievement, and reduced dementia risk.[7]

Beyond exercise, dietary choices can have profound effects on the amount of BDNF generated in the hippocampus. At the top of this list is a class of foods known as polyphenols, a type of flavonoid. Blueberries are perhaps the richest source of BDNF-generating polyphenols, but many other foods also contain these wonderful compounds.

Many published studies have examined the connection between BDNF levels and dietary flavonoid/polyphenol intake.[8] Diets high in fruit and vegetables are highly correlated with improvements in BDNF and global cognitive performance. The correlation is even higher when the diet is high in polyphenols (e.g., blueberries, cocoa, curcumin/turmeric, green tea, and grapes), DHA (an omega-3 essential fatty acid), and medium chain triglycerides from coconut oil. A diet rich in these molecules will thwart cognitive decline and reverse neurodegeneration. Polyphenol compounds are so important to brain health—and their ability to block and reverse Alzheimer's disease has been so thoroughly researched—that I have devoted several chapters (20, 24–26, 29, and 30) to them.

The essential mineral lithium has been shown to increase BDNF, stimulate neurogenesis, and reverse cerebral atrophy. Even more remarkably, lithium has been shown to prevent cognitive decline—it halts the progression of, and can even reverse, Alzheimer's disease. (See chapter 27.)

Ways To Boost BDNF Production

Here is a list of ways to stimulate BDNF production in your body. The more of these strategies you incorporate into your daily life, the more new brain cells you will grow, and the better your brain will be protected from neurodegenerative disease:

- Exercise
- Ketogenic diet (a very low-carb, high-fat diet)
- Autophagy, intermittent fasting, caloric restriction
- Lithium orotate
- Barlean's flaxseed oil (for ALA [alpha-linolenic acid] and DHA)
- DHA from Neuromins (algae-derived mercury-free DHA)
- Eicosamax molecularly distilled marine lipids (DHA and EPA [eicosapentaenoic acid])
- Curcumin (cooked in coconut oil, or as Longvida in capsules)

- Coconut oil
- B-complex vitamins, especially
  - Folic acid (as methylfolate)
  - Vitamin B12 (oral methylcobalamine or intramuscular injections)
- High polyphenol foods, such as blueberries, strawberries, raspberries, and cherries (see lists in chapter 24)
  - Green tea
  - Coffee (epigallocatechin gallate)
  - Vitamin E (mixed tocopherols)
  - Zinc
  - Resveratrol
  - Walnuts
  - Blueberries
  - Curcumin
  - Cocoa and dark chocolate

Foods and Nutrient Deficiencies That Block BDNF Production

Many of the most common dietary practices undermine our brain's ability to regenerate. To the extent you can reduce the following, you will be nurturing the neurogenesis necessary to have the healthiest possible brain:

- Sugar
- Ethanol and all alcoholic beverages
- Saturated fats
- Omega-6 oils
- Soft and white foods
- Vitamin A deficiency
- Vitamin E deficiency

EXERCISE HAS MANY BENEFITS

The hippocampus shrinks "normally" with aging at the rate of about 1 or 2 percent a year. Many studies have shown that declining BDNF, hippocampal volume, and memory loss are tightly correlated and that the rate of hippocampal atrophy is accelerated in dementia patients.[9]

To prevent this shrinkage, exercise is the single most important factor. Exercise generates a light sprinkling of BDNF throughout the brain, generally encouraging neuroplasticity and neurogenesis—but exercise deposits relatively massive quantities in the hippocampus—more there, by far, than anywhere else. Why? We don't yet know the details, but it is certainly related to the fact that the hippocampus is the brain's memory center.

Neuroscientist Kirk Erickson, an associate professor and director of the Brain Aging and Cognitive Health Lab at the University of Pittsburgh, wondered whether exercise might be able to reverse BDNF decline, so he rounded up 120 older adults and started half of them on three days a week of aerobic exercise; the other half began a placebo stretching program. At the end of one year, the two groups were compared.

The results were astonishing. The hippocampi in the aerobics group had enlarged, their BDNF levels were higher, and their memories had improved. As expected, the exercise-free control group had lost hippocampal size, their BDNF levels declined, and they were losing memory as their brains aged and shrank.

Erickson's study, entitled "Exercise Training Increases Size of Hippocampus and Improves Memory," was published in 2011 in the prestigious *Proceedings of the National Academy of Sciences of the United States of America*. The authors reported, "Exercise training increased hippocampal volume by 2 percent, effectively reversing age-related loss in volume by 1 to 2 years." This study showed that even when started later in life, aerobic exercise is neuroprotective and can dramatically enhance cognition while rekindling dormant neuroplasticity![10]

Research studies have shown that exercise enhances every aspect of a healthy high functioning brain, including neurogenesis, neuroregeneration, neuroplasticity, hippocampal volume, BDNF levels, and memory. Exercise also has been shown to reduce the generation and deposition of the two nasty proteins most intimately associated with Alzheimer's disease: amyloid beta (plaques) and tau protein (neurofibrillary tangles).[11]

TIME TO GET MOVING!

The studies are unanimous. Daily physical exercise promotes neurogenesis and specifically targets the hippocampus, the area of the brain damaged by Alzheimer's.[12] Aerobic exercise dramatically reduces the brain changes known to cause Alzheimer's. No medication can rival these effects or make this claim. A sedentary lifestyle encourages cognitive decline, while exercise protects against dementia.

Get up and shake your booty! At least that's what you need to do if you want to maintain your sharp wit and keen sense of humor—not to mention your memory.

The best scientific evidence suggests we benefit most from at least 450 minutes of exercise per week. That is a little over an hour a day, seven days a week, and that's what I recommend to my patients.

You don't have to be training for a marathon during these minutes. Almost any activity qualifies as exercise, as long as it raises your heart rate a little. The important thing is to be active and keep moving. Try different activities. Figure out what is comfortable and fun and do that. You can make it up as you go.

To optimize the benefits of exercise, we need to do it every day. Sometimes life doesn't give us a spare hour, or we are not physically ready for that level of activity, so we do what we can. Even if you can manage only twenty minutes on some days, that's far better than nothing. (But if you can't fit it in, don't stress about it; researchers have shown that stress impairs neurogenesis and neuroplasticity.)[13]

Daily walking, jogging, or running is the most important exercise. This can form the basis of your program, so if you do only one activity, let that be it. Repeating the same distance or route or intensity is fine. You can do your exercise all at once or piece it together throughout the day; it doesn't matter. The idea behind walking and jogging is to exercise the muscles in the walls of the arteries everywhere in your all-important cardiovascular system and to keep the BDNF flowing. This should happen every day.

Other than the daily walking or jogging, try to vary what you do. If you do the same routine over and over again, day in and day out, your body becomes very efficient and experiences less of a training effect.

If you choose activities you enjoy, you'll be more likely to actually *do* them. I walk or jog every day. But I also usually run and shoot baskets, play Ping-Pong with my wife, and work vigorously in the garden.

Your exercise can include any of the following for preventing Alzheimer's disease:

- Walking or jogging on a treadmill or elliptical machine
- Outdoor hiking
- Stationary bicycle
- Stair climber
- Calisthenics
- Aerobic fitness classes
- Spinning
- TV/video exercise classes
- Aggressive gardening
- Resistance exercise (weight lifting, machines, stretch bands, push-ups, etc.)
- Basketball
- Ping-Pong (but not beer pong)
- Pull-ups on a bar
- A walking desk
- Swimming

You can even make up your own exercise. Be creative. Almost any activity has the potential to become an exercise. Remind yourself that activity increases the size and health of your brain!

Biomarker Testing: Identifying the Causes of Alzheimer's

Part 2 examines the biomarker testing we use to pinpoint the root metabolic imbalances that cause Alzheimer's disease. Abnormal biomarkers identify the causes and provide a road map for prevention and reversal. To reverse cognitive decline, these metabolic errors must be restored to normal. Identifying and addressing abnormal markers early, before significant brain damage has accumulated, optimizes the effectiveness of treatment. Even late discovery, with treatment, however, can reverse (or at least arrest progression of) the disease.

Chapter 9 is about testing and provides a brief overview of the markers. The following ten chapters (10–19) discuss each specific marker. These chapters provide the information you need to understand and interpret your results and explain how to use this information to develop your individualized treatment program.

Testing Your Alzheimer's Biomarkers—Why and How

For those who want to prevent cognitive decline and eventual dementia, the markers discussed in this chapter provide valuable information as to what to do to optimize your brain power while preventing decline. They define your unique set of metabolic causes of cognitive decline and thus provide a road map for prevention.

For those who already have signs of cognitive decline, these markers provide extremely useful insight into the multiple causes of that decline. Addressing *all* the abnormal markers will slow, stop, and hopefully reverse it.

The necessary biomarkers for Alzheimer's are listed below, along with a brief explanation of how to use the test results for preventing and reversing brain disease.

Please note that the "normal" result levels provided on lab reports often differ from the optimal levels we seek in terms of preventing neurodegenerative disease. Use the normal levels provided in this book when they differ from the levels provided by the lab. For example, LabCorp gives 30–100 ng/mL as its normal range for vitamin D, but a level of 30 will do nothing more than keep most people from getting rickets (a vitamin D deficiency disease). A great body of research evidence has shown that optimum levels are considerably higher. Having studied this issue extensively, I recommend 70–100 ng/mL to prevent

Alzheimer's. The same goes for all the other markers: lab normals can vary widely from the optimum levels required to reverse dementia.

COST, PRICING, AND INSURANCE INFORMATION

Medicare will cover the blood tests. If you want your insurance to cover any test, you will need a lab order from your doctor. Be sure your test order contains the correct codes. A sample lab test order with typical ICD-10 diagnostic codes is provided in appendix 1.

Medicare covers sleep apnea testing if you have clinical signs and symptoms of sleep apnea. Medicare and most insurance do not cover hair analysis and stool testing.

Test prices can vary dramatically, so be sure to compare before ordering. Direct Labs (www.directlabs.com) offers high-quality testing at prices far below those of other major labs and at times even less than your insurance copay for the same tests. If you use Direct Labs, a doctor's order is not necessary. The company will email you a lab test order to print out. ICD-10 diagnostic codes are not necessary.

BLOOD PRESSURE

Since you will need several readings, you should plan to take your own blood pressure. For initial screening, any blood pressure device is fine. Pharmacies, department stores, and online stores sell them for $20 to $40. If your blood pressures run high, even borderline high, you might want to consider purchasing an iHealth Feel wireless blood pressure monitor (more below).

The normal range is at or below 120/80. Be concerned if your resting pressure is above 130/85. If any of your pressures are higher than these numbers—even just a little higher—you will need to do regular monitoring for a week or two to determine whether you have high blood pressure. (Stay inactive for at least fifteen minutes before taking each pressure reading.) Your blood pressure is constantly changing, so take several readings at different times of day to accurately determine whether it is high.

Above-normal readings indicate you have hypertension—and your risk of stroke, brain damage, and dementia is greatly increased. You are going to need to address this problem aggressively because the brain damage caused by high blood pressure is the most common cause of cognitive decline and Alzheimer's disease.

Hypertension's reputation as a silent killer is well deserved. In the early stages, high blood pressure does not cause symptoms. A lot of damage will be done before symptoms begin to appear.

There is no reason to learn to live with hypertension; it is a treatable, reversible disease. To understand this problem better, read chapter 10.

Follow your numbers closely until they are consistently down in the normal range. For that, you will need a good device. Since you will need to check your pressures frequently, I recommend purchasing the iHealth Feel wireless blood pressure monitor. It pairs with your iPhone or Android device. It has no tubes or wires. It will keep track of all your readings and send them anywhere, and it costs less than $100. This device makes taking blood pressures a breeze.

BLOOD TESTS

The following tests require a blood sample that is examined by a medical laboratory:

- Fasting blood sugar
- Lipid panel (cholesterol), LDL (low-density lipoprotein), HDL (high-density lipoprotein), VLDL (very low-density lipoprotein), triglycerides
- Vitamin D (25-hydroxy vitamin D)
- Homocysteine, serum
- Thyroid (TSH [thyroid-stimulating hormone], free T3 [triiodothyronine], free T4 [thyroxine], antithyroid antibody panel)
- Ferritin, serum
- Steroid hormones (testosterone, progesterone, estrogen, DHEA-S)

Fasting Blood Sugar

For fasting blood sugar the normal range is 80–90 mg/dL. Levels above 90 indicate that insulin resistance may be damaging your brain cells, causing memory problems, diminished cognition, cerebral atrophy, and dementia. (See chapter 11.)

Lipid Panel

For a lipid panel, the following levels are considered normal: cholesterol less than 200 mg/dL, triglycerides less than 150 mg/dL, LDL less than 100 mg/dL, and HDL over 40 mg/dL.

Elevated cholesterol promotes vascular dementia in several ways. It encourages strokes by causing deposition of cholesterol plaque in the walls of cerebral vessels. High cholesterol also causes the deposition of amyloid beta plaque in the brain's memory centers.

Triglycerides reflect food calories that have been consumed and absorbed through the intestinal wall and are floating in the bloodstream on the way to being either burned off or stored. Your triglyceride level is a good indicator of whether you are eating more calories than you are burning off. If your triglyceride level is above 150 mg/dL, you are consuming more calories than your body can burn off, and the excess is headed for storage as fat for later use. (See chapter 12.)

Vitamin D

You should test for 25-hydroxy vitamin D. The optimum range is 70–100 ng/mL.

Low vitamin D causes cognitive decline. Optimizing D prevents and reverses dementia. Testing—and repeat testing three months or so after any dose change—is necessary because the dose to achieve the optimum range varies from one person to another.

Vitamin D stimulates clearance of amyloid beta plaque deposits from the brain, boosts immune function, prevents oxidative damage to nervous tissue, and suppresses inflammation, the underlying cause of all neurodegenerative disease. Vitamin D also supports the production of nerve growth factor, a protein that controls the growth of new nerve cells from stem cells. (See chapter 14.)

Homocysteine

The ideal homocysteine level is less than 7.2 micromoles per liter (μmol/L).

Elevated levels are caused by B-complex vitamin deficiencies. Too much homocysteine causes cascades of toxic inflammatory reactions that damage organs and ravage the intricate inner workings of your brain. The consequence is a broad range of brain and body disorders, including strokes, heart attacks, and dementia. (See chapter 13.)

Ferritin

Iron overload causes dementia. Ferritin measures how much iron is in your system. The normal range for serum ferritin is between 20 and 80 ng/mL. Below 20 indicates iron deficiency. Above 80 indicates a surplus. The optimum range is 40–60 ng/mL. A level above 80 indicates an excess buildup of iron. Donate a unit of blood and retest in a few months to make sure levels are not creeping up again. (See chapter 18.)

Thyroid

For thyroid tests, normal ranges are as follows: free T3 greater than 3.0–5.5, free T4 greater than 0.9–1.9, and TSH 0.5–1.5.

A low thyroid predisposes one to dementia by slowing down brain metabolism, undermining neurogenesis and neuroplasticity.

Hashimoto's disease is an autoimmune disease in which antithyroid antibodies attack thyroid tissues. The antithyroid antibody panel measures levels of these antibodies. Two separate results are included: (1) ATA (antithyroglobulin antibody) and (2) TPO (thyroperoxidase antibody). (Normal ranges are supplied with the results.) The ATA is usually done just once to rule Hashimoto's disease in or out. (See chapter 17.)

Sex Steroid and Adrenal Hormones

Hormones to be tested include progesterone (males and females), estrogen (females only), testosterone (males and females), and DHEA-S (males and females). You can order these tests for yourself, but it is best to have a specialist in natural hormone replacement therapy—usually an alternative-minded MD, DO (doctor of osteopathy), or ND (doctor of naturopathic medicine)—interpret your lab results and prescribe and adjust doses.

You don't need a specialist to regulate your own DHEA. DHEA-S is a main adrenal hormone associated with stress tolerance, optimum health, and longer life span. (The sulfated form of DHEA is the most accurate measure of body levels.) Optimum is 300–500 mcg/dL in women and 500–800 mcg/dL in men. You can purchase DHEA over the counter and adjust your dose based on the lab results. For women, increments (or decrements) of 10 mg are best. For men, dose adjustments of 25 mg (up or down) work better. Wait at least a month before repeat testing. (See chapter 19.)

OBSTRUCTIVE SLEEP APNEA

OSA causes its victims to stop breathing while asleep, causing oxygen deprivation. OSA affects 30 million Americans and a majority of people over fifty-five years of age, but few victims are aware they have a problem. You can't diagnose yourself, but if your sleep partner tells you that you snore, snort, gasp, or stop breathing while asleep, you almost certainly have OSA. If you have high blood pressure, the likelihood of OSA is also high.

Your cells, tissues, and organs do not take kindly to interruptions in their oxygen supply. They churn out what I call the biochemicals of desperation—neurotransmitters, cytokines, and other pro-inflammatory compounds—a molecular biological mobilization of defenses against perceived imminent death. As the cumulative damage from months and years of these breathing interruptions mounts, arterial and neurologic disease sets in. OSA causes a range of common chronic illnesses related to neurodegeneration, including strokes, cognitive deficit, hypertension, heart problems, memory problems, foggy headedness, daytime fatigue or drowsiness, and a shorter life span.

If you snore or have difficulty sleeping, if you awaken unrefreshed or have daytime fatigue, or if you have hypertension, heart problems, or cognitive decline, get a referral from your primary care doctor for a polysomnogram. This test must be prescribed by a physician and done by a sleep specialist at a sleep lab. It is covered by Medicare and many health insurance policies. A home version of this test is now available, a welcome addition for those who don't want to sleep in a lab. For a more extensive discussion of the home test and more about sleep apnea, see chapter 15.

MICROBIOME

If you experience intestinal or digestive symptoms—food intolerance or food allergies, indigestion, heartburn, bloating, cramps, gas, loose stools—you almost certainly have a damaged and dysfunctional gut microbiome. You may have been told you have IBS or dysbiosis.

The microbiome can be severely disturbed and the intestinal tract badly inflamed without causing overt symptoms. Many people have severe leaky gut (the technical term is intestinal hyperpermeability) even though they have no intestinal symptoms.

Whether you have intestinal symptoms or not, you likely have microbiome issues and dysbiosis if you have been diagnosed with any autoimmune disease. The most common are rheumatoid arthritis, lupus, ankylosing spondylitis, chronic fatigue syndrome, fibromyalgia, allergies, multiple sclerosis, scleroderma, Hashimoto's disease, Graves' disease, type 1 diabetes, acne, and obesity. In autoimmune disease, the leaky gut wall allows undesirable chemicals to pass through the porous gut wall directly into the bloodstream, which then delivers them to far-flung target organs. (See chapter 16.)

Stool testing can help clarify the problem. You could order a Genova Diagnostics GI Effects Microbial Ecology Profile. However, this test is expensive, and standard insurance coverage is unlikely. If you have *any* autoimmune disease or if you have the typical symptoms of dysbiosis (and your healthcare practitioner has ruled out serious GI disorders), you can assume the problem is a damaged microbiome. In that case, you can proceed with the following treatment program, which addresses the causes of the disturbance using safe, natural medicines. If this program is not effective after a few weeks, see a functional medicine doctor for a more extensive workup.

The program to heal a damaged gut microbiome is as follows:

- *Probiotics*—Acidophilus, Bifidobacteria, and related species of healthy bacteria will aggressively repopulate your damaged microbiome. Forcing colonies of pathogens off your valuable gut real estate allows your microbiome to heal and function properly again so it can do its job of directing genetic traffic for the brain, the nervous system, and the rest of your body. Use Ther-Biotic Complete from Klaire Labs, four to six capsules once or twice a day.

- *Prebiotics*—These provide ideal nourishment for the probiotic organisms so they can more rapidly set up healthy bacterial colonies that will then force out the bad bugs. To feed your flora, I recommend Biotagen from Klaire Labs, three capsules once or twice a day.

- *Elimination of allergenic and inflammatory foods*—If you have food intolerances or gas (a sure sign of intestinal flora disruption), you can also take digestive enzymes; they break down food while it is still in your stomach so that it can't cause food allergic reactions or feed bad bugs (gas-forming pathogens). Take three to four capsules with each meal. In case of a severe food reaction, up to ten capsules of vegetable-derived digestive enzymes may be necessary.

- *Natural antibiotics*—These kill off the pathogens that have taken over large pieces of real estate in your gut. I recommend Tricycline from Allergy Research Group, two capsules twice a day.
- *Biofilm disrupters* (InterFase/Klaire Labs)—These contain nutrients that break down the protective barrier (known as biofilm) that bad bacteria build around their colonies to keep out threatening immune cells and antibiotics. Without their protective biofilm barrier, the bad bugs succumb a whole lot quicker. Take three or four capsules once or twice a day.

This program may seem like it requires taking a ton of pills, but I have prescribed it to thousands of people with disturbed microbiomes over the past quarter century, and it works! Fixing a damaged microbiome is a huge step toward reversing autoimmune disease, achieving optimum health, and averting cognitive decline.

For more about the microbiome and a deeper discussion of the rationale for the treatment program, see chapter 16.

TOXIC METAL HAIR ANALYSIS

In a hair analysis you want to look for elevated mercury, lead, iron, aluminum, and cadmium. These and other toxic metals cause a variety of severe health problems, not the least of which is neurodegenerative disease. Exposures are widespread and come from food, water, and our polluted environment. Mercury is in all seafood and all amalgam dental fillings. Old paint and chocolate can contain lead. Cadmium is found in batteries and almost all chocolates.

It is not possible to determine from symptoms alone whether you have been exposed to toxic metals. Hair analysis is the best way to screen for heavy metal toxicity. It is inexpensive, easy, and very accurate, I recommend it for anyone who wants to avoid cognitive decline. I suggest Doctor's Data Toxic and Essential Elements Hair Mineral Analysis. It costs less than $150.

See chapter 18 for more information about how toxic minerals damage the brain.

CHAPTER 10

High Blood Pressure Causes Vascular Dementia

Dementia is widely regarded as a disease of neurons, and when we think of Alzheimer's disease, we tend to think of damage to the brain's nerve cells. But as researchers get closer to an explanation of Alzheimer's, it is becoming increasingly apparent that damage to the blood vessels that supply oxygen and nutrients to those nerve cells is at least as important as the direct nerve cell damage.

Every nerve cell in the brain has a blood supply. If a blood vessel in the brain is compromised for any reason, every nerve that vessel supplies is affected. The more extensive the damage to the brain's blood supply, the more the brain's nerve cells will malfunction. This malfunction is that combination of damage to vessels and nerves that we call vascular dementia. This is good news because we can find the causes and reverse blood vessel damage.

The main metabolic factors that lead to vascular damage (and thus to vascular dementia) are high blood sugar, high cholesterol, and high homocysteine. Sleep apnea and low vitamin D are also causative factors in cerebrovascular injury. But uncontrolled hypertension is the most common cause of the brain blood vessel damage that leads to dementia.

WHAT IS BLOOD PRESSURE?

Let's consider a blood pressure reading of 120/80. What do the numbers mean?

When your heart contracts, it pushes blood from your left ventricle out through the aorta and into your vascular system. The *systolic* pressure (the first, higher number) is the highest pressure achieved at the end of a given heartbeat. Normal systolic blood pressure is 120 millimeters of mercury (mm Hg) or less.

After contracting, your heart muscle relaxes. The pressure in the vascular system goes down, and your ventricle fills in preparation for the next beat. The lowest pressure in the system—achieved right before the beginning of the next contraction—is called the *diastolic* pressure. Normal diastolic blood pressure is 80 mm Hg or less.

To be considered normal, both your systolic and diastolic numbers must fall at or below these limits. If either number is consistently high, you have hypertension. A systolic blood pressure consistently over 130 or a diastolic pressure over 80 will damage your vascular system, heart, kidneys, and brain—and set the stage for dementia.

In hypertension, for reasons not yet clear, the muscles in the walls of blood vessels tighten, which causes excessive resistance to the flow of blood. The heart, sensing that resistance, contracts more forcefully to push the blood through, and this drives the pressure up, damaging the blood vessels. The heart becomes a nonstop jackhammer that traumatizes blood vessels from the inside. This constant punishment causes inflammation, hardening, narrowing, plaque buildup, blockage, and even bursting of vessel walls.

The blood vessels are damaged, but the organs supplied with blood also take a beating. The three organs most dramatically affected are the brain (strokes and dementia), heart (myocardial infarctions), and kidneys (chronic renal disease and kidney failure).

High blood pressure is almost always symptom-free. Measuring your blood pressure is the only way to find out whether you have this silent killer.

MY "STROKE OF LUCK" REVISITED

In mid-2010, at age sixty-eight, I discovered I had high blood pressure. It wasn't causing any symptoms, I felt great, and I had been taking good care of my body by exercising a lot and eating a very clean diet, so at first I didn't take it seriously. That was a big mistake. For years, my brain had been accumulating exactly the kind of damage I just described: the relentless, symptom-free pounding of high blood pressure.

As I mention in chapter 7, in December 2012, I had a small stroke. Fortunately, it caused only minor, transient symptoms. It was actually a blessing because, without doing major or permanent damage, it catapulted me into an awareness that I had been traveling down a one-way road that leads to cognitive impairment.

I could just as easily have had a massive stroke with severe brain damage. I could have ended up with a physical disability or dementia, but instead I got a powerful warning. That's why I call it my "stroke of luck." You might not be as lucky.

I immediately began taking my blood pressure a lot more seriously and have worked hard to develop a program that would control it. I learned that I might be doing everything else right, but if I ignore my elevated blood pressure, sooner or later brain damage will appear.

I used to use an off-the-shelf drugstore blood pressure monitor. It worked fine, but if you have a blood pressure problem and need to take many readings, that style is clunky. A few years ago I shifted to the iHealth Feel app-based arm blood pressure monitor (around $100), and I'd never go back. It has no tubes or wires; it pairs by Bluetooth with iPhone, iPad, or Android devices; and it makes taking and recording blood pressures a whole lot easier. The cuff inflates automatically and sends the readings to your mobile device, where they can be viewed. Readings are charted to give a clear overview of your blood pressure trends and can be easily transmitted to other devices, so you can share your data with your doctor or caregiver right from your touchscreen.

When measuring your blood pressure, remember the following:

- Normal blood pressure is 120/80. Be concerned if your pressure is above 130/85.
- Several readings are necessary. If any of your readings are high, you'll need to monitor your blood pressure regularly.
- Take pressures in a relaxed sitting position at least fifteen minutes after activity.

LOWERING YOUR BLOOD PRESSURE

Getting your blood pressure under control can be challenging, but it's worth the effort. You can lower your blood pressure by getting more exercise, changing your diet, and taking supplements. Antihypertensive medications are also available.

Exercise

A comprehensive exercise regimen is recommended for anyone who desires optimum health, but for those with high blood pressure, it becomes an absolute necessity. Your vascular system can be seen as a set of muscle-lined tubes that are begging to be exercised. Daily exercise dramatically lowers pressures and decreases your risk of dementia-causing strokes. At the very least, walk an hour every day. (It doesn't have to be all at once.)

Diet and Supplements

Olive leaf extract lowers blood pressure and has a mechanism of action similar to that of calcium channel blocker blood pressure drugs. In a 2011 study, researchers gave hypertensive subjects 1,000 mg of olive leaf extract daily for eight weeks. They saw a significant dip in both blood pressure and LDL ("bad cholesterol").[1]

People with higher vitamin D levels are more likely to have lower blood pressure and are less likely to develop hypertension. Conversely, individuals with low vitamin D levels are more likely to have hypertension. Studies have shown that taking a vitamin D supplement can help reduce blood pressure in people with hypertension.[2]

Optimizing your vitamin D level doesn't just lower your blood pressure; it also protects against dementia. To learn how to determine if your vitamin D level is low and what to do if it is, see chapter 14. You will need to monitor your blood vitamin D levels and then find, through testing at two to three-month intervals, the dose of vitamin D that gets you into the optimum range.

Coenzyme QH (CoQH, the most active, reduced form of Coenzyme Q10 [CoQ10]) is a powerful antioxidant that supports optimum cellular energy production. CoQH helps lower blood pressure naturally while toning your heart and mitochondrial energy-generating system. One study showed an average reduction in systolic blood pressure of 17 mm Hg in subjects taking CoQ10.[3]

Polyphenols are nutraceuticals in food that provide a remarkable array of health benefits—including lowering blood pressure. Some of the best sources include flaxseed, walnuts, almonds, cashews, carrots, celery, beets, artichoke, kale, bell peppers, hot peppers, red lettuce, spinach, tomatoes, onions, broccoli, sweet potatoes, lima beans, blackberries, blueberries, mangos, watermelon, apples, strawberries, raspberries, cherries, plums and prunes, grapes, pink grapefruit, apricots, nectarines, peaches, citrus, cocoa, dark chocolate, green tea, black tea, coffee, pure pomegranate juice, grape seed extract, curcumin (curries), basil, and rosemary.[4]

For more about polyphenols, see chapter 24. For ideas about how to improve your diet, see chapter 20.

Medications

If, after a few months, natural methods don't seem to be moving your numbers toward the normal range, antihypertensive medications may be necessary to get you the rest of the way.

RAPID BLOOD PRESSURE REDUCTION

If your blood pressure is normally under control but shoots up because of stress, emotional reactions, or even no apparent reason, here are two methods I have found helpful to get it back down quickly:

- *Deep slow breathing*—Inhale deeply (in all the way) over four seconds, hold that breath for four to six seconds, and then exhale rapidly and completely for another four seconds. Rest a few seconds and repeat. Do this ten to twenty times. This releases nitric oxide (NO), which will quickly and dramatically lower your blood pressure.[5]
- *A hot shower or hot bath*—Use the highest temperature water that is still comfortable. Hot water causes vasodilation (opening of the small vessels near the skin's surface), which also triggers a release of NO.

The hot shower and breathing techniques are not solutions to the long-term problem of high blood pressure but are extremely useful in lowering acutely high pressures to minimize damage to your brain and kidneys while other resources (usually medication) are kicking in. I have used them often when my pressure spikes. For me, the short-term effect of a hot shower can last from one to four hours. To sustain the effects of the breathing technique, I have to repeat the ten to twenty in-out breathing cycles every fifteen to thirty minutes.

Another technique that can quickly lower blood pressure is the Emotional Freedom Technique (EFT). An EFT session takes about two minutes and involves tapping several points on the body with your fingers while repeating an affirmation to yourself that summarizes what you want EFT to accomplish.[6]

A FINAL EXHORTATION

Check your blood pressure at least twice daily for several days until you are convinced it is not elevated. If it is elevated, even minimally, see a doctor and find a way to get it under control. If you make the mistake I made by putting this off, you risk permanent damage to your kidneys and brain.

CHAPTER 11

High Blood Sugar Shrinks Your Memory Centers

For several decades, medical scientists have been aware that high blood sugar damages brain cells and that individuals with elevated levels of fasting blood sugar are at increased risk of dementia. But doctors didn't know at what level the damage began. That has changed. Recent studies now warn us that even *slight* increases in fasting blood sugar erode memory and cognition, damage the brain, and pave the road to Alzheimer's disease.

In the old system, doctors might start raising their eyebrows when fasting blood sugar levels got up over 100 mg/dL. We now know that added risk starts when your number exceeds 90. Even patients in the low 90s have insulin resistance, which means that their insulin receptors are damaged, so they have lost the ability to clear excess sugar out of the bloodstream. Anyone with a fasting blood sugar level over 90 is at significant risk of developing dementia.

Let's take a look at the evidence.

A landmark study done in 2006 at the University of California, San Francisco Medical Center scrutinized the association between chronically elevated blood sugar and the risk of developing either MCI or dementia. This study was the first to investigate the long-term association between blood sugar and the risk of cognitive difficulties. Researchers followed the blood sugar levels of 1,983 postmenopausal women for four years. What they discovered was (at the time) astonishing: subjects with *even minimally elevated blood sugar* (1 or 2 points over 90) had a dramatically increased risk of cognitive impairment and dementia.[1]

Baseline blood sugar levels were measured at the beginning of the study. Then the subjects were assessed for blood sugar level and dementia every year for four years. The study found that each 1 percent increase in glycosylated hemoglobin (HbA1C) was associated with a whopping 40 percent increased risk of developing cognitive impairment or dementia four years later. Women with a glycosylated hemoglobin of 7 percent or higher than baseline were four times more likely to develop MCI or dementia.

Aware, perhaps, that they were moving into uncharted territory, the study's authors cautiously understated the connection: "This finding supports the hypothesis that abnormal glycemic control is linked to an increased risk of developing cognitive impairment and dementia.[2]

For several years, these revelations did not set the medical community on fire, but subsequent research confirmed and extended this early study. In 2012, research published in *Neurology*, the prestigious journal of the American Academy of Neurology, linked borderline elevated blood sugar to degenerative disease not just of the brain but of the specific part of the brain assigned the task of memory and recall. In this study, entitled "Higher Normal Fasting Plasma Glucose Is Associated with Hippocampal Atrophy," Dr. Nicolas Cherbuin and colleagues used brain scans and blood sugar measurements to show that otherwise healthy people with blood sugars at the high end of the normal range (80–90) were more likely to have shrinkage of the brain in the amygdala and hippocampus, the areas most involved in memory.

This time, the authors felt no need to sugarcoat their words: "High plasma glucose levels within the normal range were associated with greater atrophy of structures relevant to aging and neurodegenerative processes, the hippocampus and amygdala. These findings suggest that even in the subclinical range and in the absence of diabetes, monitoring and management of plasma glucose levels could have an impact on cerebral health. If replicated, this finding may contribute to a reevaluation of the concept of normal blood glucose levels and the definition of diabetes."[3]

A 2013 study published in the *New England Journal of Medicine* further bolstered the concept that even minimal blood sugar elevations (above 90 mg/dL) are associated with a high dementia risk. Researchers across the country teamed up to examine blood sugar levels in more than two thousand participants in the Adult Changes in Thought study. The researchers' breakthrough finding was that *any* increase in blood sugar was associated with an increased risk of dementia. The higher the blood sugar, the greater the risk.[4]

According to author David Nathan, a Harvard Medical School professor and the director of the Diabetes Center and Clinical Research Center at Massachusetts General Hospital, "This study establishes for the first time, convincingly, that there is a link between dementia and elevated blood sugars."[5]

Another study published in 2013 pushed the envelope of understanding further by demonstrating that even marginally elevated fasting blood sugar levels damage the brain's memory areas. Published in *Neurology*, this study compared healthy people with normal blood sugars to healthy people who had slightly elevated blood sugar levels. The participants were given blood sugar tests and memory tests. Those with lower blood sugar levels scored consistently better on memory tests. One of the tests required subjects to recall a list of fifteen words thirty minutes after hearing them. The subjects with the lowest blood sugar levels remembered the most words.[6]

When the researchers measured the subjects' hippocampi (the brain's main memory center, where degeneration usually begins), they found that those with higher blood sugar levels had smaller hippocampi. To confirm that damage had in fact occurred, the researchers examined tissues in their subjects' brains under a microscope and found evidence of tissue damage, reporting that the neuronal "microstructural integrity is lower if blood sugar levels are higher." Sure enough, the hippocampal memory centers had withered under the influence of excess sugar.[7]

The researchers went on to state, "Clinically, even if your blood sugar levels are 'normal,' lower blood sugar levels are better for your brain in the long run with regard to memory functions as well as memory-relevant brain structures like the hippocampus." They suggest that changes in lifestyle strategies that lower long-term glucose levels are a "promising strategy to prevent cognitive decline in aging." Dr. Agnes Flöel, one of the study's authors, states, "These findings are important because they indicate that even in healthy non-diabetic, non-impaired glucose tolerant individuals, lifestyle choices that tend to lower blood glucose levels . . . should be recommended."[8] Other studies confirmed these findings. A 2013 study by Dr. Moyra Mortby and her team showed that even so-called normal blood sugar levels undermine cognitive function while decreasing brain volume in memory areas.[9]

The message is clear: as we approach our forties and beyond, if we wish to protect our brains from damage, shrinkage, atrophy, and cognitive decline, we need to choose foods that lower our blood sugar levels. At the end of this chapter (and in chapter 21), I'll go into detail about how to do this. For now, here are the two crucial pillars of your program: a very low-carbohydrate (5–10 percent of your calories) diet and at least one hour of daily exercise.

AN EPIDEMIC OF CARBOHYDRATE OVERCONSUMPTION AND HIGH BLOOD SUGAR

High blood sugar has reached epidemic levels. One-third of the US adult population has blood sugar regulation problems. Fifty percent of people over age sixty-five—an alarming number—have fasting glucose levels above 90.[10] Twenty-nine million persons in the United States have diabetes, and 86 million more are classified as having prediabetes (an FBS of 100–125 mg/dL). A quarter of the world's adults have metabolic syndrome. (Metabolic syndrome is a cluster of conditions that occur together, increasing your risk of heart disease, stroke, and type 2 diabetes. These conditions include increased blood pressure, high blood sugar, excess body fat around the waist, and abnormal cholesterol or triglyceride levels.) Is it surprising that an estimated 25 percent of the US population will have dementia by 2050?[11]

Glucose (from food) and oxygen (from air) are the two fuels our bodies use to generate the energy that powers everything we do. Oxygen and glucose are burned in our cells' mitochondrial energy factories to release electrons that are then stored as energy. This generates all the energy we need to drive the hundreds of thousands of biochemical reactions we call life.

Our survival depends on our energy supply. Imagine what would happen if your car's carburetor were broken. At first the engine would not run smoothly. If the problem continued, it would stop running altogether. The same is true with blood sugar control.

Eating a high-carb diet is like suddenly pressing your accelerator to the floorboard; it generates a deluge of sugar molecules that damage your insulin receptors, the gatekeepers that decide whether to allow sugar access to cells or not. The fluctuations in our bodies' fuel supply caused by damaged insulin receptors can have devastating effects. And some very sophisticated mechanisms are in place to prevent this from happening.

When we eat starch, sugars, and other carbohydrates, digestive enzymes gradually break down and release their stored energy as individual sugar molecules, which are then absorbed through the intestinal wall into the bloodstream, causing your blood sugar level to rise quickly. Within fifteen to thirty minutes of a high-carb meal, your FBS can zoom from a fasting level in the mid-80s up to 120 or more.

As you continue to absorb the carbs in the meal, your blood sugar level would continue to go up unless you had a containment system to remove extra sugar from the bloodstream so it can be stored for use later. That's what your insulin receptors do. When your pancreas detects that rise in blood sugar, it releases insulin, a hormone that tells insulin receptors (in the liver and muscles) to remove extra glucose from the bloodstream and store it as glycogen. This lowers and stabilizes blood sugar levels. Though sugars will go up after meals and down as they are stored or burned off with exercise, this system is remarkably efficient at maintaining levels within a tight normal range. When this system is working, fasting (morning) blood sugar levels will always be in the 80–90 range.

This system wouldn't work as well if it took sugar out of the blood without putting it back when necessary. So when blood sugar levels eventually drop, another hormone, glucagon, is released to convert stored glycogen back into sugar and put it back into the bloodstream. Together, insulin pushes blood sugar down and glucagon pushes it up; they cooperate to create a dynamic balance that maintains a steady, stable supply of glucose, not unlike a smooth foot on the gas pedal and a finely tuned carburetor.

CONSUMING TOO MANY CARBS CAUSES INSULIN RESISTANCE

This system works fine when we are younger, even if we habitually overdose on carbs. Eventually, however, the chronic carb overloading starts damaging our insulin receptors. By the time we get into our forties or fifties, with decades of carb overdosing under our belts, those insulin receptors have become battered and weary. Too much insulin for too long has weakened them and they can no longer handle the high carb load. They lose the ability to respond as briskly to the insulin messages as they did when they were young and strong and resilient. They begin to fail. (You can tell when this happens because this is when fat begins to accumulate around the body.)

This failure is what we call insulin resistance—literally receptor resistance to the insulin messages—and it's what causes blood sugar levels to go up. The damaged receptors can't continue to process the incoming sugar load, so excess sugar piles up in the bloodstream. (If you have ever seen the *I Love Lucy* episode where Lucy and Ethel can't keep up with the chocolate coming down the production line, you know what I am talking about.) The resulting elevated glucose levels are highly toxic to all cellular systems, especially to neurons and the blood vessels that supply them.

You won't experience symptoms in the early stages of damaged insulin receptors and insulin resistance. An elevated FBS (over 90) will be the only sign, and you can't feel that. As the decades of damage accumulate, however, the symptoms will become obvious: easy fatigue, weight gain, elevated blood pressure, elevated triglycerides and high cholesterol, and high FBS.

Remember, the probability that you have this problem is about one in three (one in two if you are over sixty-five). Unless you take action, the condition can progress to type 2 diabetes, metabolic syndrome, atherosclerosis, hypertension, stroke, and, eventually, dementia.

INSULIN RESISTANCE DAMAGES THE BODY AND BRAIN

There is no longer any doubt that insulin resistance, the metabolic breakdown that pushes blood sugar upward, causes cognitive decline, dementia, and other neurodegenerative diseases.

High blood sugar caused by insulin resistance is often accompanied by a list of other biochemical disruptions known as metabolic syndrome. The six principal signs of metabolic syndrome are high blood sugar, high blood pressure, central adiposity (*any* abdominal fat), high cholesterol, low HDL, and high triglycerides.

If your blood sugar runs over 90 mg/dL (or if you have other signs of metabolic syndrome), you would do well to lower your blood sugar levels. The first step is to remove as many carbs as possible from your diet. The second—equally important—step is to do at least one hour of moderate daily exercise. Brisk walking a few miles every day would be a good start.

Blood sugar elevations interfere with our body's energy supply, disrupting metabolism in every cell, tissue, and organ in the body, causing a broad spectrum of degenerative diseases:

- Atherosclerosis and vascular dementia
- Alzheimer's disease and other dementias
- Strokes
- Heart attacks
- Amyloid beta production
- Poor circulation in the legs and feet
- Chronic kidney disease
- Loss of vision
- Weakened immune responses
- Erectile dysfunction
- Slow wound healing
- Neuropathy (nerve damage), which causes tingling, pain, or loss of sensation in the feet, legs, and hands

For more on the dangers that carbs pose to the brain, see the two acclaimed *New York Times* bestsellers, *Grain Brain* and *Brain Makers*, by David Perlmutter, MD, which describe the intimate connection between grains, inflammation, the gut microbiome, and the brain.[12]

TESTING YOUR FBS AT HOME

If your FBS is high, you can't rely on infrequent lab testing. You need to check your fasting level every morning with your own glucose measuring device. You can purchase these online or from your local drugstore. For excellent accuracy, I recommend the Contour. Medicare will cover glucose meters with a doctor's prescription.

Whether at home or in a lab, the blood for this test must be drawn first thing in the morning before any food or drink. (Water, coffee, and tea without sweeteners or creamers are okay. Anything containing calories is not okay.)

Readings averaging over 90 indicate damage to the blood-sugar-regulating system. Beware of doctors who scoff at an FBS in the low 90s. If you show them the summary of research studies earlier in this chapter (and perhaps even the chapter references), I hope they'll start whistling a different tune.

HOW TO GET YOUR ELEVATED BLOOD SUGAR BACK TO NORMAL

Here are the basic steps to lower blood sugar, reverse insulin resistance, and restore health to your brain cells.

1. *Track your progress by testing your blood sugar level every morning.* Record your readings.

2. *Switch to a very low-carbohydrate, high-fat, ketogenic diet.* Eliminate all grains, grain products, sweetened foods, and starchy foods such as root vegetables. To spot hidden carbs, read the labels on packaged foods. Replace carb calories with high-quality proteins (eggs, lean meat) and healthy fats (coconut oil, olive oil, flaxseed oil, walnut oil, avocado oil). (See "Diet to Lower Your Blood Sugar" in the next section. See also chapter 21.)

3. *Supplement your diet with nutritional medicines that lower blood sugar and heal insulin receptors.* These include berberine, cinnamon extract, alpha-lipoic acid, banaba extract, and *Gymnema sylvestre.*

4. *Do mild aerobic exercise.* Exercise at least one hour, every day. You don't need to pump iron or run a marathon. Brisk walking is fine. Work up a light sweat. Exercise heals your broken insulin receptors, makes your muscles more sensitive to insulin, and promotes glucose uptake from the bloodstream.

5. *Practice autophagy.* Autophagy lowers blood sugar and encourages ketogenesis. (See chapter 22.)

Now let's examine these in more detail.

DIET TO LOWER YOUR BLOOD SUGAR

If your FBS is over 90, your first step is to acknowledge that your high-carb diet has damaged your insulin receptors. The next step is to remove carbs, the source of the trauma to your insulin receptors, from your diet. Replace them mostly with healthy fats and a little extra protein. This will push your metabolism toward ketogenic, fat-based energy production while protecting your insulin receptors and allowing them to heal.

Carb elimination may not be easy; after all, who isn't addicted to the rush of good feelings we get when we flood our system with the sugars from breads, chips, sugary drinks, alcoholic beverages, and sweet desserts? But you need to build your diet around fresh whole unprocessed very low-carb foods: lean meat, eggs, vegetable salads, steamed or sautéed vegetables, soups, nuts, beans, seeds, and healthy oils. Moderate amounts of less-sweet (low sugar), high polyphenol fruit (blueberries, raspberries, strawberries, cherries) are also a good idea.

Here are some low-carb-diet food suggestions:
- Salads, stir-fries, and soups (add nuts, seeds, beans, egg, meat)
- Beans and bean dishes such as chili
- Steamed vegetables
- Almond or rice milk, unsweetened
- Chicken, turkey, beef, or pork with salad and vegetables
- Eggs with ham or breakfast links and fruit
- Breakfast links (soy or pork)
- Sausage (chicken, soy, or pork) and salad or steamed vegetables
- Omelets with vegetables, meat, and cheese
- Chicken, pork, or steak with onions, bell pepper, and mushrooms
- Nuts (peanuts, almonds, walnuts, cashews, filberts, or pecans)
- Seeds (sunflower) as a snack or on salads
- Indian or Thai curries (hold the rice)

Healthy Fats

Healthy fats include coconut oil, extra virgin olive oil, avocado oil, walnut oil, flaxseed oil, hemp oil, palm oil, and algae oil.

Eliminate all omega-6 oils (soybean, sunflower, safflower, canola, cottonseed, and corn oils; margarine; and butter substitutes) from your diet. These encourage inflammation and put you at risk for all chronic degenerative diseases, including those that affect the brain.

Butter (preferably organic), in moderate amounts, is okay. A victim of the "war on fat," butter is experiencing a comeback as a healthy fat. Don't get carried away; keep it under a tablespoon a day. And it has to be real butter—not margarine and not Smart Balance or I Can't Believe It's Not Butter (these contain soy and canola oils). Read the labels on butter substitutes; if you spot any of the omega-6 oils, stay away.

Coconut oil is the ideal cooking oil because it contains 66 percent medium chain triglycerides, far more than any other food. MCTs are powerful cognitive healers because they are easily converted into ketone bodies, the preferred fuel for your brain. Ketone bodies renew neurons and restore brain function, even after damage has begun. For prevention, the optimum level of coconut oil MCTs is 20 grams per day, about two tablespoons of coconut oil. For MCI and more advanced cognitive problems, two or three times this much (40–60 grams a day) is recommended. To give your digestive system time to adjust, start at one tablespoon daily and work up gradually over a couple of weeks. (See chapter 23.)

Emphasize omega-3 oils. The body isn't capable of producing them on its own, so we must rely on our diet to supply these extremely beneficial essential fatty acids. We want more of these hard-to-come-by oils because they support healthy neurons and fight inflammation (in both brain and body). Omega-3s can be found in flaxseeds and flaxseed oil (by far the richest source), walnuts, avocados and avocado oil, chia seeds, hemp seeds, and green leafy vegetables such as kale, spinach, Brussels sprouts, and watercress.

Avocado oil has a mild taste that won't overpower dishes the way other oils might, and it's rich in monounsaturated fats, which raise levels of good cholesterol while lowering the bad. It's suitable for grilling or frying and isn't solid at room temperature (like coconut oil), so it's also a tasty choice to use in stir-fries or drizzle on salads and vegetables.

I also recommend taking brain-protective omega-3 supplements containing flaxseed oil (1–2 tablespoons daily) and DHA (600–1200 mg/day). (See chapter 28.)

No Seafood

Avoid all fish and seafood, including farmed fish. Though containing zero carbs and brimming with healthy EFAs, all seafood (even supposedly safe smaller fish and ones from arctic waters) contain unacceptably high levels of mercury, a neurotoxin for which there is *no safe dose*. Methylmercury is evenly distributed in the earth's oceans, and all seafoods grow up bathing in it. (See chapters 18 and 20.)

Foods High in Polyphenols Lower Blood Sugar

Polyphenols are especially powerful food-based medicines when it comes to fixing blood sugar problems. Polyphenols inhibit insulin resistance and boost the stabilizing effect of insulin on blood sugar. Include foods high in these powerful phytonutrients, either as fresh or frozen fruit or as supplements. Polyphenol-rich foods include blueberries, cherries, raspberries, blackberries, grapes, pomegranate, nuts, curcumin, cabbage, eggplant, greens, onions, garlic, and olives. (See a full list of polyphenol-rich foods in chapter 24.)

You may be wondering why I recommend berries, technically a high-carb food, as part of a low-carb diet. Berries do contain a relatively small amount of sugar (as fructose), but they also contain such high levels of polyphenols and other brain-boosting phytonutrient chemicals and essential minerals that we have to make an exception for them; the tradeoff works deliciously in our favor. Keep quantities to about 1 to 1-½ cups a day. Sweeter fruits such as apples, oranges, and grapes are higher in sugars and lower in phytochemicals, so use those in moderation.

Cocoa, dark chocolate, and green tea are especially desirable sources of polyphenols that—in addition to their blood-sugar-regulating properties—have been shown to reverse dementia. And they taste good!

Unsweetened chocolate is best, but the polyphenols give it a bitter taste, so sugar is added. This is two steps forward and one step back! Pay attention to the amount of sugar that comes with your chocolate by reading labels. I have found I can avoid this sugar altogether by adding unsweetened cocoa nibs to my fruit smoothies, made with almond milk, frozen blueberries, frozen cherries, frozen strawberries, flaxseeds or chia seeds, half a banana, one or two tablespoons of Barlean's flaxseed oil, and sometimes a raw egg. The fruit provides plenty of sweetness.

Unfortunately, almost all chocolate products contain cadmium or lead, which are toxic to the brain. Most nationally distributed brands and products (including most of those considered environmentally conscious and sold only in health food stores) contain levels of cadmium and lead deemed unsafe to consume as determined by state and federal law. The chocolate industry has refused to follow state and federal toxicity labeling requirements. A consumer advocacy group, As You Sow, filed suit against a long list of major producers, which are now under court order in California to move toward a solution to this problem. However, until cadmium- and lead-free chocolate products are available, I advise choosing your chocolates carefully and severely limiting the quantities you consume.[13] (See chapter 26 for more on this subject.)

Nutritional Supplements

Nutritional supplements that lower your blood sugar and heal your insulin receptors include the following:

- *Berberine*—Berberine is an extensively researched and well-tolerated herbal medicine that is extremely effective at reversing insulin resistance and lowering elevated blood sugar. In head-to-head clinical trials, berberine outperformed metformin, the most widely used blood-sugar-lowering prescription drug. Berberine plays vital roles in preventing and reversing the causes of cerebral arterial blockages that lead to vascular dementia. It reverses type 2 diabetes and metabolic syndrome, lowers cholesterol, exerts an antioxidant action, and retards neuroinflammation. Berberine reduces the accumulation of the amyloid beta and neurofibrillary tangles known to play key roles in AD. Take one or two 500 mg capsules once or twice a day. Berberine alone will usually get blood sugars below 90. If not, add one or more of the following supplements listed here.

- *Cinnamon extract*—Cinnamon contains a variety of blood-sugar-stabilizing phytonutrients including polyphenols that reverse insulin resistance. Take one or two 125 mg capsules twice a day.
- *Alpha-lipoic acid*—A coenzyme for energy production, alpha-lipoic acid helps transport blood glucose into cells, thus promoting normal blood sugar balance. Alpha-lipoic acid blood levels are usually low in those with insulin resistance and type 2 diabetes. Take one or two 100 mg capsules once or twice a day.
- *Combination products*—Combination products include varying amounts of several nutrients that synergistically support glucose metabolism and healing of insulin receptors. These may (or may not) include chromium, vanadium, alpha-lipoic acid, N-acetyl cysteine, banaba (*Lagerstroemia* species), and *Gymnema sylvestre*. Take the dose indicated on bottle.

CHAPTER 12

High Cholesterol Promotes Alzheimer's Disease

R esearch has proven beyond doubt that high cholesterol dramatically increases the risk of strokes, dementia, and Alzheimer's. If you
want to sidestep these disasters, you need to get your cholesterol under
control.[1]

If your cholesterol is above 200 mg/dL, I recommend trying natural
agents first. For modest elevations, they'll probably be strong enough.
The main natural options are red yeast rice extract, berberine, bergamot, plant sterols, and policosanol. You may need to use two or more
of these together.

Be sure to take elevated cholesterol seriously and get your numbers into the normal range. Please don't make the mistake I made.
Take the drugs if you have to. In terms of tradeoffs, I'd certainly
rather have drug side effects than another stroke! And trust me, so
would you. If diet, exercise, and supplements can lower your blood
pressure and cholesterol, great! But if, after an adequate trial (a few
months), they don't, it's time to add the medications. Before I show
you how to do that, I want to discuss the connection between cholesterol and dementia.

ELEVATED CHOLESTEROL CAUSES DEMENTIA

Contrary to popular opinion, cholesterol is not inherently evil. Cholesterol is essential for human health. Without it, your brain would be unable to function.

About 25 percent of the cholesterol in your body is found in your brain. More than 150 adrenal, testicular, and ovarian hormones are made from cholesterol. The molecule is an important component of cell walls. In the skin, sunlight transforms cholesterol into vitamin D. So we need it. But when cholesterol blood levels get a little too high, your body starts trying to get rid of the excess by shoving it into the walls of arteries, causing atherosclerotic plaque (fig. 12.1), and (in the brain) this initiates the inflammatory process that leads to strokes and vascular dementia.

Cholesterol promotes the atherosclerotic process:

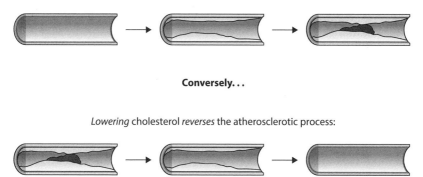

Conversely...

Lowering cholesterol *reverses* the atherosclerotic process:

Figure 12.1. Excess cholesterol promotes plaque formation

These strokes are often small and usually symptom-free. Multiple small strokes are far more likely in people whose cholesterol, fasting blood sugar (see chapter 11), and blood pressure (see chapter 10) are elevated. Repeated small strokes cause silent cumulative brain damage that accelerates the dangerous neurodegenerative process leading to vascular dementia.

CHOLESTEROL CONTROLS THE DEPOSITION AND REMOVAL OF AMYLOID BETA IN THE BRAIN

High cholesterol causes another problem: it promotes amyloid beta plaque deposition in brain tissue—not in the walls of blood vessels but sprinkled among the neurons of the brain itself. This is the telltale sign of Alzheimer's disease; it's the same stuff Alois Alzheimer spotted under his microscope one hundred years ago.

Luigi Puglielli and colleagues, in a 2003 research paper, describe the molecular mechanisms underlying the cholesterol-AD connection, stating that there is a "role for cholesterol in the pathogenesis of AD" and that "both the generation and clearance of amyloid beta are regulated by cholesterol."[2]

As recently as 2013, whether high cholesterol predisposed one to amyloid beta deposits and dementia was still unknown. A 2014 study published in *JAMA Neurology* was the first to establish a clear correlation. Bruce Reed and associates looked closely at cholesterol levels and cerebral plaques in seventy-year-olds who were early in the AD process and found a close correlation.[3]

Study leader Reed, a professor of neurology at the University of California, Davis, and associate director of its Alzheimer's Disease Center, chose what I call the "cup half full" model to frame the results: "Our study shows that both higher levels of HDL cholesterol and lower levels of LDL cholesterol in the bloodstream are associated with lower levels of amyloid plaque deposits in the brain. This study provides a reason to certainly continue cholesterol treatment in people who are developing memory loss."[4]

The "cup half empty" model would have gone something like this: "Higher LDL and lower HDL levels cause dementia." Study coauthor Charles DeCarli, also a professor of neurology at the University of California, Davis, and director of its Alzheimer's Disease Center, describes the findings as a "wake-up call" in that people can keep their brains healthy later in life by controlling cholesterol: "If you have an LDL above 100 or an HDL that is less than 40, even if you're taking a statin drug, you want to make sure that you are getting those numbers into alignment. You have to get the HDL up [to 45] and the LDL down [below 100]."[5]

HYPERTENSION PLUS HIGH CHOLESTEROL: NIGHTMARE MATERIAL

High cholesterol poses a clear threat to your brain, but what happens when you combine that high cholesterol with high blood pressure and high fasting blood sugar (like I did)?

Now you have the perfect storm. The risk of arterial damage and stroke increases exponentially because your heart is pounding hard against the inside wall of the arteries (especially in the heart, kidneys, and brain)—and these are the same arteries being damaged by excess glucose and cholesterol plaque deposition.

HOW TO LOWER YOUR CHOLESTEROL

Wheat, grain, sugar, starch, and carb addicts really don't want to hear this, but these foods provoke LDL elevation and suppress HDL. Moving to a low-carb, grain-free diet will propel you rapidly in the direction of protecting your brain. (See chapter 11.)

Take your cholesterol seriously—and keep your numbers in the normal range:

- Cholesterol below 200
- LDL below 100
- HDL above 45

The good news is that these variables are under your control. Start with one or two of these food-derived cholesterol-lowering agents:

- *Berberine*—500–2,000 mg a day. Take one 500 mg capsule once a day for the first few days; over the next two weeks gradually increase the dose to two 500 mg capsules twice a day.
- *Red yeast rice extract*—Take one or two 600 mg capsules twice daily.
- *Plant sterols* (e.g., Foresterol)—Take one or two 1.8 gram capsules twice daily.

- *Bergamot* (e.g., CholestePure Plus, containing plant sterols and bergamot)—Take two capsules twice daily.
- *Policosanol*—Take one or two 10 mg capsules twice daily.

These natural, nontoxic medicines harmonize your body's lipid management systems and are extremely unlikely to cause side effects or adverse reactions. Your body processes them like it would food because they *are* food.

If the natural approach fails after a three-month trial, you might need to add statin drugs—despite their drawbacks. Stay on the natural medicines, though (assuming they were partially successful), as they'll reduce the amount of statin needed to complete the job.

Statin side effects can include muscle aches, muscle spasms, and even memory loss. Keep in mind that lowering your cholesterol to protect your brain is, by far, the overriding concern here, so avoiding a statin because of possible side effects and leaving cholesterol (and therefore stroke) risk high is not the preferred strategy.

Regardless of the combination of cholesterol-lowering methods you use, keep testing your cholesterol every couple of months until you get it down below 200. This is a complex issue, so be sure to discuss it with your functional medicine physician.

REPLACE CoQ10 DEPLETED BY STATINS

Coenzyme Q10 is essential for mitochondrial energy production. All statins deplete this important nutrient.[6] Therefore, anyone taking any kind of statin must supplement with CoQ10, best taken as the reduced (more bioavailable, far more potent) form known as CoQH. Take 50–200 mg of CoQH a day.

Red yeast rice extract is a naturally occurring statin, so if you're using that, CoQH is necessary.

CHAPTER 13

B-Complex Vitamins Reverse Cognitive Decline

If Alois Alzheimer had known in 1905 what we know today, he would have prescribed large doses of B-complex vitamins not only to his dementia patients but to all his patients over age fifty. Why? Because all eight B-complex vitamins are crucial for healthy brain functioning, deficiency (at that age) is universal, and supplementing one's diet with the Bs has been shown to prevent Alzheimer's disease.

B-complex deficiency, high homocysteine, brain atrophy, and AD are all intimately connected. The metabolic biomarker homocysteine is a risk factor for dementia and Alzheimer's disease.[1]

An insufficient supply of dietary B vitamins causes homocysteine levels to go up and this causes brain atrophy and Alzheimer's disease. Replacing the depleted, deficient B-complex vitamins will lower homocysteine levels back to normal, reverse brain atrophy, and prevent Alzheimer's.

For those who want to sidestep cognitive decline, knowing your homocysteine level and addressing it with B-complex vitamins if it's elevated would be a very good idea. Taking Bs preventively would be even better. It's a cheap insurance policy.

Low B and high homocysteine are signs of defective methylation, an extremely common metabolic disorder. In this chapter I'll show you how a methylation disorder can damage your brain and how to use B vitamins to prevent that from happening.

B VITAMINS PROTECT AGAINST BRAIN ATROPHY

In 2010, A. David Smith and colleagues at the University of Oxford wondered whether lowering homocysteine with B vitamins could reverse the brain atrophy seen in patients with MCI. Indeed, their research showed that B vitamins dramatically lowered homocysteine and slowed brain shrinkage in such patients.[2]

But had the anti-atrophy effect been caused directly by the Bs acting on brain cells, or was something else involved? A research team led by Oxford's Gwenaëlle Douaud set out to find the answer.[3] For over two years, her research group tracked brain changes using MRIs in 156 elderly volunteers who were in the early stages of cognitive impairment. Half were given high doses of B-complex vitamins, and the other half were given a placebo. As reported in the highly regarded *Proceedings of the National Academy of Sciences* in 2013, MRIs revealed that B-vitamin treatment had reduced homocysteine levels, thus dramatically slowing the rate of atrophy. Douaud also showed that the regions of the brain that most benefitted from the Bs were those most likely to be damaged in Alzheimer's disease: the hippocampus and cerebellum. The atrophy rate in these key brain memory regions was a whopping seven times faster in the placebo group than in the group taking the B vitamins (3.7 percent versus 0.5 percent). The atrophy prevention, cognition-enhancing effects of B vitamins were further confirmed by improved performance on cognitive testing.[4]

Based on these results, and recalling that one in three of us will die with dementia, I recommend that all adults over forty take a high-potency, high-quality vitamin B-complex supplement once or twice a day. You can think of daily B-complex supplementation as a harmless, inexpensive insurance policy that protects against brain decline.

By now you may be muttering, "This can't apply to me. I've never heard of homocysteine. If I had a homocysteine problem, my doctor would surely have said something."

Ponder this: high homocysteine is not a rare disorder. The odds you have or will develop a homocysteine problem are high. Most doctors are aware of the dangers of homocysteine, but they usually don't test for it, perhaps because they aren't sure how to treat it.

Elevated homocysteine can cause a wide assortment of serious health conditions: heart disease, stroke, cancer, diabetes, abnormal immune function, chronic fatigue syndrome, osteoporosis, chronic inflammation, multiple sclerosis, macular degeneration, hearing loss, migraine headaches, autism, neural tube defects, and other neurological and psychiatric disorders. Your doctor may just not have connected the dots between your health issues and homocysteine as a possible cause.

WHY METHYL GROUPS AND METHYLATION ARE IMPORTANT

Homocysteine and B-complex vitamins are crucial parts of a very elaborate set of biochemical processes called methylation, which involves the controlled transfer of methyl groups to where they are needed to build amino acids, proteins, enzymes, DNA, and other important molecules. Methyl groups are kind of like bricks: they're simple and you need lots of them. Our bodies use these methyl group bricks in many important chemical reactions.

Methyl transfer is one of the body's most essential metabolic functions; it is necessary in the synthesis of important proteins that serve a broad variety of functions such as genetic expression of DNA, regulation of healing, cellular energy production, neurological function, liver detoxification, and immunity. Every second, more than a billion methylation reactions take place in your body.

A deficiency of B-complex vitamins impairs normal methylation and results in a buildup of the very dangerous homocysteine molecule, causing widespread damage. Homocysteine's most damaging effect is on the brain's blood vessels. Every second, like a powerful sandblaster, billions of homocysteine molecules crash into the endothelial cells lining the inside of the brain's blood vessels, ravaging crucial arterial supply lines. The endothelial lining gradually loses its integrity and becomes unable to protect the layers of artery beneath it. This results in arterial inflammation, atherosclerosis, amyloid beta deposition (plaque), cognitive decline, stroke, and dementia.

TESTING FOR HOMOCYSTEINE

Any medical laboratory can test for homocysteine. If your doctor won't order the test, or if your insurance charges you for it, use Direct Labs (www.directlabs.com). A doctor's order is not required. The test quality is identical to that of the major labs; however, the price will be substantially lower.

For screening purposes, a plasma or serum homocysteine test will suffice.[5]

Our bodies normally generate small amounts of homocysteine. The optimum level is under 6.3 μmol/L. If your homocysteine level is elevated (over 7.3 μmol/L), you need to take action.

SUPPLEMENTAL B-COMPLEX VITAMINS— USE THE *ACTIVATED FORM*

The B-complex vitamins work synergistically to block and reverse neurodegenerative disease. Take a high-quality (pharmaceutical-grade) B-complex capsule containing all eight B vitamins at the label-recommended dosage every day. Find a product containing the *activated form* of the Bs for improved bioavailability. Also be sure to take the full recommended dose of a high-quality multivitamin every day. (Although your multivitamin-mineral capsule has B-complex, the dosing is probably too low, and the active forms are not included.)

Be aware that big-box stores and food and drugstore chains do not sell pharmaceutical grade multivitamins.

Although scientific investigations into elevated homocysteine have focused on B6 (pyridoxine), B9 (folic acid), and B12 (cobalamin), the metabolic work done by B-complex vitamins is a team effort, and strong scientific evidence now tells us that adequate levels of all eight members of this group of micronutrients are essential for optimal physiological and neurological functioning—and for reversing of dementia. It's okay to emphasize some of them (like B12 and folic acid), but don't leave any out altogether.

Beware of RDAs (government recommended daily allowances), which are chosen to help guard against vitamin-deficiency diseases but are far below levels necessary to promote exceptional health. For preventing dementia, optimum doses of B-complex vitamins are several times the current RDAs.

B vitamins are extremely safe; in fifty years of family practice specializing in nutritional and molecular medicine, I have never seen a case of B-complex vitamin overdose. On the other hand, I have treated a great many patients damaged by insufficient B vitamins (especially vitamin B12 in vegans) and elevated homocysteine.

Homocysteine levels change slowly, so wait at least two months before retesting. Getting homocysteine to optimum (under 7.3) is not the immediate goal; that could take up to a year or more. Any movement in the downward direction would indicate that the combination you are taking is working and that you should stay the course.

If you see no decline, a deficiency of other nutrients could be blocking the removal of excess homocysteine. The following supplements can sometimes solve the problem when the B-complex vitamins alone fail:

- CDP-choline—Take two to four 250 mg capsules daily. (See chapter 31.)
- SAMe (S-adenosyl methionine)—Take 200–800 mg daily.
- TMG (trimethylglycine or betaine HCl)—Take one to six 500 mg capsules in divided doses. TMG is mildly acidic and helps digest protein but can upset the stomach, so take it only with meals.

- Zinc (as citrate, picolinate, or aspartate)—Take 30–90 mg daily. (Dose per capsule varies.)
- Vitamin C—Take 1,000–8,000 mg daily of buffered C or Ester-C. (Dose per capsule varies.)
- Vitamin E—Take 400–1,200 IU (international units) daily only as mixed tocopherols. (Dose per capsule varies.)

You still need the extra Bs, so keep taking them while trying these other possibilities.

In some individuals, homocysteine levels inexplicably refuse to budge, regardless of the supplement program. This does not mean the Bs are not working! An elevated homocysteine always tells us that extra Bs are needed. In these cases I recommend continuing to take all the B-complex vitamins because they will still support optimum brain function and protect against dementia.

CHAPTER 14

Vitamin D Defeats Dementia

Vitamin D is necessary for healthy brain function. A low level of the vitamin dramatically increases your risk of dementia and a long list of other serious health problems.

Most people with Alzheimer's disease have a vitamin D deficiency. Individuals with the lowest vitamin D levels have a twenty-five-fold risk of developing MCI (the earliest stage of Alzheimer's) when compared to those with the highest levels of D.

Vitamin D influences about three thousand of your twenty-five thousand genes, and thus plays crucial roles in virtually every aspect of nervous and immune system health and responsiveness. It affects a broad range of human metabolic activities. Virtually every organ and tissue type in your body—kidney, heart, lung, blood vessel, skin—listens closely when vitamin D talks. Your central nervous system, which is loaded with vitamin D receptors, listens most closely of all.

A VITAMIN D DEFICIENCY EPIDEMIC

We are in the midst of a national—and international—vitamin D deficiency epidemic.[1] Worldwide, at least 1 billion people are thought to have health-eroding low vitamin D levels.[2]

Chances are high that you are part of this epidemic. Achieving and maintaining optimum levels of vitamin D is a powerful strategy for preventing and reversing cognitive decline, MCI, Alzheimer's disease, and other dementias (not to mention cancer and a vast array of vascular, immune, autoimmune, and other chronic disorders).

OUR CHANGING APPRECIATION FOR THE IMPORTANCE OF VITAMIN D

Vitamin D is a misnomer. Vitamin D is actually not a vitamin but a hormone. And it's not just any hormone; D is a powerful steroid hormone made from—would you have guessed it?—cholesterol.

In 1921, Sir Edward Mellanby showed that dogs left in the dark developed rickets, the prototypical vitamin D deficiency disease, characterized by weak bones.[3] The dogs needed sunlight so their bodies could manufacture the vitamin. How D works seemed simple and straightforward: it promotes the absorption of calcium and phosphorus needed for stronger bones and teeth. D's importance for preventing weak bones (rickets and osteoporosis) motivated the US government to mandate its presence in the milk supply in the 1930s.

In 1936, researchers began to discover that D's effects were far more complicated, and vitamin D's official biochemical designation was gradually upgraded from vitamin to hormone.[4] What's the difference? Vitamins do molecular piecework: they work on one molecule or one chemical reaction at a time. Hormones, on the other hand, act like switches that activate large groups of chemical reactions. That's why, with the discovery that D is a hormone, the list of diseases caused by vitamin D deficiency became very long.

We now know that optimum vitamin D is essential for protection against virtually all cardiovascular diseases, including diabetes, metabolic syndrome, hypertension, heart attacks, and strokes. These are the metabolic disorders that cause vascular dementia, a disease that affects 90 percent of Alzheimer's patients. Also, virtually all types of cancer are much less likely in people with healthy vitamin D levels.

LOW VITAMIN D MORE THAN DOUBLES YOUR RISK OF DEMENTIA

In 2012, noted neurodegenerative disease specialist Cédric Annweiler and his team asked whether a low dietary vitamin D intake could predict dementia. His group followed 498 women for seven years and found that higher dietary D intake was associated with a lower risk of developing Alzheimer's disease.[5]

But does consuming extra D protect you? In 2014, University of Oxford researcher Thomas J. Littlejohns and his team did the first large study to investigate the relationship between vitamin D dose and dementia risk. In a study published in *Neurology*, they followed 1,658 healthy dementia-free elderly patients for over six years to determine whether sufficient vitamin D protected against dementia. They found that subjects with the lowest vitamin D levels were more than twice as likely to become demented as those with optimum levels. Those who were moderately deficient in vitamin D had a 51 percent increased risk of dementia, which increased to 122 percent for those who were severely deficient.[6]

Study author David Llewellyn, of the University of Exeter Medical School, said, "We expected to find an association between low vitamin D levels and the risk of dementia and Alzheimer's disease, but the results were surprising—we actually found that the association was twice as strong as we anticipated."[7]

HOW VITAMIN D PROTECTS AGAINST DEMENTIA

The discovery that D can prevent and reverse cognitive decline is only a few years old now, and molecular biologists and nutritional biochemists haven't yet unraveled the entire puzzle as to exactly how D does it. Because the neurological impact of D is so widespread and so fundamental, researchers don't doubt that a detailed biochemical explanation is just over the horizon.[8] The answer will most likely involve the vitamin D receptors (proteins that are like little locks for which vitamin D is the key) that can be found on every cell in every organ and every tissue type—but are especially dense in the brain. Alzheimer's patients have fewer vitamin D receptors in the hippocampus.[9]

Another piece of the puzzle relates to D's neuroprotective effect. As a neurohormone, vitamin D stimulates the production and release of neurotrophins, a family of proteins that control neurogenesis. The most potent neurotrophin is nerve growth factor (NGF). Vitamin D is a potent upregulator of both NGF and NGF receptors, promoting the growth, development, functionality, and survival of all nerve cells. This facilitates neuroregeneration and neuroplasticity. Researchers have shown that vitamin D regulates the release of NGF in hippocampal neurons, those most closely connected with memory.[10]

Amyloid beta is the harbinger of Alzheimer's disease first seen by Alois Alzheimer over one hundred years ago. Optimum D levels stimulate removal of amyloid beta plaque deposits from the cerebral cortex and increase the rate of excretion of amyloid beta from the brain. (The spice curcumin has been found to boost this effect.)[11]

Vitamin D suppresses inflammation, the underlying cause of all neurodegenerative diseases, and prevents oxidative damage to nervous tissue by regulating anti–free radical activity. D also serves as a catalyst for the synthesis of our main antioxidant, glutathione.[12]

D controls the manufacture of well over two hundred antimicrobial peptides, small protein-like molecules that fight off infection, an important consideration because microbial CNS infections appear to be an important piece of the Alzheimer's puzzle.[13]

Vitamin D regulates blood sugar, blood pressure, and nitric oxide synthesis. D deficiency is associated with hypertension, left ventricular hypertrophy, increased arterial stiffness, and endothelial dysfunction— all critical factors in the health of the vascular system, and important for prevention of high blood pressure, strokes, renal vascular disease, and vascular dementia. (See chapter 10.)

D also protects brain cells by supporting the effectiveness of glial cells, the supporting cells of the nervous system. Glial cells form myelin, the thick sheath that surrounds axons. They hold neurons in place, insulate one neuron from another, supply nutrients and oxygen to neurons, nurse damaged neurons back to health, and destroy and remove the carcasses of dead neurons.

D regulates calcium homeostasis inside nerve cells. Problems with calcium regulation are intimately associated with Alzheimer's. Vitamin D regulates calcium channels in brain cells, the doorways that allow calcium to flow into and out of nerve cells.

Though usually not associated with obvious symptoms, a deficiency of vitamin D (less than 70 ng/mL) undermines well-being and vitality, weakens immunity, and increases one's susceptibility to colds and flus and a vast array of chronic diseases. Osteoporosis, multiple sclerosis, autoimmune disease, diabetes (types 1 and 2), depression, and breast and colon cancers are closely linked to low vitamin D levels. All chronic diseases are either caused or worsened by low D levels.[14]

So even though we haven't yet discovered all the mechanisms of vitamin D's dementia-protective effect, we know it exerts a multiplicity of influences on the health of the nervous system and that keeping it in the 70–100 ng/mL optimum range will dramatically lower dementia risk and reverse the disease process if it has already begun.

ACHIEVING OPTIMUM D LEVELS

Do not assume that your level is okay because you take D supplements. Some need a little; others need a lot. Blood testing for 25-hydroxy vitamin D is the only way to determine whether your vitamin D level is optimum.

Any standard medical laboratory can do this test. Double check to make sure you are getting the correct test. (Doctors sometimes erroneously order a 1,5-hydroxy vitamin D test. Though the name is similar, this is not the same test and its results will be misleading.)

Optimum D is 70–100 ng/mL. If your level is below 70, adjust your daily dose upward. If your level is over 100, lower your dose. Work in 5,000 IU dose increments using 5,000 IU capsules of vitamin D3 (cholecalciferol), the only supplemental form that is bioavailable. Wait three months after any dose change and then test again. Adjust the dose up or down, as needed, to keep yourself in the 70–100 range. When you are in the optimum range on two successive testings, you need to test only every six to twelve months.

Keep in mind that because the half-life of vitamin D in your body is measured in months, level changes will happen slowly. You may need up to a year to find your optimum dose.

Normal ranges provided by labs and health publications usually run in the 20–50 ng/mL range. These are much too low! These may be acceptable for preventing rickets or osteomalacia, the severe D deficiency diseases of yesteryear, but they do not reflect our modern, research-based understanding of vitamin D. Individuals who settle for a normal vitamin D level of less than 50 will be not only depriving themselves of the protective, preventive rewards available from optimum D but also choosing to significantly increase their likelihood of contracting one or more D-deficiency diseases—including Alzheimer's.

On the other end of the spectrum, having a vitamin D level over 100 ng/mL has no known benefits. Levels of between 100–150 ng/mL aren't toxic and aren't usually harmful but are thought to be unnecessarily high.

DON'T WE MAKE OUR OWN VITAMIN D
FROM SUNLIGHT?

Some may argue, "Why take supplements if we can make our own vitamin D for free from sunlight?" Ultraviolet light from the sun bounces off our skin cells, triggering the manufacture of vitamin D. But we can't depend on the sun to supply optimum levels because sunlight is not always available, varies by season, and is in short supply at higher latitudes. Even with abundant sunshine, we don't usually run around outside with our clothes off.

CHAPTER 15

Sleep Apnea Increases Dementia Risk

"Last night you were snoring pretty heavily, Tim." It was a sunny Saturday morning a few years ago. My wife, Dellie, and I were savoring our favorite antidementia breakfast treats: blueberries and hot chocolate.

"Hmm," I murmured, and left it at that.

A couple of weeks later, she brought it up again. "You know, last night your snoring woke me up. In fact, you snore just about every night. Isn't snoring bad for you?"

"Not as far as I know," I replied, slightly irritated. (Was she questioning my superior medical wisdom? If sleep apnea posed a dangerous health risk, I surely would have heard about it.)

A couple more weeks went by and then she said, "Tim, I've been reading about snoring, and it is not a pretty picture. Snoring almost certainly means you have sleep apnea, and if you have sleep apnea, that can lead directly to a lot of serious health problems."

"Like what?" I said, again with some irritation. Here she was, questioning my medical invincibility again. "Oh, like stroke, for example," she paused—"Or sudden death, Tim. Also diabetes, hypertension, and daytime sleepiness—all of which you have."

"Hmmm."

"Oh, and sleep apnea triples your risk of dementia. Aren't you writing a book about that?"

"Yes."

She hauled out a printout of some research she had found.

"Tim, in the concluding remarks of his extensive review article, 'The Epidemiology of Adult Obstructive Sleep Apnea,' in *Proceedings of the American Thoracic Society*, Naresh M. Punjabi states"—Dellie paused for dramatic effect—"and I quote, 'There is now a wealth of information indicating that untreated obstructive sleep apnea is associated with an increased risk of fatal and nonfatal cardiovascular events, a higher propensity of sudden death during sleep, and a greater risk for stroke and all-cause mortality.'"[1]

My wife is very intelligent and is rarely wrong, so I checked the scientific research on sleep apnea and was appalled. Sleep apnea is a well-kept medical secret—even though it is often deadly, most doctors don't take it seriously.

She had also found some data about prevalence. "You probably didn't know that most people your age [I was seventy] have OSA."

I gulped. "Most?" I said.

"Yes, most."

"No, I didn't."

Why hadn't my cardiologist, my neurologist, and my family doctor thought of this? At my next visit, we asked my cardiologist (an affable, wise, and caring guy) about it. He agreed it was a possibility and (without apologizing for overlooking it) promptly wrote a referral to a sleep specialist, who ordered a polysomnogram.

The polysomnogram is an easy, painless overnight test in a sleep lab that is very much like your own bedroom. They really go out of their way to make you comfortable. You can bring your favorite jammies, comforter, pillows, bedtime treats, medications, electronic devices—even your teddy bear, if you have one.

Repeated oxygen starvation night after night is guaranteed to cause extensive damage to organs, tissues, and cells everywhere in your body. Inadequate oxygen delivery to your tissues is a huge stress. (If you doubt this, try holding your breath for a while.) Chronic, low-level oxygen starvation—like that in OSA—is even more stressful. Adrenaline levels go up, and widespread inflammatory reactions ravage the blood vessels supplying the body and brain.

The chronic oxygen deprivation of OSA compromises sleep patterns and causes sleep loss, which damages brain cells, enhances amyloid beta plaque deposition, and debilitates nerve impulse transmission, all of which set the stage for neurodegeneration and dementia. Restoring continuous oxygen delivery to starved blood vessels and the brain, on the other hand, removes the disruption and the body heals. Once the endothelial membranes that line the inside walls of your blood vessels start getting enough oxygen, they stop sending those SOS chemical messages that warn your entire body of impending doom, and they start healing.[2]

The sleep patterns revealed on my polysomnogram were classic for OSA. My sleep medicine specialist, prescribed a CPAP device. It generates a steady stream of air that is gently introduced into my mouth and nostrils while I am sleeping to keep the sides of the pharynx from collapsing and cutting off my air supply. Voila! No more obstruction to air flow, no more snoring, and no more brain damage.

The CPAP machine took a little getting used to, but I'm fine with it now. I first tried the type with a mask that covers the mouth and nose, but that tickled my mustache. The nasal-pillow type worked better for me. It's a smaller device that rests on the upper lip and has two soft plastic pillows that sit below and outside the nostrils and gently emit air. After a couple of years using the nasal pillow, I switched to a third device, with a different design, called the DreamWear Nasal mask by Philips Respironics. This is the most comfortable and easy to use because the air supply line is at the top of the head, so you can move your head (and even your body) around in your sleep without pulling the mask off.

Now, several years later, I am here to tell you that diagnosing my OSA and treating it with a CPAP machine has greatly improved my health, wellness, and pizzazz. It helped lower my blood pressure. My head is clearer in the daytime. And since curing the sleep apnea dramatically reduces the risk of several deadly diseases, it possibly saved (or at least extended) my life.[3]

And Dellie doesn't mention the topic anymore.

If you experience snoring of any kind, choking or gasping during the night, insomnia, sleep that is not restorative, daytime fatigue despite sleeping well, or hypertension, you may well have obstructive sleep apnea. Get tested!

Since there is a powerful connection between sleep apnea and brain health, anyone with brain fog, memory issues, or MCI also should be tested. Sleep apnea dramatically increases the risk of dementia.

OSA CAUSES SEVERAL SEVERE DISORDERS AND PREMATURE DEATH

Sleep apnea causes or exacerbates many severe diseases, including hypertension, stroke, atrial fibrillation, other arrhythmias, elevated fasting blood sugar, metabolic syndrome, chronic heart failure, diabetes, and chronic unexplained fatigue or depression. If you suffer from any of these, tell your doctor you need a polysomnogram to determine whether sleep apnea might be causing or contributing to your problems.

Because it is silent, asymptomatic, and therefore insidious and subversive, OSA contributes to premature death in a significant percentage of the population. In fact, a 2008 University of Wisconsin study published in the journal *Sleep* followed subjects for eighteen years and revealed that death (from any cause) is three times as likely in people with severe sleep apnea compared to those without the disease.[4]

WHAT IS OSA?

Sleep apnea is an involuntary cessation of breathing that occurs while one is asleep. In fact, the Greek word apnea means "without breath."

The three types of sleep apnea are obstructive (caused by narrowing of the pharynx), central (caused by a brain breathing-center malfunction), and mixed. Of the three, the obstructive type (OSA) is the most common, but any sleep loss, regardless of cause, results in brain damage.

People with untreated sleep apnea stop breathing repeatedly during their sleep, often hundreds of times during the night, usually for a minute or longer. The sleeper is rarely if ever aware of these breath stoppages because they don't trigger a full awakening.

Obstructive sleep apnea occurs when the pharyngeal muscles that surround the upper airway collapse. This narrows the airway opening, which cuts off the air supply, and breathing stops for a few seconds to a minute or more. Normal breathing then restarts, sometimes with a choking sound or loud snort. This sequence may occur up to thirty times or more per hour. OSA is diagnosed when apnea episodes occur more than five times per hour.

Each apneic episode (each sleep interruption) produces arousal—not enough to wake one up but sufficient to put one's body, especially the central nervous and vascular systems, on high alert. It's a Paul Revere–like warning of impending oxygen deprivation.

The collapsing pharynx and pauses in breathing choke off the body's oxygen supply. Each apnea event causes the entire body to secrete cascades of alarm molecules that scream at the brain's breathing centers, "If you don't start breathing really soon, I will die."

Imagine what would go on in a person's mind and body during strangulation or drowning; sleep apnea is like that but subtler and more chronic. Of course, you don't die during an apneic episode; you just rise to a shallower level of sleep with no conscious awareness of the event.

COMPROMISED SLEEP QUALITY DAMAGES THE HIPPOCAMPUS AND ACCELERATES THE ONSET OF DEMENTIA

Sleep quality is a critical component of AD risk for older adults. Poor sleep quality, like that seen in OSA, predicts cognitive decline. It's pro-inflammatory and associated with increased risk of developing metabolic and cardiovascular diseases, independent risk factors for AD. Sleep apnea has been shown to injure the brain by causing inflammatory damage to hippocampal memory circuits that results in impairments in cognition, learning, and spatial memory.[5] Conversely, good sleep quality protects against AD by reducing inflammation and increasing amyloid beta clearance from the brain.[6]

Undetected OSA greatly accelerates the onset of dementia. Among people destined to get Alzheimer's disease, researchers have found that people with untreated OSA develop the early symptoms about ten years earlier than those who do not have sleep apnea.

SLEEP APNEA IS NOT A RARE DISEASE

Sleep apnea affects an estimated 30 million Americans. Roughly 25 percent of men have it and about 15 percent of women. It is as common as type 2 diabetes. Worldwide, about one in five adults has at least mild OSA, and about one in fifteen has the illness in a moderate to severe form. But because this disease stays below the radar and eludes diagnosis so much of the time, the actual numbers may be much higher.

The frequency of sleep-disordered breathing goes up dramatically with age. Epidemiologic surveys reveal that OSA affects a majority of people over fifty-five.

Because of lack of awareness by both the public and healthcare professionals, most sleep apnea patients remain undiagnosed and therefore untreated. Remarkably, 95 percent of people who have moderate to severe sleep apnea do not know they have it. As a member of the medical profession, I find this appalling. Doctors need to be better educated about the disease, and patients need to remind their doctors to test for OSA.

OBLIVIOUS VICTIMS

Like most victims, I was oblivious to the fact that I suffered from OSA.

OSA might be causing your high blood pressure. It might be setting you up for a stroke. It might be the cause of your daytime fatigue, your lack of energy, your lack of focus, and even your memory problems and cognitive impairment—but you remain clueless. Why? Because OSA is an asymptomatic disease.

I've always needed a lot of sleep—eight and a half to nine hours a night—and I was making sure I got it. Even with that much sleep I had some daytime fatigue, but like most people, I learned to live with it. A few years ago, I developed hypertension and metabolic syndrome. The research articles I read (after my wife suggested it) made it abundantly clear that sleep apnea is extremely common in hypertensives and in folks with blood-sugar-regulation problems (type 2 diabetes, insulin resistance, metabolic syndrome). A person with any of these diagnoses should be tested for OSA.

My only symptom was snoring, but who is aware that they snore? Almost nobody. Your sleep partner has to tell you. Or if you sleep alone, you can record your sleep. If you snore, you probably have sleep apnea, and the probability is very high that it is wreaking havoc on your metabolism and damaging your central nervous and vascular systems.

OBLIVIOUS DOCTORS

Very few doctors routinely ask about patients snoring or sleep apnea (medical lingo for this is "low index of suspicion"), and it usually goes undiagnosed. Two cardiologists and two neurologists missed it in me. Most doctors are oblivious to how common sleep apnea is and how serious its consequences are. Your doctor is probably unaware of the tight link between snoring and sleep apnea. He or she probably never considered (until you mentioned it) that your hypertension or your blood sugar problems, fatigue, headaches, heart disease, or other problem might be caused by OSA. But it might. This is a medical tragedy waiting to happen. What if my wife hadn't read about the connection between snoring, hypertension, and sleep apnea?

The possibility of OSA should be on every physician's checklist. Help me spread the word to all doctors that every patient with these diagnoses needs screening for OSA:

- Hypertension
- High blood sugar
- Type 2 diabetes

- Stroke
- Metabolic syndrome
- Coronary artery disease
- Atrial fibrillation
- Headaches
- Impotence
- Memory impairment
- Cognitive decline
- Daytime drowsiness
- Unexplained fatigue

Because undiagnosed and untreated OSA exacerbates all the above conditions, doctors who miss the OSA diagnosis also inadvertently contribute to the progression of these conditions in their patients. By posing a few additional questions during the routine clinical interview, doctors can easily identify patients in need of further diagnostic testing and, if appropriate, refer them to a sleep center.

On top of all that, people with OSA are much more likely to have accidents while driving and during other activities. Missing this diagnosis on such a large scale creates a public safety crisis.[7]

"THAT'S NOT ME"

You may be saying "That's not me. I sleep fine. I awaken refreshed, and I am not especially tired in the daytime." Keep this in mind: *There is absolutely no way you can diagnose yourself.*

We count on symptoms to tell us whether our bodies are working right. That approach does not work with OSA. This diabolical disease often has no symptoms—at least no obvious ones. Some patients do experience daytime sleepiness, foggy headedness, fatigue, morning headaches, depression, or a lack of vitality. But lots of other health issues can cause these symptoms; they are not specific to OSA. And OSA can coexist with other diagnoses that also cause these symptoms.

The bottom line here is that your doctor doesn't know everything—sometimes you have to take care of yourself. If your doctor missed this diagnosis and you are sure you snore, show him or her this chapter and ask for a referral to get tested. If you have hypertension or mild cognitive decline or early dementia—or any of the other diseases in the list above—a polysomnogram is an absolute must.

HOW CAN I TELL WHETHER I HAVE SLEEP APNEA?

Snoring, gasping, or choking sounds during sleep are the most common signs of sleep apnea. But how do you know you're making these sounds if you are asleep? You can ask your sleep partner if you snore. In addition, smart device apps are available that are designed to find out if you are snoring (whether you sleep alone or not).

Factors that increase the likelihood of sleep apnea include hypertension, excess body weight, daytime drowsiness, daytime fatigue, a narrow airway, or a misaligned jaw. If you have any of these, a workup is in order.

Sleep apnea should be at the top of the list of diagnoses considered and tested for in every patient with memory or cognitive complaints or even just foggy headedness. The diagnosis is best made by a sleep specialist at a sleep disorder center who will help you decide on your need for further evaluation. The testing possibilities include the following:

- *A polysomnogram*—This is the standard diagnostic test for OSA and the only definitive diagnostic tool for determining the presence of sleep apnea. During this painless overnight test done in a sleep laboratory, you're hooked up to equipment that monitors your heart, brain-wave activity, respiration patterns, arm and leg movements, and blood oxygen levels while you sleep. Simultaneous recordings of multiple physiologic signals during sleep generate a graph of the data called a polysomnogram that is then analyzed and interpreted for you by a physician sleep specialist.
- *Home sleep tests*—In case the idea of spending the night in a strange sleep lab while hooked up to dozens of monitors sounds

less than appealing to you, your doctor may provide you with simplified tests to be used at home to diagnose sleep apnea. These tests usually involve a portable monitor that measures your heart rate, blood oxygen level, airflow, and breathing patterns. If you have sleep apnea, the test results will show drops in your oxygen level during apneas and subsequent rises with awakenings. Home kits cost around $300 (compared with about $1,500 or so in a sleep lab) and will diagnose OSA but may miss other sleep disorders. If the results are abnormal, your doctor may be able to prescribe therapy without further testing. Talk with your doctor about whether home testing is right for you.

The only nonsurgical treatment for OSA in adults is the CPAP machine. Wearing the mask takes some time to get used to, but considering the alternatives, including stroke, AD, and early death, I'd say the choice is obvious.

CHAPTER 16

The Human Microbiome and the Gut-Brain Connection

If you thought you were thoroughly human, think again. Only 10 percent of the 100 trillion or so cells in your body are actually yours. The other 90 trillion are not human in any sense. They are microbes, mostly bacteria, that have colonized your body. They occupy real estate provided by us and eat food supplied by us. They make many chemicals we need for survival. In fact, we'd be dead without them.

The microbes living on and within us (mostly within our GI tracts) compose a complex and dynamic community that has different genomes from ours and is thus truly foreign. These bugs profoundly influence the health of our brains and bodies.

Say hello to your microbiome.

A REVOLUTION IN MEDICAL THINKING

Investigations into the diversity of the human microbiome started with Anton van Leeuwenhoek (fig. 16.1), the Father of Microbiology, who in 1676 designed powerful single-lens microscopes through which he was the first to see microorganisms. He called them *animalcules* and described at length their peculiar lives. Later, he was the first to use the microscopes to scrutinize his own oral and fecal microbiota.

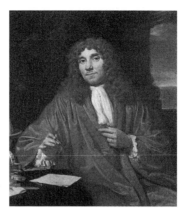

Figure 16.1. Anton van Leeuwenhoek, the Father of Microbiology

Over three hundred years later, scientists are finally beginning to appreciate the importance of this vast community of microbes. Recent advances in genetic technology have provided a glimpse into the powerful and populous world of microbial life inside us. Cutting-edge DNA sequencing technology combined with computing power and massive international research partnerships have put medical science on the cusp of the biggest revolution in medical thinking in 150 years. Our somewhat paranoid view of microbes as the enemy is being replaced by the more sensible view that they are essential allies that we depend upon for our very survival. Gut microbiome (GM) bugs are busy partnering with us behind the scenes—processing food, micromanaging immune responses, turning human genes off and on, and otherwise generally helping us do the work of being human.

SOME TERMINOLOGY

Before going any further, let me clarify some terminology. Technically, the term *microbiome* refers to the various genes associated with the resident microbes, while *microbiota* refers to the actual bugs themselves. The problem is, the word *microbiota* hasn't caught on. Just about everybody incorrectly uses the word *microbiome* to refer to the bugs (rather than their genome), and so will I.

Human microbiome (HM) populations inhabit virtually every inner and outer surface of our bodies. Each region has its own distinct community of microbes. The *gut microbiome* (GM) is the microbiome that resides in our gastrointestinal systems. Because it is chock-full of food and has a very large surface area, it contains most of our microbiome organisms. The skin, eyes, mouth, nose, ears, respiratory system, and urogenital system also support significant microbiome populations.

AN EIGHT-HUNDRED-POUND GORILLA LIVING IN YOUR GUT

The old joke asks, "Where does an eight-hundred-pound gorilla sit?" The answer: "Anywhere it wants to." It's an entity so powerful it can do whatever it pleases.

Your gut microbiome is your eight-hundred-pound gorilla.

Ninety-five percent of your HM bugs live and thrive on the inner pink mucosal surface of your intestinal tract. They're there because that's where they want to be. It's a great place to reproduce, raise a family, and create a community. And every day, a couple of pounds of tasty human food slides past the GM's bacterial colonies, from which that hungry gorilla and all those trillions of baby gorillas can pick and choose exactly what they need.

The intestinal mucosal surface is a huge chunk of real estate: flattened out, it would be the size of a football field. So if a bug wants to start a large family (a colony), it has plenty of space to accommodate its offspring. (And it does possess the capacity to generate billions of children in minutes!)

The balance and composition of the HM and GM are influenced by your microbial exposures, what you eat, where you live, your genetic makeup, your hormones, and even your behaviors. The makeup of your microbial populations changes every time you pet an animal, kiss someone, eat a meal, apply a cosmetic, or touch a doorknob. Bathing, shampooing, hand-washing, and toothbrushing remove some microbes, but they quickly grow back.

Consider these interesting facts:

- A ten second kiss transfers about 80 million bacteria.
- There are more bacteria on your scalp than people in North America.
- A typical hand can harbor more than 150 different bacterial species, only 17 percent of which are common to both hands of the same person and only 13 percent of which are shared by different persons.
- Some of the bacteria living on you can move as fast as cheetahs, when their relative size is considered.
- Your belly button contains over two thousand species of bacteria.

OUR BODIES USE THE GM AS A KIND OF EXTERNAL HARD DRIVE

What makes these microbiome bacterial populations so interesting, and important, is that they are the repository for over 99 percent of the DNA we use. One would expect DNA to be located in our own cells. Not so.

The Human Genome Project was launched in 1990 to identify and map all the genes of the human genome. Based on the level of complexity of human metabolism, researchers had expected to find millions of genes—but they found only about twenty five thousand.[1] "Where," they wondered, "are the rest?" (By way of comparison, a grain of rice, *Oryza sativa*, has around forty thousand functional genes. A worm, *Caenorhabditis elegans*, contains nineteen thousand genes. A typical *E. coli* bacterium living in your GI tract carries about five thousand genes.)

A few years later, the astonishing answer emerged: the missing genetic material was hiding in our gut microbiome.[2]

We now know that more than 99 percent of the total DNA we use comes from bacterial genes living in our gut microbiome. Here's how that works. Humans are only one species, so our maximum contribution to our gene pool is a paltry twenty-five thousand genes. We borrow the remainder of our genetic material from the ten thousand different species of bacteria in our GM, each of which has a different genome.

Let's do a little math. Ten thousand different species of bacteria multiplied by five thousand genes each expands our available gene pool to roughly 50 million. Some of these bacterial genes are duplicates, so let's round the number down to 20 million genes that we can draw from. The vast majority of chemicals circulating in human blood depend on these microbiome-derived genes in our microbiome for their synthesis. The genes we borrow from microbes are critical for metabolism, immune health, and most of the work done by the central nervous system.

Via this leveraging process, the human GM's incredibly large and diverse gene pool can accomplish tasks our own genes could never dream of. The GM plays important roles in nutrition, growth, inflammation, repair, and protection against foreign pathogens. GM bugs help us break down food and extract nutrients from it to generate energy, as well as produce vitamins and bolster immunity.

The gorilla in your gut doesn't really weigh much or take up much space. At about three pounds, the average adult microbiome weighs roughly as much as an average human brain. Bacterial cells are much smaller than body cells, so a hundred times more DNA is packed into that three-pound gut microbiome than in the entire rest of the human body.

Your GM controls the health and destiny of your brain. GM microbes exert powerful control over important aspects of brain function, including nerve impulse transmission, neuroinflammatory reactions, and neuroimmunity. No organ in the body is more sensitive to changes in the gut microbiome than your brain.[3]

MODERN PRACTICES ARE DAMAGING OUR MICROBIOMES

Researchers have begun to search for a causative connection between gut microbial infections and neurodegenerative brain disease. They are asking why people in modern society have become so prone to inflammatory, autoimmune, and allergic diseases. Could it be that society-wide shifts in our microbial communities have contributed to our seemingly hyperreactive immune systems and thus to neurodegenerative brain disease? Could it be that certain modern practices are driving this shift?

Several factors undermine our microbiome's ability to protect us—and our brains—from disease:

- The widespread overuse of antibiotics in humans and livestock
- Sanitary practices that are aimed at limiting infectious disease but that also hinder the transmission of symbiotic microbes
- Our high-sugar, high-carbohydrate, refined, processed, and preserved modern diet, which throws our gut microbiome out of balance by encouraging undesirable pathogenic microbes while discouraging symbiotic microbes

BAD BUGS CAN DISRUPT THE MICROBIOME AND DAMAGE THE BRAIN

Researchers are unraveling the mysteries of how pathogenic microbes cause neurological dysfunction and cognitive decline. They have studied virtually every known class of microbe, including bacteria, viruses, fungi, and prions. They have found that the human central nervous system is under constant assault by a vast array of microbes and pathogens. The changes seen in Alzheimer's disease closely resemble those seen when an infection affects the brain. In both contexts we see inflammation, brain cell atrophy, plaque formation and deposition, altered gene expression, immunological aberrations, and cognitive deficits. Because of these similarities, researchers have begun searching for a connection between infections that disrupt the gut microbiome and neurodegenerative brain disease with an eye toward discovering a causal connection between gut pathogenic microbes and Alzheimer's disease.

In an ambitious attempt to catalog these effects, James M. Hill and colleagues, in their 2014 paper entitled "Pathogenic Microbes, the Microbiome, and Alzheimer's Disease (AD)," published in *Frontiers in Aging Neuroscience*, enumerate several "highly specific and illustrative insights into the potential contribution of pathogenic microbes, altered microbiome signaling, and other disease-inducing agents to the development of AD."[4]

SUPPORT BRAIN HEALTH BY PROTECTING AND HEALING YOUR MICROBIOME

Science has so far only scratched the surface of how the gut-brain connection works, but even at this early stage of our understanding, it is clear that nurturing the health of your GM is a powerful strategy for preventing and reversing cognitive decline.

Keeping pathogenic microbes under control is something your microbiome does well. Occasionally, however, these disease-causing bugs—very much like invasive weeds in a flower garden—can get the upper hand. This happens most often as a result of dietary neglect: eating foods that encourage the proliferation of bad bugs (junk food, fast food, processed foods, high-carb foods, grains, sugars, allergenic foods). The result is an upset in the sensitive balance among colonies of microbes in our gut microbiome—an infection called dysbiosis. (Mainstream doctors almost always misdiagnose dysbiosis as IBS.) Chronic or recurring dysbiosis—regardless of whether it causes gut symptoms—sets the stage for dementia.

How can you tell if pathogens are getting the upper hand? If you have intestinal symptoms such as gas, bloating, food sensitivities or intolerances, sluggish digestion, loose stools, or even an upset stomach, your gut microbiome is trying to tell you "There's trouble down here."

But often, symptoms do not appear in the gut. Evidence of microbiome disruption instead might manifest as an allergic reaction or auto-immune disease, with the symptoms appearing in relatively faraway places such as joints, blood vessels, the skin, and the brain. Autoimmune reactions can cause inflammation in the brain, heart, pancreas, liver, kidneys, thyroid, skin, muscles, joints—just about any tissue. The list of autoimmune diseases is long,[5] but every single one traces back to a disturbed gut microbiome and a damaged, leaky intestinal mucosal inner lining. When an infected or allergically reactive intestinal lining loses its integrity, it leaks antigenic/allergenic partially digested proteins, called polypeptides, into the bloodstream. Immune cells (lymphocytes) recognize these polypeptides as foreign and make antibodies that attack them. These antibodies go through the bloodstream to various healthy target organs and tissues, where they cause inflammatory reactions—joints in arthritis, skin in psoriasis and eczema, the thyroid in Hashimoto's disease, and so on. Healthy brain tissue also becomes a target for these antibodies, resulting in neuronal damage and increased dementia risk.

Every single autoimmune disease is caused by the combination of a leaky gut and a disturbed microbiome. The list includes rheumatoid arthritis, ankylosing spondylitis, lupus, celiac disease, psoriasis, scleroderma, Hashimoto's thyroiditis, Graves' disease, type 1 diabetes, multiple sclerosis, Sjögren's syndrome, Cushing's disease, alopecia, Addison's disease, polycystic ovary syndrome, inflammatory bowel disease, ulcerative colitis, Crohn's disease, antiphospholipid syndrome, Guillain-Barré syndrome, Raynaud's disease, Ménière's disease, pernicious anemia, myasthenia gravis, autoimmune pericarditis, polyarteritis nodosa, polymyalgia rheumatica, and sarcoidosis. The complete list is much longer; there are over one hundred autoimmune diseases.[6]

If you have any autoimmune disease, you have a significantly higher risk of eventual cognitive impairment. Start learning how to address your disturbed microbiome now, before significant damage has been done.

For many years I was in denial about my own recurring dysbiosis. Like many, I had learned to live with the symptoms. I knew better but still found it extremely difficult to give up wheat, other grains, sugar, and other carbs. When I finally did, I experienced a dramatic improvement in my gut health and my general health as well. I also began taking the supplements mentioned below. My foggy-headed feeling went away, my energy zoomed, and my gas, bloating, and heartburn became things of the past.

THE PROBLEM WITH CARBS, GRAINS, AND STARTS IN THE GUT

Dr. David Perlmutter—an expert on the neurodegenerative effects of gluten, grains, starchy high-carb diets, and sugars—has written two books, *Grain Brain* and *Brain Makers,* that describe how and why grains and carbs are disastrous for the gut, the immune system, and the brain.[7] He explains that virtually all grains contain gluten and other allergy-causing, immune-system-damaging proteins. When we eat grains, we expose the lining of our gut to these proteins, which *always* activate a local immune reaction. This reaction, in turn, triggers the production of zonulin, a chemical that causes a local breakdown in the gut lining such that it becomes excessively permeable. This allows partially digested proteins and inflammatory debris to leak through the inflamed intestinal wall and into the bloodstream, which carries them far and wide. Immune cells in the bloodstream recognize the allergenic food debris as a foreign invader and release targeted antibodies to dispose of it. These antibodies are then attracted to areas of inflammation throughout the body, causing autoimmune allergic reactions that are most commonly seen in the joints (autoimmune arthritis, ankylosing spondylitis, rheumatoid arthritis, lupus), tendons and ligaments (fibromyalgia), blood vessels (Raynaud's disease, lupus), skin (discoid lupus, scleroderma), kidneys, heart (pericarditis, lupus), and central nervous system (AD).

In the short run, the symptoms will be brain fog, fatigue, and painful muscles, tendons, and joints, but long-term exposure to those grain-based allergenic proteins causes chronic changes in the intestinal tract and brain that lead to neurodegeneration and dementia. The allergic inflammation of the gut wall caused by grains also disrupts the intestinal microbiome, setting the stage for a long list of chronic degenerative diseases. And cognitive decline is at the top of that list.

ANTIBIOTICS DAMAGE YOUR GM

Antibiotics are sometimes necessary to combat pathogenic bacterial invaders. Broad-spectrum antibiotics, however, target broad swaths of normal microbiota as well, causing collateral damage—a kind of anti-microbial "friendly fire." Even in very small doses, antibiotics can kill significant quantities of beneficial GM bacteria along with the bugs that are causing the infection.

Antibiotics appear to be the single most important disrupter of the human genome–microbiome symbiosis. Their use has been shown to cause long-term GM repercussions that can take months or years to reverse, and are sometimes not reversible. The introduction of mass antibiotics coincides with the dramatic increase of a whole series of modern plagues, all of which have been experimentally linked to microbiome disturbances: atopic diseases, autoimmune diseases, allergies, asthma, and even multiple sclerosis and Parkinson's disease. Scientists are now also exploring links between the disturbance of microbes and some cancers.

For life-threatening bacterial infections, antibiotics can't be avoided, but they should be used only when absolutely necessary as their use always comes with microbiome damage and heightened long-term risk of immune dysfunction, cancer, and dementia.

DIET FOR A HEALTHY GUT MICROBIOME

Your diet profoundly affects the structure, organization, and function of your gut microbiome. Unhealthy dietary choices damage the GM and brain. (In part 3, we'll discuss in detail the diet that protects against dementia and reverses it.)

Sugar and carbohydrates feed undesirable microbes and thus encourage overpopulation of the GM by colonies of pathogens. A high-carb diet also discourages the beneficial, probiotic species. To protect your brain, you will need to remove grains, breads, pastas, baked goods, chips (all kinds), snack foods, most desserts, beer, wine, and all those other carb-laden foods we have come to know and love. (Beyond carb content, other chemicals in grains and high-carb foods directly damage the brain and its blood vessels. See chapter 11.)

Eat only whole fresh foods: vegetables, fruit, lean meat, eggs, nuts, seeds, and beans. These shift the composition of the gut microbiome away from gas-forming pathogens.

Avoid processed (packaged) foods. These will damage your microbiome, as will GMO (genetically modified organism) foods, fast foods, junk food, chlorinated water, fluoridated water, antibiotics, pesticides, artificial flavoring, and preservatives.

Whenever possible, choose organic foods.

REESTABLISHING A HEALTHY MICROBIOME AND TREATING DYSBIOSIS—THE "PILLARS" OF TREATMENT

Most conventional health practitioners fail to appreciate gut symptoms as signs of a disturbed ecosystem. Thus, patients with dysbiosis are usually not helped by these doctors, who tend to prescribe antibiotics or symptomatic medicines that not only fail to address the underlying causes of the problem but can make the situation worse. Functional medicine physicians, on the other hand, have experience treating intestinal dysbiosis. They apply the following standardized principles that guide the understanding and treatment of a disrupted GM:

1. *Use digestive enzymes*—Enhanced digestion is a powerful tool for protecting the gut microbiome and immune system from bad bug invasions and reducing the load of food-derived allergens. In patients with dysbiosis, digestive enzymes should be taken with every meal.

    Digestive enzymes eliminate the problem of incompletely digested leftovers in the gut that feed pathogens and allow their colony size to increase. Incompletely digested food also creates allergens (mostly partially digested proteins) that slip through the inflamed leaky gut wall and generate a systemic immune response.

The enzymes can also be used to abort acute digestive upset accompanied by cramps, bloating, and gas. In these situations, I recommend six to ten plant-based digestive enzyme capsules. These work very fast—usually within fifteen minutes—to shut down the reaction and restore balance. For long-term use to reestablish gut health, take them with every meal: two capsules with a snack, four with a normal meal, and six with a large meal.

2. *Repopulate the gut with probiotics* (*Lactobacillus acidophilus, Bifido-bacterium*, etc.)—Probiotics are the good bugs, the acidophilus-like microorganisms that repopulate the gut to force pathogenic invaders out. Repopulating the diseased and depleted intestinal tract with beneficial microorganisms is a very important, widely used, and incredibly effective way to accelerate its healing. These bugs strengthen the immune system, assist digestion, provide essential vitamins, neutralize dietary carcinogens, bolster immune function, heighten resistance to infection, and protect against autoimmune disease, neurodegeneration, and aging itself. The beneficial health effects of probiotics all trace back to the fact that they dramatically enhance the health of the microbiome.

   Be extremely careful when purchasing acidophilus products; most of them are ineffective despite fancy labels, high prices, and claims of tens of billions of microbes per capsule. In a huge market saturated with substandard products, Klaire Labs is the acknowledged industry quality leader. I recommend its Ther-Biotic Complete, the most potent and effective acidophilus product available. Take two to six capsules a day. These can be taken all at once or in divided doses, with or without food. The only caveat is to not take them within two hours of a natural antibiotic such as Tricycline (see below), berberine, or grapefruit seed extract, as the antibiotic will kill some of the acidophilus.

3. *Use biofilm disrupters* (e.g., InterFase from Klaire Labs)—The pathogenic microbes that destroy the microbiome and cause dysbiosis secrete a slippery protein that surrounds and protects their

colonies. This biofilm wall insulates them from the immune cells and antibiotics that would otherwise be able to kill them. Biofilm disrupters break down the biofilm. Take two to four capsules twice daily. They are more effective if taken at least a couple of hours before, during, or after meals.

4. *Use prebiotics* (Biotagen from Klaire Labs)—Prebiotics are fiber compounds that pass undigested through the upper part of the gastrointestinal tract and travel to the large bowel, where they selectively enhance the growth and activity of beneficial bacteria, especially *Lactobacillus* and *Bifidobacterium*. Prebiotics also inhibit the growth of potentially pathogenic microbes such as *Clostridium*. By encouraging the growth of Bifidobacterium species, prebiotics enhance the production of short-chain fatty acids, the main energy source for colonic epithelial cells. Take two to four capsules twice daily.

5. *Use natural antibiotics*—Natural antibiotics kill offending pathogens without damaging the GM. My favorite is Tricycline (Allergy Research Group), which contains the natural antibiotics berberine, citrus seed extract, black walnut hull, and artemisinin. Take one to three capsules once or twice a day, at least two hours away from probiotics.

6. *Identify and remove food allergens*—Everyone has food allergies, but most people don't know it. Food allergens cause inflammation that damages the microbiome and the gut wall, causing it to leak antigenic materials into the bloodstream, which takes them to target tissues around the body where they can cause foggy headedness, arthritic pain, headaches, skin rashes, bloating, water retention, gas, heartburn (acid reflux), and other intestinal symptoms. Digestive enzymes help with food allergies by breaking foods down into nonallergens. More thorough digestion also allows nutrients to be absorbed higher in the digestive tract, and this discourages dysbiotic infections by reducing the amount of food available to the pathogens.

Food allergy testing helps identify the allergenic foods in your diet. I recommend Meridian Valley Lab's E95 and E90. (Eliminate or rotate [every fourth day] all allergenic foods.)

7. *Repair and rebuild the integrity of the intestinal mucosa*—Only a healthy gut can host the microbiome's probiotic microbes and immune cells—and, of course, your microbiome. A damaged mucosa becomes host to pathogens and, because it is damaged, it leaks. This leads to autoimmune disease. L-glutamine, inulin, acacia, and N-acetyl-N-glucosamine heal the gut wall. A healthy gut wall no longer leaks, and provides a welcome environment in which probiotic microbes can thrive. Take nutritional combination products such as GastroThera (Klaire Labs) that heal the mucosal surface and restore the damaged villi. Take six caps once or twice a day.

OBTAINING MEDICAL HELP FOR GUT PROBLEMS

Dysbiosis tends to be chronic and recurring. If you have acute or severe symptoms, be sure to see your primary care physician. You may be fortunate to have an alternative-minded doctor who will know how to address your gut issues. Conventional doctors, however, are not up to speed on current gut developments. They'll usually prescribe medicines that merely suppress symptoms and don't address underlying causes. If you are lucky, you might get a prescription for acidophilus, but don't get your hopes up. The conventional medical diagnostic system is not yet capable of diagnosing and treating ecological disturbances in the gut microbiome.

Your first choice should be to find a doctor who practices functional medicine and who understands and will follow the standardized principles described above. This healing work can be started while the mainstream diagnostic workup is being done (blood work, antibody testing, cultures, other lab testing, upper or lower GI tract imaging, ultrasound, etc.).

CHAPTER 17

A Healthy Thyroid Prevents Cognitive Decline

Untreated hypothyroidism is a very common health problem that impairs brain function, undermines cognitive health, and serves as a launchpad for dementia.

MY THYROID STORY

My entire life I had been cold and tired—and more or less constipated. And my immune system was weak; I had frequent infections. If a cold was going around, I'd get it. I had multiple allergies, dry skin, and cold hands and feet. No doctor ever suspected my thyroid might be the cause because the kind of borderline low thyroid function I had—now known as subclinical hypothyroidism—hadn't yet been discovered.

Finally, as a family doctor in my forties, I realized I was probably hypothyroid. When blood tests revealed low levels of thyroid hormone, I began taking a small dose every morning. At first, I didn't notice any difference (which, by the way, is fairly typical). After a month, however, I started feeling better. Two months in, my fatigue had pretty much disappeared, and I wasn't cold all the time. The improvement was so gradual that I barely noticed it, but when I thought back to all the symptoms that had improved or disappeared, I became convinced. My hands and feet were warm, I didn't need to bundle up anymore, my energy and immune system improved, and my brain fog cleared.

If you are among the large percentage of the population with hypothyroidism, you, too, may be amazed at how much younger and better you feel once your thyroid health is restored. But be advised—thyroid hormone replacement works slowly over several months. The results are worth the wait.

My healing from hypothyroidism inspired me to carefully study all aspects of endocrinology, especially the alternative approach that uses bioidentical hormone replacement and avoids synthetic wannabe hormones that are notorious for disrupting our sensitive systems. When I started testing for hormonal deficiencies in my patients, I began to see how common deficiencies of estrogen, progesterone, testosterone, pregnenolone, and DHEA were. The most frequent—by far—was a low thyroid.

AN UNUSUAL SUSPECT

Most people go to their doctors with some idea of what's wrong with them. "My neck hurts." "This wart won't go away." "My allergies are acting up." I've yet to have a patient say to me, "Dr. Smith, my thyroid gland is bothering me." It's always something else.

For example, Ellen said that she felt cold all the time. Herb had high blood pressure. Mary complained of constant fatigue. Joe's eczema drove him crazy. Sue couldn't lose weight. Al suffered from chronic headaches. Alice struggled with severe premenstrual syndrome. Mel had lost all interest in sex. Jenny couldn't get pregnant (and no, she isn't married to Mel). Jeff couldn't shake his allergies. Carol was plagued by recurrent infections. Michael didn't have any symptoms at all—just elevated cholesterol. When tested, every one of these people had an underactive thyroid.

Certain symptoms serve as fairly accurate predictors of hypothyroidism. In my medical practice, I always test for the condition whenever a patient has one or more of the following: high cholesterol, anemia, allergies, constipation, fatigue, foggy headedness, infertility, premenstrual syndrome, hair loss, dry skin, chronic infection or illness, cold hands and feet, a need for extra layers of clothing when others don't, or other temperature intolerance.

AGING AND HYPOTHYROIDISM ARE OFTEN CONFUSED

Thyroid function declines with age. Most people over sixty have some degree of hypothyroidism, which often causes cognitive decline. The diagnosis of hypothyroidism is commonly overlooked in this age group.

Declining thyroid function is especially difficult for doctors to diagnose because its symptoms are identical to the physical and mental changes seen in aging. Normal aging and hypothyroidism do have a lot in common. In fact, the symptoms of both aging and low thyroid include fatigue, circulatory problems (feeling cold), dry skin, depression, digestive problems, memory loss/forgetfulness, and muscle weakness. Doctors often erroneously attribute these signs to normal aging when in fact they are caused by a low thyroid. This may not seem important until you consider that a low thyroid is easily treated and reversed, unlike aging.

This reminds me of Sam. A retired business executive in his seventies, Sam had been healthy all his life. But then he started to experience a puzzling array of symptoms. He felt cold and tired most of the time. He had trouble remembering things. He no longer cared about sex. He was constipated. His entire body seemed to be shutting down. He mentioned all of this to his doctor, who replied, "You're getting up there, Sam. It's normal aging. What do you expect?"

Needless to say, the doctor's remarks didn't sit well with Sam. That's when he came to see me. Sam's laboratory tests checked out fine. But his basal metabolic temperature was running about one half degree low, a good indicator of hypothyroidism.

I started Sam on a trial dose of thyroid hormone. Within a few weeks, he reported improvements in his stamina, memory, and libido. I continued to monitor Sam's treatment for a few months, adjusting the hormone dose a couple of times. Within six months, his initial symptoms had all but disappeared.

Clearly, Sam's problems had nothing to do with normal aging. They were the handiwork of an underactive thyroid gland. And Sam is not alone. Because their doctors don't suspect it, millions of folks suffer from undetected hypothyroidism that comes on as they get older and might also be an early warning sign of Alzheimer's disease. Unfortunately, very few get tested for hypothyroidism. (And, as you will see, even when they are tested, the diagnosis is often missed.)

AN EPIDEMIC OF HYPOTHYROIDISM

Hypothyroidism is responsible for a great deal of human suffering and disability and plays a major role in causing and perpetuating cognitive decline, dementia, and Alzheimer's disease. Of all the health problems I discuss in this book that undermine health, accelerate aging, and cause dementia, none is more easily corrected than a low thyroid.

According to the American Thyroid Association, the world's leading professional association of thyroid specialists,[1]

- An estimated 20 million Americans have thyroid disease.
- Up to 60 percent of those with thyroid disease are unaware of their condition.
- More than 12 percent of the US population will develop a thyroid condition during their lifetime.
- Women are five to eight times more likely than men to have thyroid problems.
- One woman in eight will develop a thyroid disorder during her lifetime.

You'd be hard-pressed to find a condition more thoroughly misunderstood, misdiagnosed, and just plain missed. Doctors miss this diagnosis so often that untreated hypothyroidism has reached epidemic proportions. A big part of the problem is that doctors often believe they know everything they need to know about the thyroid and are extremely resistant to upgrading their approach.

Hypothyroidism usually presents with a long list of vague symptoms that impersonate scores of other ailments. Most people who have the condition don't realize it, and most physicians who see it don't recognize it for what it is. In fact, the American Association of Clinical Endocrinologists estimates that only half of those afflicted have actually been correctly diagnosed. No wonder hypothyroidism was dubbed "The Unsuspected Illness" by legendary endocrinologist Broda O. Barnes, MD, PhD, whose work brought us a deeper understanding of the thyroid gland's pivotal role in human health.[2]

HOW YOUR THYROID GLAND WORKS

The thyroid is a butterfly-shaped gland that sits in the front of your neck, just below and to either side of the Adam's apple. Its diminutive size—it weighs less than an ounce—belies its importance. The thyroid manufactures thyroid hormone and releases it into the bloodstream, which carries it to every cell in the body.

Once a molecule of thyroid hormone has reached its target organ, it finds a target cell. It then passes through that cell's outer membrane and docks on the wall that surrounds the cell's nucleus (the nuclear membrane). From there it sends a signal directly to the cell's DNA, telling it at what rate to translate into messenger RNA—in other words, the thyroid hormone molecule is setting that cell's (and *all* cells') level of activity.

By releasing varying amounts of hormone, your thyroid thus regulates the rate of metabolism in all 100 trillion of your cells. Thyroid hormone doesn't tell your cells what to do; it tells them how fast to do it. If your thyroid is underactive and thyroid hormone is in short supply, cellular activity will slow down. When the thyroid is low, your body's cells don't get their proper marching orders. They don't know what level of activity is appropriate, so they slow way down.

WHAT HAPPENS WHEN THYROID HORMONE IS LOW?

Because all your cells contain thyroid hormone receptors, impaired thyroid performance can cause a surprisingly broad range of health problems. Symptoms vary from one organ or tissue type to another and are tissue-specific. In muscle cells, strength declines. In intestinal cells, gut motility may slow down, causing constipation (one of the most common symptoms of a low thyroid; digestion of food and absorption of nutrients may also be compromised. In skin cells, acne, eczema, hair loss, and dryness may occur. In the immune system, there'll be more colds and flus and persistent infections, as well as more allergies. Vascular system symptoms may include cold extremities, circulatory problems, and atherosclerosis.

In the central nervous system, hypothyroidism causes fatigue and low energy—and cognitive decline. And researchers have documented size decreases in the hippocampal memory centers in patients who are hypothyroid.[3]

Our gray matter is arguably the most metabolically active body part, so it is especially vulnerable to a shortfall of thyroid hormone.

A low thyroid hormone level causes hippocampal memory centers and processing speed to slow to a crawl, so cognition plummets. Neuroplasticity and neuronal resilience—the ability to learn and grow and change—become severely hampered.

BLOOD TESTS FOR THYROID FUNCTION

Three blood tests are necessary to assess thyroid function and determine the optimum thyroid dose: free T3, free T4, and TSH.

Your body makes two thyroid hormones, T3 and T4. (TSH is a pituitary hormone.) Over 99.5 percent of your T3 and T4 is attached to and carried around by thyroglobulin, a large protein molecule. The small remainder is the free fraction that is not attached to the carrier protein and is therefore available to attach to receptor sites and go to work. We are interested in measuring only the free fractions: free T3 and free T4.

Free T3—the single most important thyroid test—is by far the most active and most bioavailable form of thyroid hormone. Free T3 exerts a receptor effect that is estimated to be ten times more potent than that of free T4. Many researchers believe that free T4 serves primarily as a precursor for T3 and itself has almost no hormonal acitvity.[4] The optimum range for free T3 is 3.5–5.5 picograms per milliliter (pg/mL).

If your free T3 is below 2.9 pg/mL and you have symptoms of a low thyroid, you are hypothyroid. It doesn't matter what your doctor says. It doesn't matter if your TSH and free T4 are low or high or normal— your level of the active, bioavailable free T3 hormone is low and you are therefore hypothyroid.

Free T4—the other main thyroid hormone—is the weak, minimally active storage form of thyroid hormone and serves as the precursor from which T3 can be made. As you will see in a moment, this crucial T4 to T3 conversion is easily disrupted, and when this occurs it can undermine proper thyroid function, causing a shortfall of the all-important free T3.

The pituitary gland regulates thyroid hormone levels by monitoring blood thyroxine levels and secreting TSH if levels go down. TSH released from the pituitary gland stimulates increased thyroxine production everywhere in the body. Because the pituitary cranks out more TSH when thyroid (T3 and T4) levels go down, a higher TSH level indicates lower thyroid activity (lower levels of T3 and T4) and is thus a good rough barometer of thyroid activity. TSH, however, is an indirect and imprecise and often unreliable marker on its own. Because it is a pituitary hormone (not a thyroid hormone), it is vulnerable to fluctuations in the pituitary environment that may be completely unrelated to body-wide thyroid status. Using the pituitary gland's TSH hormone to determine thyroid function is kind of like trying to determine how much money is inside a bank by watching how many people go in and out. You're going to be wrong a lot of the time.[5]

About 80 percent of free T3 is made not in the thyroid gland but in the various peripheral organs and tissues where it will be used.

Many doctors make the mistake of ordering only TSH and free T4 tests. They omit the all-important free T3 test. Free T3 is crucial because it is the most prevalent, most active, most potent form of thyroid hormone; without knowing a patient's free T3 level, a clinician cannot accurately diagnose a low thyroid, determine thyroid status, or accurately adjust thyroid hormone dosage. Proper diagnosis—and proper adjustment of dosage—always requires all three tests: free T3, free T4, and TSH. Additionally, all three must be done on the same sample of blood.

Following is a guide to interpreting the results of your thyroid tests:

- *Free T3*—The ideal range is 3.5–5.5 pg/mL.
  - Low free T3 (<3.0) indicates hypothyroidism.
  - High free T3 (>6.0) indicates hyperthyroidism or excess thyroid replacement.
- *Free T4*—The ideal range is 0.9–1.9 ng/dL (nanograms per deciliter).
  - Low free T4 (<0.9) indicates hypothyroidism.
  - High free T4 (>1.9) indicates possible overcorrection with thyroid replacement or hyperthyroidism.
- *TSH*—The ideal range is 0.1–2.0 μIU/mL (micro–international units per milliliter).
  - Low TSH (<0.1) indicates excess thyroid hormone. This is hyperthyroidism, and it can be caused by a body malfunction (in which case you should see an endocrinologist) or by taking too much thyroid hormone.
  - High TSH (>2.0) indicates probable hypothyroidism.

DOCTORS OFTEN MISS THIS DIAGNOSIS

When it comes to hypothyroidism, otherwise good doctors often miss the diagnosis. They might not pay attention to symptoms. They might order the wrong combination of tests, use incorrect normal ranges provided by the labs, or misinterpret the meaning of the test result numbers. A low thyroid may be difficult to diagnose but is dangerous to miss because hypothyroidism causes brain and body-wide malfunctions. More than one in three US adults has some degree of hypothyroidism. Millions of Alzheimer's disease patients are wandering around in a cognitive fog because their doctors failed to understand how much a healthy brain depends on optimum thyroid functioning and failed to make the diagnosis of hypothyroidism—a mistake that could lead to preventable dementia, dramatic lowering of the quality of life, and even premature death. That's a lot of disease that doesn't need to happen.

Even when common symptoms of hypothyroidism are staring them in the face, most doctors manage to miss the diagnosis. I am talking about low energy, easy fatigue, a constant cold feeling, constipation, an inability to lose weight (even on a low-calorie diet), frequent colds and allergies, anemia, and elevated cholesterol.

Perhaps the most grievous error of all is that doctors incorrectly assume that a TSH reading applies to the entire body and gives them a clear read on whether the thyroid is working properly. It does not. They fail to appreciate the fact that 80 percent of T3 is made in the peripheral tissues (rather than in the thyroid) and that the enzyme that accomplishes this conversion (5'-deiodinase) resides locally in peripheral tissues and organs (as opposed to centrally in the thyroid gland).[6] They are oblivious to the reality that, in the same person, the rate of conversion of T4 to T3 can vary dramatically from one organ or tissue type to another, which translates into far-flung variations in thyroid hormone levels.

If your doctor dismisses your symptoms, tells you that they are a normal part of aging, or says that your thyroid is fine, find another doctor who will take your concerns seriously. It may take a bit of legwork, but it's important. We're talking about your health and longevity here.

If you believe you are hypothyroid and your doctor will work with you, you'll need to hold his or her feet to the fire. You may have to diagnose your own low thyroid, order the proper tests, and then convince your doctor you are right. Before you attempt that, please educate yourself. The following sections contain additional technical information about what goes wrong and how to diagnose yourself. I offer this information not so that you can treat yourself (not a good idea) but to provide the information you need to work with your provider to get your thyroid back on track.

T4-TO-T3 PERIPHERAL CONVERSION PROBLEMS

In medical school, we were taught that TSH from the pituitary gland tells the thyroid gland to make more thyroxine. But now we know that most T4-to-T3 conversion (and T3 production) happens not centrally in the thyroid gland but in local peripheral tissues where it will be used, such as the skin, liver, brain, and GI tract.

Our bodies use the much weaker "carrier" form of thyroid hormone, T4, to make T3, the main, most active, and most potent thyroid hormone. Our cells convert T4 to T3 by removing one atom of iodine from the T4 molecule. The enzyme that is responsible for this is called 5'-deodinase. Many hypothyroid patients are unable to generate this enzyme, so their cells can't perform the peripheral conversion of T4 to T3. Their peripheral conversion pathways could have been damaged by inflammation, injury, illness, trauma, stress, caloric restriction, exercise, hepatic or renal pathology, toxic metal exposures, chemical poisons, and several drugs. There is no way that the pituitary gland, in setting the TSH level, can monitor these peripheral influences and provide meaningful information. Hypothyroidism is most likely to be missed or mistreated in such paients.

Most physicians are unaware of peripheral conversion issues and continue to assume that the thyroid makes all the T3 and that TSH accurately reflects what is going on in the thyroid system. As a consequence, they misdiagnose and continue to ignore the need for T3. They incorrectly prescribe even more of the pure T4 medicines (levothyroxine, Synthroid, Levoxyl, etc.), which can't be converted to T3 and therefore can't address these patients' most important deficit, the shortfall of T3. This perpetuates the patient's thyroid deficiency and exacerbates the conversion problem.[7]

Patients who can't convert T4 to T3 will do much better on natural bioidentical hormones, such as Armour Thyroid and Nature-Throid, because they contain both forms of the hormone. I have seen hundreds of thyroid patients in whom Synthroid, Levoxyl, or other versions of levothyroxine didn't work or made them sicker—but when I changed the prescription to natural Armour Thyroid or Nature-Throid, they started feeling much better.[8] These patients will also respond to pure T3 medications such as Cytomel.

Lack of physician awareness of T4-to-T3 conversion issues has caused millions of thyroid patients to receive improper treatment and has contributed significantly to the epidemic of hypothyroidism. Many of these patients will needlessly go on to experience cognitive decline and dementia.

AUTOIMMUNE THYROID DISEASE

Our immune system is usually very good at identifying, attacking, and destroying foreign matter—toxins, viruses, bacteria, and allergens. But at times it struggles, and sometimes it gets lost, and when this happens it can turn its weapons—T cells, B cells, natural killer cells, cytotoxic T cells, and cytokines—on ourselves, a kind of "friendly fire" in which the immune system attacks and destroys our own healthy tissues. We call this *autoimmune disease*, and these attacks cause widespread inflammation.

Autoimmune thyroiditis (also known as Hashimoto's disease) is one such condition in which the immune system makes antibodies that attack either the thyroid gland cells or thyroglobulin (the protein that carries thyroid hormone in the bloodstream). The inflammation from these attacks blocks the conversion of T4 to T3 (both in the gland and in peripheral tissues) and interferes with the thyroid's ability to communicate with the pituitary gland. The result is a lowered activity of the gland and its hormones—and lab test results that even less accurately reflect what is going on.

The basic test used to detect thyroid autoimmune disease is the antithyroid antibody (ATA) panel, which contains two tests: (1) the ATGA (antithyroglobulin antibody) and (2) the anti-TPO (antithyroperoxidase) antibody. This very reliable ATA panel is usually done just once to confirm or rule out the presence of Hashimoto's.

You do not need a doctor's order to get these tests. You can order them from Direct Labs (www.directlabs.com). The results will be sent directly to you.

INFLAMMATION: A MAJOR DISRUPTER OF THYROID FUNCTION

Inflammation exerts profound effects on all aspects of thyroid metabolism and physiology and is arguably the single most effective way to disrupt the thyroid gland's ability to make and regulate its hormones. Inflammation—caused by Hashimoto's or another autoimmune disease—disrupts important hormone-regulating communication between the hypothalamus, pituitary, and thyroid. But the damage isn't limited to just the thyroid gland: inflammation decreases the number and sensitivity of thyroid hormone receptors throughout the body. As Chris Kresser puts it, "If there aren't enough receptors, or they aren't sensitive enough, it doesn't matter how much thyroid medication we take. The cells won't be able to use it. It's like when my grandpa used to turn down his hearing aids while he was watching the football game. It didn't matter how much my grandma yelled at him—he couldn't hear a word she said."[9]

When a physician gives a T4-only medication (Synthroid, Levoxyl, levothyroxine) to someone with inflammation, regardless of its cause, it is not going to work because inflammation blocks the conversion of T4 to T3—so these patients continue to be T3 deficient. They desperately need T3-containing medication.

HOW TO DETERMINE WHETHER YOU ARE HYPOTHYROID

You owe it to yourself—and to the future health of your brain—to make sure that your thyroid gland is in good working order. If it's not, you need to be able to confidently confront your doctor to help him or her make the correct diagnosis. Your symptoms, lab test results, and body temperatures will provide all the information you need to determine whether you are hypothyroid.

First, generate a list of your symptoms to show to your doctor. Below is a list of hypothyroid symptoms:

- Allergies
- Anemia
- Angina
- Atherosclerosis (hardening and clogging of the arteries)
- Brittle nails
- Chronic or frequent infections
- Cold hands and feet
- Constipation
- Depression
- Difficulty losing weight
- Digestive problems
- Dry skin
- Fatigue
- Foggy headedness
- Hair loss
- Headaches
- Heart rhythm disturbances
- High cholesterol
- Immune dysfunction (allergies and infections)
- Infertility
- Irregular menstrual periods
- Lethargy
- Loss of appetite
- Loss of libido
- Low resistance to colds and flu
- Memory problems
- Mental sluggishness
- Muscle weakness and atrophy
- Osteoporosis and osteopenia
- Premenstrual syndrome
- Slowness of movement

- Slow wound healing
- Sluggish feeling
- Stiff joints
- Weight gain

Second, get tested. Ask for free T3, free T4, and TSH testing. If your insurance covers these tests, fine. If your copay is more than $89, you might want to consider using Direct Labs, which offers the same high-quality testing as you would receive from your doctor's order, minus the need for a doctor's order.[10]

To determine whether you have Hashimoto's disease, the first time you get tested include a thyroid antibodies panel (thyroid peroxidase and antithyroglobulin antibody); Direct Labs calls this a "Free T's Plus TSH & Thyroid Antibodies" test. (You don't need to retest for the antibodies because they almost never go away if they are present, and whether or not you take thyroid hormone doesn't affect them.)

Third, do the Barnes Basal Metabolic Temperature Test (BMTT). Developed in the 1950s by Broda O. Barnes (mentioned earlier), the BMTT is an extensively researched, widely used, easy, and remarkably accurate at-home method for diagnosing low thyroid. It does not, however, replace the free T3, free T4, and TSH testing.

The BMTT is based on the idea that your thyroid sets your rate of metabolism, which, in turn, determines your body temperature. If your thyroid is low, you'll have a slow metabolism, and a low temperature. Many doctors believe that the BMTT is the most sensitive and accurate measure of thyroid function. (It is useful in detecting hypothyroidism; it is not used to follow progress or to make dose adjustments once treatment has been initiated.)

To conduct the BMTT, use an ordinary body thermometer, whether the old-fashioned mercury type or a newer digital model. Take your armpit (basal) temperature before you get out of bed in the morning. (That is when your temperature has not yet been raised by any activity.) The night before going to sleep, put your thermometer within easy reach, right next to your bed. If you use the mercury kind, be sure to shake it down the night before, as that activity in the morning would raise your temperature and spoil the test.

Place the thermometer deep into your armpit. Leave it there for ten minutes; then read and record your temperature.

I want to stress that even a little movement, like getting out of bed or going to the bathroom, will raise your temperature and give a false reading.

Repeat this process for at least three consecutive days.

The BMTT normal range is from 97.8°F to 98.2°F. Dr. Barnes checked over ten thousand people this way and found that hypothyroid people always test below 97.8°F. If your temperatures are below 97.8°F—even if all your blood tests are normal—you are hypothyroid.

Please note that fever and menstrual periods will falsely raise your temperature and skew the results. If you have an infection of any kind, or if you are having your period, you should wait until these pass before performing the test.

TREATMENT, FOLLOW-UP RETESTING, AND DOSE ADJUSTMENT

If your basal temperatures, symptoms, and lab tests indicate your thyroid is low, you will need a doctor's prescription for (natural) thyroid hormone replacement. Getting one can be tricky. As already discussed, you will need to work with a physician who is familiar with functional medicine and the thyroid concepts presented here.

Thyroid hormone is available only by prescription. Over-the-counter thyroid glandular support formulas will not correct a thyroid hormone deficiency, nor will taking iodine.

Always take your thyroid hormone replacement first thing in the morning. Take it with water only. All other foods, medications, and drinks will interfere with its absorption, so no coffee, tea, juice, or even lemon juice is allowed. The only acceptable fluid is water. Wait at least fifteen minutes before consuming anything else; thirty minutes is even better.

Your ideal dosage can be determined by monitoring your hormone levels and adjusting the dosage as needed. The optimum dose can't be determined without repeat testing, so you or your healthcare provider will need to monitor your serum levels of TSH, free T3, and free T4. As thyroid hormone (free T3 and free T4) levels rise, your TSH will fall.

The thyroid changes slowly, so be patient. For all the same reasons you wouldn't jam your gas pedal to the floor when you accelerate, it's best to increase thyroid dosing in small increments—usually ¼ to ½ grain (15–30 mg) at a time—to give your body a chance to get used to each change. Your body needs three to four weeks to adjust to any dose change, so there is no advantage to changing the dose or testing more often than that.

The BMTT won't usually return to normal with hormone replacement, so it is useful only for the initial diagnosis, and not for adjusting your dose.

Most people tolerate natural, bioidentical thyroid hormone. (After all, this is exactly the same hormone your body would be making if it could.) Side effects are exceedingly rare. If you are getting too much T3 thyroid hormone, you might experience jittery feelings or heart palpitations (a rapid heart rate). If either of these symptoms happens the first day or two after starting the thyroid hormone or changing the dose and it is mild, just persevere; it will disappear in a few hours or a day as your body adjusts. If your heart rate is over 90 or you are more than a little jittery, discontinue the thyroid hormone for a day or two and then resume at a lower dose.

Once your thyroid health is restored, you might be amazed at how much younger you feel and how much better your brain works. Correcting your hypothyroidism dramatically reduces the probability that you will get Alzheimer's.

CHAPTER 18

Neurotoxic Metals Can Ravage Your Brain

Toxic metals pose a threat to brain health. Are they lurking in your tissues, insidiously setting the stage for dementia? If you eat one or more servings of fish a week, I can assure you that enough mercury has already accumulated to cause damage. But other brain-eroding heavy metals can also easily get into your cells, riding in on water, food, air, and drugs. Most toxic metal exposures are due to chronic exposure: a dental filling that leaks mercury into your bloodstream, antacids taken regularly for heartburn (aluminum), chocolate consumption (cadmium), lead in drinking water, or your antiperspirant (aluminum).[1]

A hair analysis (less than $150) that you can do from home will identify your risk.

TESTING TO IDENTIFY YOUR NEUROTOXIC METALS RISK

Hair analysis is the best way to determine whether your brain is being exposed to toxic metal elements. As hair grows, toxic metals in the body are incorporated into it in direct proportion to amounts in other tissues. Scalp hair thus provides a temporal record of element metabolism and exposure to toxic elements. Analyzing a sample of hair will reveal how much mineral has been deposited over the weeks or months when that hair was growing. (Blood and urine testing are of limited value because they detect only very recent acute exposures, in hours or days.)

In addition to measuring levels of all potentially toxic metals, hair mineral analysis looks at levels of the good stuff—important essential mineral nutrients such as magnesium, zinc, chromium, selenium, lithium, and cobalt, which are necessary for optimum brain function.

Toxic elements may be two hundred to three hundred times more highly concentrated in hair than in blood or urine. Therefore, hair is the tissue of choice for detection of recent exposure to toxic elements such as arsenic, aluminum, cadmium, lead, antimony, and mercury.

Iron, however, is a special case. Iron is an essential element (needed to make hemoglobin) and becomes toxic only at high levels. Hair analysis is not the best way to find toxic iron levels; a serum ferritin level is required.

The Centers for Disease Control and Prevention has acknowledged the value of hair mercury levels as a maternal and infant marker for exposure to neurotoxic methylmercury from fish. The US Environmental Protection Agency stated in a report, "If hair and nail samples are collected, cleaned, and analyzed properly with the best analytical methods under controlled conditions by experienced personnel, the data are valid. Human hair and nails have been found to be meaningful and representative tissues for biological monitoring for most of these toxic metals."[2]

MERCURY

Mercury is one of the most potent neurotoxins. Even minute exposures are poisonous. The brain and central nervous system are especially vulnerable to mercury toxicity, and many studies have established a clear causal connection between mercury exposure, brain levels of mercury, and Alzheimer's disease.[3]

Mercury disrupts neurogenesis and neuroplasticity, thus blocking the ability of nervous system tissue to repair damage and to grow. The brains of Alzheimer's patients have been found to contain high mercury levels.[4]

When I see my friend Jack slurping down buttery oysters on the half shell, I want to say, "About those brain cells you are destroying, you might be needing those down the road," but I don't want to ruin his meal. There is no denying, however, that about fifteen minutes post-slurp, when the mercury arrives at his brain cells, neurons will start shriveling and dying. Mercury blocks the assembly of tubulin, a structural protein that acts as a scaffold providing structural integrity for newly forming neurons, causing misshaped tubules that collapse.[5] These are the "neurofibrillary tangles" observed by Alzheimer and seen in 80 percent of Alzheimer's patients' brains on autopsy.

Researchers at the University of Calgary shot a fascinating video of a growing neuron through a microscope.[6] A long thin tube of protoplasm (a neurite process) juts out of the main body of this healthy nerve cell. A new axon is growing and developing. Then one drop of water is dripped onto the slide. That drop contains a small number of mercury ions at about the same concentration as in a small bite of fish. What happens next is astonishing. The entire protoplasmic arm stops growing and then, within seconds, rapidly shrivels up, as if the life is being sucked out of it. A single mercury atom in that drop is enough to sabotage the enzyme that assembles the microtubules that serve as the scaffold for new axonal growth, so the entire structure collapses in minutes. The "rubble," the clumps of unused, damaged tau protein left behind, are the same as those first observed by Alois Alzheimer one hundred years ago.

Mercury impairs brain functions such as reaction time, judgment, and language. Exquisitely minuscule levels of mercury can cause psychological, neurological, and immunological problems, memory loss, vision loss, sensory impairment, lack of coordination, and trouble with blood pressure regulation. They can also cause extreme fatigue and neuromuscular dysfunction. At high exposures, mercury can affect your ability to walk, speak, think, and see.

A single mercury atom can cause neurological damage, triggering the formation of a single neurofibrillary tangle. I regard mercury's level of toxicity as comparable to that of ionizing radiation. Mercury is the Whack-a-Mole of supertoxins; it keeps popping back up over and over again and is extremely hard to get rid of.

Most doctors and even nutritional medicine experts fail to appreciate how toxic mercury is. They believe that small doses from fish are not a problem. This worries me a lot. People need to know how incredibly toxic mercury is and that no type or amount of seafood has a place in a healthy diet.

Sources of Mercury Exposure

Sources of mercury include the following:

- Fish
- Dental amalgams
- Coal-fired power plants
- Polluted water
- Vaccines
- Pesticides
- Fungicides
- Landfills
- Latex marine paint
- Broken thermometers
- Release of a vast reservoir held in melting polar ice

The nightmarish process begins with the burning of coal to generate electricity, which releases thousands of tons of mercury vapor into the atmosphere. Rainwater deposits the metal onto the soil and it washes into waterways, which dump it into the ocean. Along the way, bacteria convert most of it into methylmercury, a particularly dangerous form, which then finds its way into the fish. Roughly 75 percent of all human exposure to mercury comes from methylmercury in fish.

FISH AND FISH OILS

If it weren't for the mercury that contaminates all of it, fish and seafood would be a near-perfect food. It's high in protein and full of essential nutrients like the omega-3 essential fatty acids DHA and EPA. But mercury is a neurotoxin at any dose, and higher mercury concentrations are found in the brains of fish eaters and Alzheimer's patients.

I see a lot of otherwise intelligent medical scientists dancing around the mercury-in-fish issue. Here's their dilemma: mercury is clearly bad for you and your brain. We all know that. But fish, which *all* contain mercury, are the best source of the DHA and EPA that are very good for your brain and body. So what to do? The only reasonable solution is to get your omega-3s somewhere else. (See chapters 20 and 28.)

Eating smaller fish has been suggested because they are lower on the food chain and have thus accumulated less mercury. Charts have been created that show which fish are safer. Some people say eat only North Sea or wild Alaskan salmon. Hogwash! The earth's oceans are uniformly contaminated with methylmercury, and all fish contain levels that damage the brain. Big fish do bioaccumulate more mercury than little fish, but that's just because they are bigger and older and have been accumulating mercury longer. There is no safe dose of mercury or safe type of fish.

Aren't North Sea or Arctic Ocean fish safe? The Arctic Ocean is becoming a toxic nightmare as global warming melts the ticking time bomb of accumulated mercury hidden beneath the earth's permafrost. Human greenhouse gas emissions are causing climate change, and as the ice melts 15 million gallons of mercury are being released from permafrost and dumped into the Arctic Ocean, from which it quickly spreads to the rest of the planet's oceans. Permafrost regions contain twice as much of the world's mercury as all the soils, atmosphere, and oceans of the rest of the planet combined.[7]

The best option is to avoid all fish and seafood products—whether from ocean, lake, river, or farm—including fish oils.

AMALGAM DENTAL FILLINGS

Dentists are the largest users of mercury. Dental amalgam fillings are 50 percent mercury by weight and are the second major source of human heavy metal toxicity. The mercury in fillings is the pure (non-methylated) metal. If your hair mercury level is elevated, find a biological dentist and have your amalgams removed.[8] Biological dentists have special training in proper removal procedures.

A "Safe" Level?

Mercury exposure is ubiquitous in modern society. We are all exposed, via seafood, amalgam dental fillings, vaccines, water, and the atmosphere.

Is there a safe level of mercury? No. As noted, many authors and so-called experts will try to convince you otherwise, but toxicologists have established that, as with lead, ionizing radiation, PCBs, and DDT, there is *no safe level* of mercury. Every atom of mercury that comes into contact with your nerve cells damages them. Extremely small amounts of mercury—trace levels—can cause the cellular damage found in Alzheimer's disease.

Chronic low-level mercury exposure (e.g., a serving of fish a week, of even the small species such as sardines, or a single dental filling) can slowly damage neuronal structures without causing overt symptoms. The FDA and EPA use the appearance of symptoms as a marker for damage, but this is bogus, because (as any molecular biologist or toxicologist can tell you) by the time symptoms appear, a huge amount of irreversible cellular damage has already been done.

CADMIUM

Cadmium is a toxic mineral that causes damage at very low levels of exposure. Exposure to cadmium is a known risk factor for Alzheimer's disease.[9]

Cadmium exerts adverse effects on all body systems. The brain and central nervous system are especially sensitive. The mechanisms underlying cadmium neurotoxicity are not completely understood. Cadmium causes oxidative stress and inflammation. Exposure to cadmium damages the brain, damages the brain's systems for healing and regeneration, and enhances neurofibrillary tangle production, deeply implicating it as an Alzheimer's disease causative factor.[10]

Cadmium also weakens the body's immune system, causes prostatic enlargement and lung cancer, and is linked to a broad assortment of reproductive problems, including an increased incidence of premature birth, low birth weight, stillbirth, deformity and mutation, and spontaneous abortion.

Sources of Cadmium Exposure

Cadmium is widely distributed at low levels in the environment. Problems arise when plants such as the cocoa plant take it up from the soil and concentrate it. Chocolate consumption poses the largest problem, but cadmium is also present in water supplies, plant material, fish, and air (as smoke). Cadmium's low rate of excretion from the human body is responsible for the fact that its biological half-life exceeds twenty years. Once it gets into your body, it is extremely difficult to get back out.

CADMIUM IN CHOCOLATE

Despite chocolate's remarkable array of polyphenol-driven dementia-reversing properties, virtually all chocolate products—even the highest quality, priciest ones—contain toxic levels of cadmium. The consumer group As You Sow has confronted the chocolate industry about this problem, accusing it of exposing customers to toxic food and breaking the law by omitting label disclosures for dangerous cadmium and lead levels. Limit your exposure and choose wisely. An extensive list of chocolates that have been tested for lead and cadmium content is available at the As You Sow website.[11]

See chapter 26 for more on this subject and an extensive discussion of chocolate's amazing brain benefits as well as its "dark" side (pun intended).

OTHER SOURCES

Besides chocolate, cadmium exposure may also come from tobacco products, nickel-cadmium batteries, soil near highways, water from galvanized pipes, sewage sludge, refined flour or rice, metal rustproofing material, some carpet backing, high-phosphate fertilizers, West Coast oysters, mining and smelting activities, pigments and paints, electroplating, electroplated parts, plastics and synthetic rubber, photographic and engraving processes, old drums from some copy machines, photoconductors and photovoltaic cells, and some alloys used in soldering and brazing.

LEAD

After the water crisis in Flint, Michigan, we all know how bad lead can be. But did you know that lead is not just a problem in Flint? Lead is everywhere. Lead used to be commonly found in paint, gasoline, and factory emissions. It also was used to make water pipes and the solders that held them together. Once we discovered how poisonous lead is, laws were put in place to limit its use, but unfortunately, our environment still contains a whole lot of lead, hiding under old paint jobs and along roadways where it was deposited for decades.

Lead has no necessary role in the body, and there is no safe dose. If you are unwittingly being exposed, this terrible poison can slowly and silently change your life.

Lead is a well-known neurotoxic pollutant. At very low levels, lead mimics and disrupts essential brain molecules, causing irreversible brain damage. It shrinks the brain and erodes IQ while undermining learning, cognition, and recall. Victims of lead poisoning are less able to define words, identify objects, and remember. Lead poisoning is also linked to aggressive behavior, criminal activity, and neurological disease.

Chemically, lead looks a lot like the essential element calcium, so lead uses this "phony ID card" to sneak into the body. Once inside, lead releases a barrage of cellular carnage that could be likened to a cluster of cyclones. It disrupts the movement and storage of calcium inside cells and hijacks calcium's roles in the brain, triggering apoptosis (neuronal death) and excitotoxicity (excessive stimulation by neurotransmitters), disrupting neurotransmitter storage and release and destroying cellular mitochondrial energy factories. Neurogenesis and neuroplasticity are not possible in the presence of lead.[12]

Lead in the brain changes the way genes are turned on or off. For example, it increases the expression of genes programmed to make amyloid beta plaque and tau protein neurofibrillary tangles, hallmarks of Alzheimer's.[13]

Neurotransmitters need calcium to function properly; when lead replaces some of their calcium, neurons release fewer neurotransmitters, sending a weaker signal to the following neuron. Lead can also bollix thinking up by triggering spontaneous unpredictable neurotransmitter release, so neurons receive inappropriate signals.

BDNF, the key to neuroregeneration and neuroplasticity, is produced in the neuron's nucleus and then transported as cargo in a railroad-car-like vesicle along a track called a microtubule toward sites of release in the axon and dendritic spines. Lead exposure, even in small amounts, impedes or even derails the BDNF train.

Lead also damages the hippocampus, blocking BDNF production and neurogenesis.[14] BDNF is critical to the creation of new synapses in the hippocampus, the brain's center for memory and learning. Lead scrambles BDNF signaling in the hippocampus, causing a breakdown of ability to think and remember.[15]

Using magnetic resonance imaging, researchers examined how lead exposure altered total brain size, as well as the size of specific brain regions. They found that higher lead exposure was associated with a smaller prefrontal cortex in young adults.[16] Since the prefrontal cortex is responsible for attention, complex decision-making, and regulation of social behavior, differences in its size and function could explain the cognitive and behavior problems seen with lead exposure.[17]

Sources of Lead Exposure

Lead exposures are often from dust in houses with lead paint, from water contaminated with lead (by passing through old pipes, which is what happened in Flint), and from toys, jewelry, tableware, and ceramics. Common sources include the following:

- Lead-based paint (chips, sanding dust)
- Drinking water
- Batteries
- Lead-glazed pottery and cookware
- Industrial pollution
- Welding and soldering fumes
- Plastic miniblinds
- Some fertilizers
- Candy and spices from Mexico
- Ayurvedic herbs

If your home was built before 1978, it almost certainly contains old lead paint. If you are going to have lead paint removed or do renovations to an older house that may have lead paint under layers of other paint or wallpaper, make sure that the work is done by people who are certified in lead removal.

Your tap water could contain lead. Lead leaches into water from old pipes in your house or leading to your house. If you think your house or city lines might be old and contain lead, have your water tested. National Testing Laboratories (https://watercheck.com) is one option.

For much more information about lead—who is at risk, where it is found, its health effects, how to detect sources and reduce your exposure, and information about reproductive risks—visit the EPA website (https://www.epa.gov/lead/learn-about-lead).

For a referral to a specialist in removing lead from the body, contact the American College for the Advancement of Medicine (https://www.acam.org, 1-800-532-3688).

IRON

Iron is essential for life. It is found at the center of the hemoglobin molecule in the red blood cells that carry oxygen to your cells.

However, too little or too much iron causes problems. If your iron is low, you might experience iron-deficiency anemia with weakness, fatigue, and decreased immunity. The body doesn't have enough red blood cells, and this can be serious if left untreated.

At the other end of the spectrum, too much iron presents an altogether different set of risks. Iron can accumulate in body tissues as a consequence of excess consumption of iron or because the body has a hard time excreting it. Aging is also sometimes accompanied by accumulation of iron.

Excessive iron is consistently seen in the brains of people with Alzheimer's, Parkinson's, and other neurodegenerative diseases. Iron's effect on cognition starts early, however; older adults who have higher brain iron accumulations (but not overt dementia) perform poorly on cognitive tests when compared with people whose brain iron concentrations are normal. Is the declining cognition seen in people with high iron levels caused by the iron, or is it just an incidental finding? A recent groundbreaking UCLA study conclusively showed that excess iron in brain tissue causes neurodegenerative brain disorders such as Alzheimer's.[18]

George Bartzokis, a researcher and professor of psychiatry at the Semel Institute for Neuroscience and Human Behavior at UCLA, has devoted his career to understanding the role that iron plays in human brain development, function, and aging. He and his colleagues have generated a detailed picture of iron metabolism across the human life span. They used a noninvasive MRI to measure iron levels in living human brains and discovered significantly larger amounts of stored iron in the brains of Alzheimer's patients than in control subjects. These increased iron levels were present from the earliest onset of disease, indicating that they were a potential cause (rather than a consequence) of brain degeneration.[19]

Researchers have shown that iron accumulates selectively in the areas of the brain most vulnerable to AD—specifically in the hippocampal brain regions associated with memory and thought processes. This iron causes amyloid beta and tau protein deposition in these areas. Lowering the iron lowers these deposition levels to normal.[20]

Bartzokis went on to show that people with the highest brain iron accumulations had the earliest age at onset of neurodegenerative disease. The presence of excess iron in affected brain areas was directly involved in triggering neurodegenerative disease. Bartzokis's research demonstrated for the first time that limiting one's lifetime exposure to iron lowers the risk of neurodegenerative brain disease.[21]

Sources of Iron Exposure

Sources of excess iron include drinking water high in iron, eating too many iron-rich foods, or cooking in iron pots or pans. (Cooking acidic foods such as tomatoes in iron pots or skillets will increase iron levels because the acid dissolves iron from the pan; the iron is then absorbed into the food.)

One of the most common causes of excess iron is the regular consumption of alcohol, which increases the absorption of iron. A regular diet of steak plus wine, for example, can cause problems.

Genetic predisposition can also cause a tendency for excess iron absorption or impaired excretion.

Regardless of the source, too much iron in the body is toxic. A high iron level leads to the production of free radicals—highly reactive oxygen species that damage cell membranes, DNA, mitochondria, and multiple tissues and organs. Free radical excess causes serious health problems. Iron overload is a causal contributor to a broad spectrum of degenerative diseases, significantly raising the risk of liver fibrosis, cardiovascular disease, cancer, and Alzheimer's.

Even though it is easy to test for iron overload, most doctors do not inform their patients of the dangers of high iron levels, nor do they test for iron status.

Testing

To detect excess iron, blood testing is best. Serum ferritin levels should be between 20 and 80 ng/mL. The optimum range is 40–60 ng/mL. Below 20 indicates iron deficiency. Above 80 indicates a surplus.

You can also spot high iron content via a hair mineral analysis by Doctor's Data (www.doctorsdata.com), a reputable laboratory that has specialized in lead and heavy metal testing for several decades (less than $150 for a complete toxic and essential hair elements test). If your hair iron level is high, you still need a serum ferritin level as a baseline for treatment.

What to Do If You Have High Levels

If you need to lower your iron levels, here are several options:

- Donate a unit of blood. If a blood donor center is unable to accept your blood for donation for some reason, you can obtain a prescription for a therapeutic phlebotomy (same as blood donation but the blood is not used for transfusion). Check your ferritin level in a few months to make sure it has been reduced into the normal range, repeat the ferritin test once a year, and repeat blood donation if indicated.
- Get rid of your iron skillet.
- Do not take multivitamins that contain iron (the best ones leave it out).
- Use a water softener if you live in an area where the water contains a lot of iron.
- Supplement with nutrients that are potent antioxidants or those that bind (chelate) the iron: curcumin, quercetin, green tea, N-acetyl cysteine, milk thistle (silymarin), alpha-lipoic acid, cranberry, and pomegranate. You may need to consult a specialist for help with this.

ALUMINUM

Aluminum, an element abundant in the earth, occurs naturally in food and water and is widely used in cans, cookware, medications, and cosmetics. This well-documented neurotoxin damages living systems by sabotaging key metabolic pathways. It causes oxidative stress and damages our mitochondrial energy factories.

Aluminum has been found in the neurofibrillary tangles and senile plaques of AD patients.

Many studies have shown a statistical association between elevated exposure to aluminum and Alzheimer's disease. When the metal shows up in drinking water supplies, for example, AD occurrence goes up. Other researchers have loaded up experimental animals with the metal and have seen brain disease that looks a lot like AD. Researchers are still working on this problem, and they will solve it. In the meantime, it's best to steer clear.[22]

Sources of Aluminum Exposure

Municipal drinking water supplies and antiperspirants are the two most common sources of aluminum exposure. Regardless of whether the metal enters the body through these paths or through antacid medications, vaccine adjuvants, aluminum pots and pans (many nonstick cookwares are aluminum), processed foods, aluminum welding or machining, environmental pollution, or any other route, it passes right through your blood-brain barrier and attacks your brain.

CHAPTER 19

Bioidentical Estradiol Prevents Neurodegeneration in Women

Estradiol, a form of estrogen and the major female sex hormone, has been much studied in recent years. Researchers have made tremendous progress toward understanding the molecular and cellular mechanisms by which estradiol affects the brain. The controversy is over, and the results are in.

Strong scientific evidence supports the fact that transdermal bioidentical estradiol enhances cognition and protects against Alzheimer's disease. And giving horse hormones (Premarin) to perimenopausal women (instead of bioidentical hormones) has been found to be ill-advised.[1]

Real estradiol does not increase breast cancer risk. Real estrogen is clearly beneficial to the body and brain. So why are doctors and patients so afraid to use it? Because a failed 2002 research study, the Women's Health Initiative (WHI), based its fear-mongering conclusions on the effect of foreign, toxic horse hormones.[2] The researchers made a series of glaring errors that could have been spotted by an observant high school chemistry student. The most egregious of these may have been to focus their research on women taking horse hormones rather than bioidentical human hormones. The researchers misled readers by using the word estrogen to describe the horse hormones used in the study. This caused confusion because people were led to incorrectly assume the word referred to real, bioidentical estradiol (the main hormone made by human females).

In the eighteen years since the WHI debacle, we have learned a great deal about the molecular mechanisms by which estradiol exerts its neuroprotective and neurotrophic effects. The focus has fortunately shifted from "Does estradiol affect cognition and memory?" to "How does estradiol enhance cognition and protect neurons from neurodegenerative disease?"

THE FAILED STUDY THAT FOMENTED
WIDESPREAD FEAR OF HORMONES

Many women (and many doctors) have irrational fears about hormone replacement therapy (HRT). The most prominent reason for these fears, by far, is the 2002 Women's Health Initiative study, a fiasco in which researchers misinterpreted their own data and incorrectly assumed estrogen was causing heart disease in the study population. Fearing (incorrectly) that continuing the study would cause deaths, they then compounded their errors by abruptly discontinuing it, in effect announcing to the world (again, incorrectly) that: "hormones are dangerous."[3]

Then they reexamined their original data and realized they had gotten it all wrong. Two years later a revised study admitted the errors, stating that the risk of heart disease was not higher, breast cancer risk decreased in women using the hormones, and women who took "estrogen" (it was actually the horse hormone Premarin) within ten years of menopause had a reduced risk of death compared to those who did not. But by then it was too late. The misinformation and damage had been done. Millions of worried women around the globe had flushed their Premarin down the toilet, fearing that hormones were dangerous.

Irresponsible research caused widespread damage that adversely affected women for decades. Out of unfounded fear, and for no better reason than misguided scientists making bad assumptions and mislabeling the hormones used in their study, millions of women unnecessarily suffered hot flashes, night sweats, depression, and other menopausal symptoms.

WOMEN ARE NOT HORSES

In addition to misinterpreting their own data, these researchers made another grievous error: they failed to take into consideration the actual chemical structure of the hormones they were investigating! They lumped together the thirty different estrogenic compounds in Premarin and called them "estrogen." Only a small fraction of Premarin is estradiol, the main human estrogen molecule. The rest were other hormones found in the urine of pregnant horses.

In the world of hormones, very small changes in molecular structure can translate into huge changes in function. For example, the addition or removal of a single atom of oxygen or hydrogen can turn estradiol into a radically different hormone. Hormone receptors are so structurally finely tuned that they won't work properly if they are presented with the wrong hormone.

So what did these researchers do? They gave the wrong hormone. They ignored (and many researchers continue to ignore) the fact that horse estrogen and other horse hormones are chemically very different from what the human body makes and uses. They failed to see the obvious: the jumble of foreign hormones decanted from *pregnant mares'* ur*ine* (thus Pre-mar-in) is guaranteed to confuse the finely tuned human estrogen receptor system.

Natural human bioidentical estrogen (estradiol) never harmed anyone (or even any lab rat)—but instead, the researchers chose to study the effects of the very toxic set of horse molecules called Premarin.

And they doubled down on this error by also studying another very toxic, nonhuman bio*in*compatible molecule, medroxyprogesterone acetate (Provera) in their research. They called it "progesterone," but (as with their "estrogen") Provera is chemically and functionally very different from real human bioidentical progesterone.

Neither real estradiol nor real progesterone causes cancer or heart disease. If you look only at Premarin and Provera studies, though, you see a little cancer risk and significant cognitive decline. However, when you look only at the natural alternatives, real estrogen and real progesterone, not only do you see no cancer risk, you see these hormones teaming up to enhance and protect the brain!

BIOIDENTICAL ESTROGEN PREVENTS AD

Bioidentical estradiol, the most important molecule for making a woman a woman, serves to maintain and protect brain structures in ways that improve cognitive function and decrease dementia risk.

Brain tissue has a high concentration of estrogen receptors. Prior to menopause, the natural estradiol supplied by a woman's body supports brain health through her life, but cognitive function begins to decline when the menopausal estradiol shortfall kicks in. Natalie Rasgon, MD, PhD, director of the Stanford Center for Neuroscience in Women's Health, wanted to know why some women taking replacement hormones experienced cognitive decline and others didn't. Her Stanford team looked at two specific variables: the type of hormone used and when treatment was begun. Her team found that if natural hormone replacement is begun during or shortly after menopause (not more than five years after), the estradiol will continue its job, protecting women from dementia.[4] However, to be effective, the hormone had to be bioidentical. (In other words, Premarin didn't work.) Rasgon states it plainly. "Hormone therapy's neurological effect on women at risk for dementia depends critically on when they begin therapy and on whether they use estradiol or Premarin."[5]

HOW ESTROGEN ENHANCES BRAIN HEALTH

Now let's take a look at several of the ways in which estrogen (natural bioidentical estradiol) enhances brain health.

Estradiol Supports Attention, Learning, Memory, and Mood

Estradiol exerts a powerful influence on the brain's hippocampal memory centers.[6]

Your hippocampus is densely populated with estrogen receptors. When these receptors are stimulated by estradiol, neurons grow there.

A greater density of hippocampal neurons means there will be more dendritic spines (the protrusions from dendrites that connect with nearby axons to relay electrical impulses from one nerve cell to the next), and these generate the increased synaptoplasticity so intimately linked to improved memory. Estradiol thus improves memory and protects against memory loss.[7]

Estradiol has also been shown to increase BDNF in the brain's memory areas (prefrontal cortex and hippocampus). In a 2012 study Victoria Luine and Maya Frankfurt showed that estradiol enhances memory function by increasing BDNF (the brain hormone that triggers growth of new nerve cells) and dendritic spines in the hippocampus.[8] (For more about BDNF, see chapter 8.)

Estradiol Facilitates Major Neurotransmitter Systems in the Brain

The brain's major neurotransmitters—acetylcholine, serotonin, dopamine, and norepinephrine—are all involved in attention, learning, and memory, as well as in the declining cognitive functions of AD. Estradiol enhances the activity of these neurotransmitters. The sharp fall in estrogen at menopause contributes to a decline in the neurotransmitter system, which results in the cognitive decline that predisposes one to AD.[9]

Estradiol Protects the Brain from Inflammation–Induced Injury

The protection from brain damage provided by estradiol has been shown to apply to injury from a broad range of sources including toxins, trauma, infection, stroke, and free radical damage. The underlying molecular mechanisms for this protection are not yet understood and are currently the subject of intense scientific scrutiny.[10]

Estradiol Protects against Amyloid Beta

A deficiency of estrogen accelerates the formation of amyloid beta plaque in the brain. Estradiol enhances the breakdown of amyloid beta and increases its clearance from brain tissues and the cerebrospinal fluid that bathes the brain. Estradiol has also been shown to reduce the inflammatory response to amyloid beta and thus to protect against amyloid beta mediated toxicity.[11]

Estradiol Benefits Blood Vessels and Improves Cerebral Blood Flow

Any woman who has taken estrogen for menopausal hot flashes, mood swings, and depression has firsthand evidence of estradiol's ability to protect the vascular system and boost blood flow to the brain.

Estrogen receptors are found in both the smooth muscle and the inner endothelial lining of the brain's blood vessels. Estradiol improves the effectiveness of these receptors and this, in turn, improves control of brain blood flow.

Estrogen provides protection from coronary artery disease (heart attacks) by incorporating itself into LDL particles (so-called bad cholesterol), where it slows the rate of oxidation. Estrogen also decreases damage from strokes. If a stroke does occur, damage is less likely, and estradiol increases the repair rate.[12]

DELIVERY SYSTEMS MATTER, AND TRANSDERMAL ESTRADIOL IS BEST

Numerous research studies tell us that, for a variety of reasons, transdermal bioidentical estradiol (cream or patch) supports cognitive enhancement, whereas oral estradiol (pills) does not.[13]

When a hormone is consumed orally, it must be absorbed through the intestinal wall and processed by the liver before it is sent out to its target tissues (in this case, the brain). During this "liver first pass," the liver alters and dilutes the hormone and sometimes generates toxic and inflammatory metabolites that are released back into the general circulation. When a hormone is administered directly through the skin—as in transdermal creams, patches, or sublingual drops—it avoids liver first pass, traveling directly through the bloodstream to the brain (and other tissues), so it is not removed or altered by the liver before it reaches its target.

DECIDING WHETHER TO TAKE NATURAL HORMONE REPLACEMENT THERAPY

A shortfall of estrogen can cause pathological brain changes that lead to Alzheimer's disease. This can begin decades before clinical symptoms become evident. Strong research evidence tells us that women can significantly improve their chances of avoiding cognitive decline by taking supplemental estradiol and progesterone and that starting early, at the earliest sign of menopausal decline in estradiol production, offers the highest probability of success. Beginning estradiol during the menopausal transition will delay—and may prevent—the onset of Alzheimer's disease.[14]

A woman entering menopause therefore has a complex decision to make regarding natural hormone replacement therapy (NHRT). Many factors must be considered.

Most women don't need extra estrogen while they are still ovulating. As menopause approaches, however, levels of estradiol decrease precipitously to approximately one-tenth that of menstruating women. Ovarian estrogen production begins to decline one to two years before menopause (during perimenopause) and reaches a stable low level about two years after the final menstrual period. As described above, the brain is rich in estrogen receptors. The steep drop in estrogen levels during the menopausal transition is closely linked to cognitive decline and subsequent dementia.

Timing is important. Several studies have shown that HRT-induced Alzheimer's protection in postmenopausal women is far more likely to be successful if estrogen is started within five years after menopause. When NHRT is initiated this way, the results are often dramatic.

Consider, for example, the Cache County Study on Memory in Aging, a longitudinal, population-based study of Alzheimer's disease and other dementias from 1995 to 2013, following more than five thousand elderly residents of Cache County, Utah, for more than twelve years. Women who initiated hormone replacement therapy within at least five years of menopause had a 30 percent reduced risk of developing Alzheimer's disease.[15]

Though early estrogen replacement provides the greatest neurocognitive benefits, estrogen has also been shown to be effective in women who have already begun to display cognitive decline. Again, this effectiveness appears to depend on the choice of estrogen (bioidentical) and the route of administration (transdermal cream or patch).

Every woman is unique. There is no one-size-fits-all formula for determining whether estradiol replacement is the optimum choice. However, the preponderance of evidence tells us that most women can safely benefit from natural estrogen therapy and that women who start early and use transdermal bioidentical estradiol can expect improved cognition and a greatly reduced risk of Alzheimer's disease.

Women entering menopause should not make this complex and crucial decision alone. Professional guidance from a well-informed healthcare provider is essential. Even with such guidance, the answers are not always clear-cut. My suggestion to women is that they work with an integrative or functional medicine doctor or alternative endocrinologist trained in bioidentical hormone replacement therapy who is familiar with NHRT and its role in neurodegenerative disease.

Family history, personal medical history, risk factors, symptoms, and concerns must be taken into consideration. The doctor will need to complete a physical exam and laboratory analysis to make optimal recommendations. The risks of osteoporosis, cardiovascular disease, cancers (breast, uterine, and ovarian), and dementia must all be carefully weighed.

PART 3

Your Anti-Alzheimer's Diet

Your dietary choices have everything to do with your dementia risk. Suboptimal nutrition causes Alzheimer's disease; optimum nutrition enhances repair, neurogenesis, and neuroplasticity and reverses the disease. Part 3 is a comprehensive guide to the anti-Alzheimer's diet—eating practices and food choices that have been shown in research studies to prevent and reverse the disease.

You'll discover why a very low-carb diet is so important and how autophagy (collapsing the time frame in which you consume food) activates longevity genes. We'll examine why a ketogenic (high-good-fat) diet enhances neurogenesis and protects nerve cells and is a major key to brain longevity. You'll learn which foods help repair a damaged hippocampus and enhance cognition—and which foods encourage brain disease and must be avoided. Part 3 closes with four chapters that focus on the most amazing and powerful anti-Alzheimer's foods of all: coconut oil, polyphenols, blueberries, and cocoa.

CHAPTER 20

Eating to Reverse Cognitive Decline

A wealth of research studies tells us that the foods you eat—and those you avoid—exert powerful control over your cognitive health.[1] Suboptimal nutrition causes Alzheimer's disease.[2] Conversely, preventing AD requires optimum nutrition. Optimum nutrition is necessary for neuroplasticity, neurogenesis, and repair.

Every bite counts. Every food choice you make directly affects your brain's chemical structure and function. When you choose not to eat a brain-enhancing food, you are losing an opportunity to nudge your brain health and level of cognition in a positive direction.

The damage done by eating the wrong foods begins decades before signs and symptoms of cognitive decline appear, so it's important to develop the habit of making healthy food decisions now, while you're still in prevention mode. These are not casual recommendations; each is based on published, peer-reviewed research.

Following are the principal features of an Alzheimer's-prevention diet:

- *Autophagy*—This process involves intermittent fasting and morning fasting.
- *Very low-carbohydrate and grain-free diet*—5–10 percent of calories should come from carbohydrates.
- *High-fat ketogenic diet*—About 60–75 percent of calories should come from good fats. The *type* of fat is extremely important.
  - *Omega-3 oils*—The best source of omega-3s by far is flaxseed oil. Other sources include olive oil, avocado oil, and walnut oil, as well as all beans and nuts.

- *Medium chain triglycerides*—Coconut oil is the best source of MCTs and the best oil for cooking.
- *No omega-6 oils*—Omega-6 oils promote neurodegenerative disease. Avoid safflower, sunflower, soy, canola, cottonseed, and corn oils; hydrogenated oils; and margarine and butter substitutes. The high levels of omega-6 fatty acids in these oils fan the fires of inflammation.
- *Low-protein diet*—15–30 percent of calories should come from protein. This includes small to moderate amounts of clean, simple, high-protein foods such as lean meat and eggs.
- *Fresh, whole, pure, simple foods*—To the extent possible, consume only foods that are unprocessed, additive-free, preservative-free, pesticide-free, hormone-free, non-GMO, heavy-metal free, BPA-free, and organic.
- *Polyphenol-rich foods*—Vegetables and fruits should make up the largest component of your diet because these offer the highest concentrations of antidementia compounds. (See the lists in chapter 24.) Fruits—especially berries—are loaded with polyphenols, so emphasize blueberries, blackberries, strawberries, raspberries, plums, pomegranates, red grapes, and cherries.

Now let's discuss the details.

AUTOPHAGY

Autophagy is the waste removal and recycling system in our cells. It's the mechanism by which cells remove unnecessary, redundant, and/or dysfunctional components. The process of autophagy is turned on by shrinking the daily time span in which you consume foods. This has powerful effects on the body and brain because it gives them the extra time needed to clean up and heal. When autophagy is switched on, your cells dramatically shift into "cellular housekeeping."

Autophagy is neither a trendy diet craze nor a vague philosophical concept; it has been extensively researched by cell and molecular biologists, and thousands of research articles can be found in the cell biology literature. Good science has clearly shown that an autophagic lifestyle promotes optimum health and longevity and shuts down neurodegenerative brain disease.

Autophagy facilitates healing and repair everywhere in the body, but especially in neurons. Autophagy enables the removal of debris that would otherwise accumulate and damage sensitive neuronal systems, causing neurodegenerative disease.

Dr. Ralph Nixon of the New York University School of Medicine examined how the failure of autophagy in neurons can cause Alzheimer's disease and how inducing autophagy may reverse the disease by clearing undesirable molecules from diseased neurons. In a 2013 article entitled "The Role of Autophagy in Neurodegenerative Disease," published in the journal *Nature Medicine*, Nixon states, "The autophagy pathway has been a completely overlooked aspect of Alzheimer's." He explains why it is important to enhance autophagy to protect the brain from toxic damage and to provide extra cleanup and repair time so diseased brain tissue can heal.[3]

Autophagy is switched on by shrinking the time frame in which you consume food to less than ten to twelve hours a day. Fasting a few hours a day, every day allows your cells to shift into cleanup and organize mode. You can easily accomplish this by finishing your last meal by nine or ten o'clock in the evening and then postponing breakfast for a couple hours in the morning.

Chapter 22 delves deeply into how autophagy works.

A VERY LOW-CARBOHYDRATE AND GRAIN-FREE DIET

Put carb avoidance at the top of your anti-AD diet list.

High-carb foods damage insulin receptors and cause inflammation in your brain cells, diverting them from healthy functioning onto a dead-end road leading to dementia. Carbs gum up your metabolism, feed pathogenic microbes in the gut, jump-start autoimmune diseases, shred the sensitive inner endothelial lining of your blood vessels, and cause toxic and allergic reactions in your brain.

Conversely, a very low-carb, grain-free diet is linked to a dramatically lower risk of dementia. Mayo Clinic researchers have shown that individuals on a high-carbohydrate diet had a remarkable 89 percent increased risk for developing dementia. In the same study, those whose diets contained the most fat had a reduction in risk for developing dementia of over 40 percent.[4]

To preserve brain health, you will need to avoid all grains and cereals, including wheat, oats, barley, rye, rice, and corn—and the breads, cereals, crackers, pastas, cakes, cookies, flours, and other goods made from them. Avoid pizza, refined potato products, snack foods, sugary drinks, candies, jams, preserves, and sweetened foods. All alcoholic beverages are pure carbohydrate; in fact, beer (since it is derived from grains) has been referred to as liquid bread.

Dr. David Perlmutter, author of the two breakthrough *New York Times* bestsellers *Grain Brain: The Surprising Truth about Wheat, Carbs, and Sugar* and *Brain Maker: The Power of Gut Microbes to Heal and Protect Your Brain for Life*, puts it this way: "It may seem draconian, but the best recommendation I can make is to completely avoid grains."[5]

A food does not have to taste sweet to add to your sugar load. All grains—even those wonderful-tasting organic grains, whole-grain pastas and cereals, and beer and wine—are the sources of glucose overloading that fuels high-carb brain damage.

Modest amounts of colorful (high polyphenol) carrots, beets, and squash are okay, but don't overdo starchy vegetables. These, too, are converted to glucose in the bloodstream. Eliminate corn, rice, and potatoes altogether, as they will quickly undermine your otherwise conscientious low-carb dieting efforts.

Eliminate white sugar and refined flour and sweeteners. Use dates, coconut sugar, honey, stevia, or molasses in limited quantities. (How carbs and sugars damage the brain is discussed in greater detail in chapter 11.)

A HIGH-FAT KETOGENIC DIET

Ketogenic diets are high in fat, adequate in protein, and extremely low in carbohydrates. (The exact amount of fat and protein is a function of individual body responses and activity levels.) It's best, if you're on a ketogenic diet, to consume no more than 5 percent of calories from carbohydrates.

The idea behind a ketogenic diet is to protect your brain from damage by removing carbs. The other main reason for a ketogenic diet is that fats and oils—if chosen correctly—not only protect the brain but also reverse brain damage.[6]

How does it work? Removing carbohydrates forces your metabolism to use fat as its main source of energy. Burning fat generates ketone bodies (thus, ketogenic). These build up in your bloodstream, causing a state of ketosis.

Ketosis is a very desirable state. It protects neurons from injury. Ketones increase the production of neurotrophic factors such as BDNF that enhance neurogenesis and protect nerve cells. Ketones reduce brain inflammation and improve neuronal mitochondrial energy production.

The fat your body uses as fuel can be derived either from dietary fat (fat you have just eaten) or from body fat stores. All dietary fats need to be drawn from the pool of high-quality fats described in this book. Replacing carb calories with damaging pro-inflammatory fats would move you in the direction of brain damage.

Ketogenic dieting is so important that I have devoted a full chapter to it (chapter 21). That's where I'll delve into details on which fats are best and which to avoid.

A LOW-PROTEIN DIET

A low-protein diet consists of 15–30 percent of daily calories from clean, simple, high-protein foods such as meat and eggs. Eating meat is fine. Fatty meats, however, are chock-full of pro-inflammatory omega-6 fatty acids that you don't want or need, so stick to the leanest cuts and keep the quantities modest: 100–200 grams (4–8 ounces) daily.

Think of chicken, pork, or beef as a complementary side dish rather than the main course. Humanely raised, pastured chicken and grass-fed beef are preferable.

Eggs are a wonderful food, packed with goodies that nourish the brain: B-complex vitamins, choline, and healthy fats. Eggs from pastured chickens or ducks are best. The average chicken egg contains about 6 grams of protein, so you could have quite a few without pushing the limits for protein. For those worried about too much cholesterol from eggs, the science is clear that up to three whole eggs per day are perfectly safe for healthy people. Eggs consistently raise HDL cholesterol.

THE MOST POWERFUL ANTIDEMENTIA SUPERFOODS

Here's a list of the best of the very best—foods that protect the brain from dementia and reverse the neurodegenerative disease process if it has begun.

- *Polyphenol-rich foods*—These include blueberries, blackberries, raspberries, strawberries, cherries, green tea, black tea, coffee, citrus, onion, garlic, beans, nuts, spinach, tomatoes, eggplant, olives, apples, grapes, pomegranates, nectarines, peaches, cranberries, plums and prunes, walnuts, sunflower seeds, and curcumin (turmeric, curry). Polyphenols stimulate the secretion of BDNF, the hormone that stimulates the growth of new neurons from stem cells in the hippocampus and elsewhere, protects the brain from damage, and reverses the changes that lead to Alzheimer's. (See extensive lists of polyphenol-rich foods in chapter 24.)
- *Chicken or duck eggs*—Eggs are packed with high-quality protein and B-complex vitamins. They are also high in the omega-3 essential fatty acid ALA.
- *Vegetables*—Vegetables contain a brain-enhancing bonanza of B-complex vitamins, minerals, enzymes, and antioxidants.
- *Curcumin*—Think curry and other Eastern dishes. Derived from the herb turmeric, curcumin exerts a broad spectrum of antidementia effects. It is a cleanser and anti-inflammatory, and it

dissolves amyloid beta plaque in the brain. The kind of curcumin you take matters. Unprocessed curcumin powder sprinkled on food is ineffective because it will not be absorbed by the body. Curcumin must be prepared by cooking it at high heat in oil. Specially processed products (Meriva and Longvida) have been developed to enhance curcumin's bioavailability. For lots more about this wonderful and amazing compound, see chapter 29. Take 2,000 mg a day (or more) in capsule form.

- *Flaxseed oil*—The best source of brain-nourishing essential omega-3 EFAs is flaxseed oil (FSO). You can't cook with it (the unsaturated fatty acid molecules are damaged at heats above boiling), but you can stir 1–2 tablespoons into any hot or cold dish. Add 1–2 tablespoons daily directly to salads, or make salad dressing with FSO and vinegar.

- *Coconut oil*—Coconut oil contains medium chain triglycerides, important fats that enhance ketogenesis and stimulate the secretion of BDNF. Use coconut oil as your main oil for cooking. Two tablespoons a day is a reasonable dose. (See chapter 23.)

- *Avocado and avocado oil*—These are high in omega-3 oils.

- *Walnuts and walnut oil*—These are rich in omega-3 oils.

- *Coffee* (decaf or regular)—Our favorite drink gets a big reprieve. Not only does coffee give us pizzazz and delay the onset of Alzheimer's,[7] but it contains another active antidementia ingredient: epigallocatechin gallate (EGCG), which may be a lot easier to pronounce after you've drunk some of it.

- *Green and black tea*—Green tea also contains EGCG and other polyphenol compounds that offer powerful proven protection for neurons and are strongly associated with reversal of neurodegenerative diseases.[8] Green tea catechins can be obtained from hot or iced tea, as an extract, or in capsules. (See chapter 30.)

- *Chocolate and cocoa*—Though they contain ingredients that have been shown to protect against—and even reverse—Alzheimer's disease, almost all chocolate and cocoa products also contain brain-addling levels of cadmium and lead. So far, no one has figured out a way to get them out. Once the cadmium and lead have been removed, however, chocolate products can be added back to the safe foods list. The heavy-metal-free versions will be incredibly good for the brain because they reverse cognitive decline and dementia. Be sure to check out chapter 26 before indulging.

Now that we've discussed brain-healthy foods, let's take a look at the dark side.

FOODS AND PRODUCTS THAT DAMAGE THE BRAIN, INDUCE MEMORY LOSS, AND INCREASE THE RISK OF ALZHEIMER'S

Memory-hampering foods are staples in the American diet. White breads, pasta, processed cheeses and meats—all are linked to an increased incidence of Alzheimer's disease. The most common are listed here, as are damaging food-related products:

- *Processed cheese*—This is a food product made from cheese, but the manufacturers have added undesirable ingredients such as sodium phosphate, vegetable oils, dairy substitutes, extra salt, food colorings such as yellow 6 and tartrazine (banned in European countries because they promote kidney and adrenal tumors), and sugar. All those additional ingredients are bad for your brain.

- *Processed meats*—These include bacon, smoked turkey from the deli counter, and cold cuts. Health food stores offer products that are free of processing, additives, and nitrates.

- *Other processed foods*—These include instant meals, microwave meals, snack foods, chips, and crackers. Much of the food value has been removed and replaced with unnatural chemicals that are not listed on the label. Packaged and/or processed foods almost always contain brain-damaging additives. Pesticides, fungicides, unnatural flavoring and coloring agents, preservatives, and fillers in processed foods promote neuroinflammation and neurodegeneration.

A major shortcoming of the labeling laws is that they require listing only the principal ingredient in a barrel of source material; they do not require listing all the other ingredients, even though many are toxic. Replace processed and packaged foods with fresh organic unprocessed fruit and vegetables, frozen fruits, nuts, carrots, and other healthy simple snacks. Purchase organically grown foods as much as possible. In terms of snacking, skip the chips and have a handful of almonds and a tangerine or some blueberries.

- *Beer*—Even one beer weakens the junctions between intestinal cells, altering gut wall permeability and allowing undesirable chemicals into the bloodstream, which then trigger autoimmune inflammatory attacks on the brain and other organs. The grains in beer also trigger autoimmune allergic responses. Ethanol, an active neurotoxin and all-purpose cellular toxin, is metabolized as a sugar; in fact, beer derives all of its calories from carbohydrates. All beers contain nitrites, which have been linked to Alzheimer's.

- *All grains and white foods*—These include pasta, cakes, white sugar, white rice, and white flour. Whole-grain breads and other whole-grain products are no less dangerous than white flour because both cause blood sugar spikes and consequent brain inflammation (see chapter 11). All grains damage the intestinal mucosal surface, cause leaky gut and consequent autoimmune disease, and interfere with nutrient absorption.

- *Foods packaged in containers lined with BPA*—Bisphenol A is a nightmarishly neurotoxic hormonally active chemical used in almost all plastic bottles and as a sprayed-on liner in metal cans (beans, tomato sauce) and cardboard cartons that hold packaged and processed foods (almond milk, soy milk, cow milk, half and half, juice—almost anything that comes in a cardboard container). Conscious producers are switching to BPA-free cans and cartons.

- *Foods cooked in aluminum, Teflon and other nonstick-coated, and chemically treated cookware*—Cook with stainless steel, glass, or ceramic pots and pans. Under high heat Teflon breaks down into its component chemical polytetrafluoroethylene (PTFE), which is highly toxic. The PTFE is released into the food and air and can cause polymer fume fever (Teflon flu). Every year, thousands of cases of this disease are treated in the United States. The disease mechanisms include pro-inflammatory cytokine release, neutrophil activation, and oxygen radical formation.[9] A few years ago, after much research, my wife and I settled on the DaTerra Cucina Vesuvio ceramic frying pan. We continue to be pleased with the performance of this fine Italian cookware and feel safe knowing it is free of unwanted toxic chemicals. It's available at the company's website and at Amazon.com.

- *Impure water*—For drinking and bathing, avoid water to which chlorine or fluorine has been added or that which has been drawn from wells in rural agricultural areas (contains glyphosate and other neurotoxic pesticides). Install a point-of-use combined carbon filter and reverse osmosis at your kitchen sink and an in-line filter for your shower.

- *Seafood*—Since all seafood contains mercury, it should be eliminated from your diet, even though it contains brain-enhancing essential fatty acids.

  Mercury, like radiation, is a potent neurotoxin. Mercury is normally safely encapsulated in the earth, but mining and coal burning dump it into the environment, and it finds its way into the ocean. It accumulates in fish and wildlife at concentrations up to a million times higher than the levels found in the environment. As it travels up the food chain—from plankton to fish to marine mammals to humans—mercury becomes more concentrated and more dangerous.

  Because mercury is evenly distributed throughout the world's oceans (as methylmercury), *all* seafood contains brain-addling amounts. There is no "safe" or "acceptable" or "normal" amount. A single atom of mercury will corrupt the synthesis of a single neurofibril, resulting in a neurofibrillary tangle (the hallmark of Alzheimer's disease seen by Alzheimer under his microscope one hundred years ago).

In humans, mercury causes cardiovascular damage, neuro-logical damage, and developmental malformations in fetuses and children. The developing fetal nervous system in a pregnant woman is especially sensitive and vulnerable to mercury damage at exceedingly minuscule doses. To protect their babies, preg-nant women must avoid all seafood. For more about the dangers of mercury, see chapter 18.

You can get mercury-free, cognition-enhancing essential fatty acids from algae-derived DHA, which is grown in a mercury-free environment. (I use Ecological Formulas' Neuromins.) You can also purchase omega-3 fish oils that have undergone molecular distillation, a low-temperature vacuum distillation process that removes heavy metals, PCBs, and pesticides. A good daily dose of DHA would be 300–2,000 mg. (See chapters 18 and 28.)

- *Artificial sweeteners*—Aspartame shortens memory response, impairs memory retention, and damages hypothalamic neurons. It acts as a chemical stressor by elevating plasma cortisol levels and triggering production of free radicals that damage the brain.

Animal studies have linked even low doses of aspartame to dementia and brain tumors. Research scientist H. J. Roberts, in a 1997 letter published in the *Lancet*, warns, "I have documented other severe neuropsychiatric reactions to aspartame products—most notably headache, seizures, confusion and depression, and the probable acceleration of Alzheimer's disease by aspartame products. I believe that our society faces a preventable medical disaster if aspartame products are not promptly removed from public use."[10]

- *Monosodium glutamate*—Monosodium glutamate (MSG) is another neurotoxin used to enhance the flavor of processed foods. Avoid this ingredient by reading food labels and asking at restaurants.
- *Soy, including tofu*—Higher consumption of tofu at midlife has been correlated with low brain mass. Cerebral shrinkage may occur naturally with age, but men who consumed more tofu showed an exaggeration of the usual patterns seen in aging. One well-designed epidemiological study showed that men who ate tofu at least twice weekly had more cognitive impairment compared with those who rarely or never ate the soybean curd, and their cognitive test results were about equivalent to what they would have been if they were five years older than their current age.[11]

Those who wish to maintain healthy brain function should avoid unfermented soy products including tofu, soy milk, soy burgers, soy ice cream, tofu, edamame, and all those vegan products with added soy. All soybeans (even organic, non-GMO ones) naturally contain antinutrients, toxins, and plant hormones. These are removed by fermentation. Fermented products include miso, natto, tempeh, and tamari.

The next chapter delves into the specifics of ketogenic dieting.

CHAPTER 21

The Very Low-Carb Ketogenic Diet

I loved my carbs and had overdosed on them most of my life. As a child and through my early adult life, I consumed large quantities of white flour, sugar, and other high-carb foods—very much like the average American. The US Department of Agriculture (USDA) reports that the average American consumes between 150 and 170 pounds of refined sugars in one year! That's ¼ to ½ pound of sugar each day.[1]

I'd start in the morning with coffee sweetened with sugar and a sweet roll or toast with jam. Lunch would be a sandwich with a soda and maybe some chips. In the middle of the afternoon, I'd perhaps have a candy bar or some chips. Before dinner, a beer or a glass of wine. Dinner would include plenty of bread, potatoes, and pasta. Dessert would be something lovely and sweet and filled with carbs. Later on, I'd eat more chips. I squeezed in a few token vegetables, but almost all my calories were coming from carbs.

Back then (the 1970s–'90s), Americans were fat phobic. We thought we could safely eat all the carbs we wanted as long as we avoided saturated fats.

In the early 2000s, I discovered my fasting blood sugar was high. I wasn't alone: half the people over fifty in the United States have this problem. When I started trying to whittle away at my carb consumption, the cravings fought back, and I began to realize how addicting carbs are and how hard it is to stop eating them.

At the same time, I was reading the latest studies and discovering how metabolically damaging carbs are and how important it is to replace them with healthy fats and protein. My high-carb diet was taking a huge toll on the health of my body, especially my brain. The evidence from study after study was shouting at me that I needed to fix my diet.

The best research of recent years tells us that a grain-free, sugar-free, very low-carbohydrate diet—in other words, a ketogenic diet—lowers blood sugar and improves cognition while protecting against neurodegeneration.

It took a lot of work, but I gradually eliminated almost all carbs. My two mantras were "The fewer carb calories, the better" and "Use coconut oil and omega-3s."

BENEFITS OF MCTS AND A KETOGENIC DIET

A ketogenic diet includes the following benefits:
- Protects against most neurodegenerative diseases
- Enhances neuronal energy reserves, which improve the ability of neurons to resist metabolic challenges
- Protects insulin receptors and heals the blood-sugar-regulating metabolic system
- Increases the health and efficiency of our cells' mitochondria and protects them from damage
- Provides antioxidant and anti-inflammatory effects
- Enables weight control
- Increases glutathione, a naturally occurring antioxidant that protects the hippocampus, our seat of memory
- Reduces the beta-amyloid plaques associated with Alzheimer's while blocking the damaging effects of beta amyloid on cortical neurons

The main reasons for being on a ketogenic diet is to optimize cognitive health and minimize brain damage. A ketogenic diet also supports weight loss by dramatically reducing carb intake and replacing carb calories with high-quality good fats that support healthy cognition. Replacing as many carbs as possible with healthy fats and oils stimulates neurogenesis and prevents inflammation in the brain. But what does this mean in terms of food choices? First we need to know what carbs and healthy fats are. Then I'll show you how to choose the right replacement fats—the ones that improve cognition and enhance overall brain health.

LIMIT YOUR CARBOHYDRATES AND CHOOSE YOUR FATS CAREFULLY!

All foods contain some combination of the three macronutrients—carbs, fats, and protein—that make up 100 percent of the calories in your diet. Adopting a low-carb diet—the ketogenic diet—automatically means that you will have to consume more fats or proteins or both. Too much protein is not a good idea. A high-fat diet, however, can be extremely beneficial, especially if you choose your fats carefully. Here, again, are the ratios to shoot for:

- 5–10 percent calories from carbs
- 60–75 percent of calories from fat
- 15–30 percent of calories from protein

HIGH-CARBOHYDRATE DIETS CAUSE COGNITIVE IMPAIRMENT

A recent Mayo Clinic study funded by the National Institute on Aging and published in the *Journal of Alzheimer's Disease* provided some deep insights about how damaging carbs are to your brain.[2] Research subjects who consumed high-carbohydrate diets were almost twice as likely to develop mild cognitive impairment or early dementia than those with the lowest carb intake. Participants with the highest sugar intake were 1.5 times more likely to experience mild cognitive impairment than those with the lowest levels. On the other hand, those whose diets were highest in fat were more than 40 percent less likely to face cognitive impairment. When total caloric intake (including fat and protein) was taken into account, people with the highest carbo-hydrate intake were a whopping 3.6 times more likely to develop mild cognitive impairment. The authors concluded that "high caloric intake from carbohydrates and low caloric intake from fat and proteins may increase the risk of MCI or dementia in elderly persons."[3]

A plethora of similar statistical studies reinforces what basic science has been telling us all along: excess carbs cause the inflammation that messes up our metabolism and batters the blood vessels that nourish our brains. In recent years, as the studies have gotten better and better, it has become crystal clear that even small amounts of carbohydrates in our diet—especially ones from refined grains or sweeteners but even those from more respectable sources such as root vegetables, noodles, and whole grains—undermine brain health and increase the risk of dementia.

WHAT ARE CARBOHYDRATES?

So you'll know what foods to avoid, I want to go into a little more detail about what carbs are. They are the sugars, starches, and cellulose fibers found in fruit, grains, nuts, beans, root vegetables, and milk products. Meats and eggs do not contain carbohydrates. Salad vegetables and leafy green vegetables contain almost none. Starchy root vegetables such as potatoes, squash, sweet potatoes, beets, and carrots are almost entirely carbohydrates.

Sugar is the generalized name for carbohydrates that are soluble and sweet. Single sugar molecules are monosaccharides; these are the most basic unit of carbohydrates in that they cannot be further broken down into simpler compounds. Examples of monosaccharides include glucose (dextrose), fructose (levulose), and galactose.

Monosaccharides are the building blocks for disaccharides, which contain two sugar molecules. Maltose and lactose are examples of disaccharides.

Sucrose is a naturally occurring disaccharide that consists of a molecule of fructose bonded to a molecule of glucose. Present in many plants and plant parts, sucrose is often extracted and refined from either cane or beet sugar. Modern refinement processes often involve bleaching and crystallization, producing a white, odorless, crystalline powder, commonly referred to as table sugar or just sugar. Sucrose plays a central role as an additive in food production and food consumption all over the world. About 175 million metric tons of sucrose were produced worldwide in 2013.[4]

Starches are polysaccharides made up of glucose units bonded together in very long chains. Starches are found in corn, wheat, rice, other grains, potatoes, beets, sweet potatoes, and other root vegetables. Our amylase digestive enzymes break down all starches and carbs—whether from bread, potatoes, corn, or soda pop—to monosaccharides, which are then absorbed into the bloodstream.

Artificial sweeteners are not sugars; even though they taste sweet, they are chemically different. The most commonly used sugar substitute, aspartame, is extremely damaging to the brain.

CARBS BATTER THE BODY AND THE BRAIN

Here's an explanation of how high carb intake, high insulin, and insulin receptor damage spell trouble for the brain. (For a more thorough discussion, see chapter 11.)

Insulin receptors are proteins positioned on the surface of cells. Insulin hormone molecules in the bloodstream dock on these receptors and signal glucose transport mechanisms inside the cell to move sugar into the cell, where it can fuel energy production. Sugar and carb overloading damages the insulin receptors. Broken receptors cause insulin resistance, a condition in which cells cannot transfer sugar molecules out of the bloodstream, so sugar accumulates there, forcing blood sugar levels upward. High blood sugar levels damage blood vessel walls, causing plaque and atherosclerosis and vascular dementia.

Insulin resistance causes problems everywhere in the body but is especially problematic in the brain because it starves the brain of its primary fuel: glucose. This brain starvation causes neurodegeneration and cognitive impairment and is a hallmark of Alzheimer's disease.

Another problem with carb overloading is that when insulin receptors are damaged, insulin also builds up in the bloodstream. Excess insulin increases amyloid beta deposition in the brain.

These problems do not happen overnight; the gradual damage to insulin receptors accumulates over months and years of carb overloading, but once a person's FBS has climbed up over 90 mg/dL, you can be certain insulin resistance, metabolic syndrome, and type 2 diabetes have arrived.

LOW-CARB DIETING

Low-carb dieting means eliminating all grains, grain products, sweetened foods, and starchy foods, including root vegetables. To spot hidden carbs, read the carbohydrate content on packaged-food labels. (Better yet, eliminate packaged foods altogether.) Replace carb calories with healthy fats and high-quality protein: lean meats, eggs, vegetables (raw and cooked), nuts, seeds, beans, coconut oil, avocado oil, and olive oil.

When you switch to a high-fat, low-carbohydrate diet, you are making an important metabolic adjustment. Deprived of carb calories, your body must switch over to fats as its primary source of fuel. This causes ketone production, and ketones are really good for the brain.

GETTING THE RIGHT COMBINATION OF FATS AND OILS

Your fat choices really matter. I've mentioned healthy fats several times, and I'll now elaborate on what they are.

Your primary mission with fat choices is to consume more of the hard-to-find healthful omega-3s while reducing the easily gotten pro-inflammatory omega-6s. Most people are already consuming way too many omega-6s and not enough omega-3s. The ratio should be 1:1. To balance that ratio, increase your omega-3 oil choices by emphasizing flaxseed oil, olive oil, walnuts and walnut oil, other nuts, avocados and avocado oil, and beans. And be sure to take supplemental flaxseed oil and DHA every day.

In chapter 28 I discuss EFAs, omega-3s and omega-6s, flaxseed oil, and DHA. I explain what they are, why they are so important, and why we need to take supplements to get enough of them.

Keep Omega-6 Fats to a Minimum

Avoid soybean, corn, sunflower, safflower, cottonseed, and canola oils. Avoid margarine, butter substitutes, and hydrogenated oils. These are high in those pro-inflammatory omega-6 fats that undermine brain health.

Replace polyunsaturated vegetable oils with healthy fats that support the brain and blood vessels: coconut oil, flaxseed oil, olive oil, walnut oil, avocado oil, and (modest amounts of) butter.

Add MCTs to Your Diet

Medium chain triglycerides are saturated fats your body can digest very easily and quickly transform into cognition-enhancing ketone bodies. Coconut oil (see chapter 23) is the single best source of MCTs. Smaller amounts of MCTs are also present in butter and palm oil.

Include Monounsaturated Fatty Acids

Monounsaturated fatty acids are found in avocados, olives, beef, nuts (almonds, cashews, pecans, macadamias), and nut butters. MUFAs lower your risk of heart and cardiovascular disease by improving serum lipid profiles (cholesterol, LDL, triglycerides, etc.). Use MUFAs to replace those unhealthy omega-6 oils.

WHAT ABOUT SATURATED FATS?

Pretty much everybody except Robert Atkins, MD, got it wrong on saturated fats. For fifty years, from the 1950s to the 2000s, almost every expert believed that saturated fat and cholesterol were the major causes of coronary heart disease and obesity. The lipid hypothesis, which posited that the epidemic of heart attacks and strokes was caused by too much saturated fat, was based on bad science—the flawed and fraudulent research of Ancel Keys. We now know that small amounts of saturated fats are not only okay but actually good for you, a necessary part of a healthy diet.

Your saturated fat intake should come from small amounts of eggs, meat, butter, ghee, cream, coconut oil, or palm oil. Be sure to use the forms of these oils that are organic, from sustainable agriculture, and free of hormones and GMOs.

Now that you know *what* to eat, let's discuss *when* to eat it.

CHAPTER 22

Autophagy: A Powerful Anti-Alzheimer's Weapon

Our bodies don't like trash lying around. They prefer a clean house. Junk in our cellular house causes metabolic dysfunction and neurodegenerative disease.

Autophagy, or autophagocytosis (from the Greek *auto*, "self," and *phagein*, "to eat"), is the waste removal and recycling system in our cells—a combination of mechanisms by which cells remove unnecessary, redundant, or dysfunctional components. Through autophagy, our cells process and recycle or eject an enormous hodgepodge of different kinds of cellular debris—used-up or broken biomolecules, faulty or broken cell parts, and cancer-causing chemicals. These may include proteins, carbohydrates, lipids, nucleic acids, viruses, and bacteria.

Optimum autophagy is necessary for maintaining a healthy brain. It slows brain aging, prevents cognitive decline, accelerates neuroregeneration, protects and heals the brain, and increases one's life span. It even reverses dementia. This chapter will explain how it works and how to switch it on.

The link between autophagy and brain aging is so strong that if a competition were staged between autophagy and all other known strategies for enhancing brain health and longevity, autophagy would win it hands down.

INITIATING AUTOPHAGY

Our cells start cleaning house after the body has fully processed and assimilated its most recent meal. This takes about eight hours. Assuming no more food is eaten, autophagy kicks in at the eight-hour mark and our cells begin cleaning up—busily scrubbing, detoxifying, and spiffing up.

This process—autophagy—screeches to a halt the moment the next batch of food rolls in. Our cells must then redirect their metabolic attention to processing that food. Cleanup time is over.

HOW AUTOPHAGY WORKS

Autophagy is accomplished through the actions of spherical vesicles in our cells called autophagosomes, sometimes referred to as the garbage disposal units of the cells. As shown in figure 22.1, autophagosomes start out as a small, flat piece of cell membrane material that elongates, wraps itself around unwanted material, engulfs it, and forms a cyst-like vesicle to encapsulate it in a Pac-Man-like process known as phagocytosis. The autophagosome-containing cellular waste matter then merges with another cyst-like vesicle called a lysosome to form a third type of vesicle, the autolysosome. Autolysosomes release over fifty different kinds of enzymes that rapidly digest the waste material, breaking it down into its component parts, which are then recycled into new cell parts, burned for energy, or tagged for expulsion.

When autophagy is impaired, or blocked because of frequent eating, toxic molecules accumulate, and this pushes the body toward a variety of pathological conditions, including cancer, insulin resistance, diabetes, infections, heart disease, inflammation, myopathies, cognitive impairment, Alzheimer's, and other neurodegenerative disorders.

AUTOPHAGY PERFORMS IMPORTANT TASKS

Autophagy can clear just about any kind of cellular trash, including intracellular viruses, bacteria, organelles, particulate structures such as

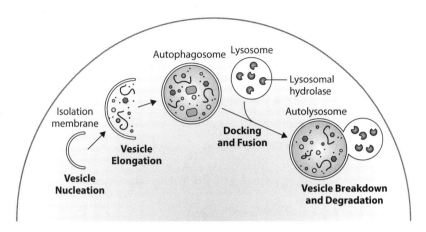

Figure 22.1. The autophagy process

protein aggregates, and damaged, dysfunctional, or misfolded proteins (such as amyloid beta and tau proteins). Autophagy can also clear out damaged cytoplasm, endoplasmic reticulum, peroxisomes, Golgi apparatuses, and even damaged parts of the nucleus, including DNA. If some of these names seem like Greek to you, just think of autophagy as a very powerful, very selective Shop-Vac inside your cells.

One of autophagy's most important jobs in nerve cells is to remove damaged or defective mitochondria, the body's energy-producing factories. Maintaining a healthy population of mitochondria is essential to the well-being of cells because damaged or worn-out mitochondria will produce copious amounts of cell-debilitating free radicals that cause mutations to mitochondrial DNA. Mutated DNA doesn't perform well, and cellular energy production is compromised. Once it has been activated (by fasting or caloric restriction), autophagy clears out dysfunctional mitochondria, shuts off the flow of free radicals, and reverses the damage they have done.

Autophagy also contributes to the removal of potentially damaging intracellular brain pathogens: bacteria, herpesviruses, Epstein-Barr virus, and prion-like proteins. This takes stress off of the immune system and frees it up to do other important work.

Many of the neurodegenerative effects we associate with aging are driven by dysfunction of the brain's stem cells. Autophagy protects the viability and vitality of the brain's pool of stem cells so they can differentiate into new healthy brain cells.

Autophagy's cleansing, detoxifying action resonates throughout the body, dramatically reducing the number of damaged cells and reversing many of the negative effects of aging.

Enhanced Autophagy Reverses Cognitive Decline

Researchers have theorized that compromised autophagy drives the abnormal protein aggregation of dementia. In 2013, research scientist Dr. Per Nilsson and his colleagues at the RIKEN Brain Science Institute in Japan bred Alzheimer's-prone mice (genetically programmed to generate abnormally high levels of amyloid beta) with mice that were incapable of autophagy. In effect, the researchers created rodents with ramped-up amyloid beta production but a dialed-down ability to remove it. The researchers showed that intracellular amyloid beta is toxic and the accumulation within neurons is what kills nerve cells.[1] In mice deprived of the protection provided by autophagy, amyloid beta accumulated inside brain cells and caused the typical Alzheimer's pathology: neurodegeneration and memory impairment.

Autophagy Clears Out Protein Aggregates

Of particular interest to those of us who wish to stave off cognitive decline, autophagy removes protein aggregates, clumps of misfolded proteins that damage nerve cells (fig. 22.2).

Dementias are considered by many experts to be diseases of misshaped proteins. The amyloid beta, tau protein, and Lewy bodies that collect in the brains of dementia patients are prime examples of misshaped protein aggregation. They are seen in all the neurodegenerative diseases, including Alzheimer's disease, Parkinson's disease, Huntington's disease, ALS, and chronic traumatic encephalopathy. Autophagy digests and removes these misshaped proteins. Recent research suggests that

Protein Aggregate

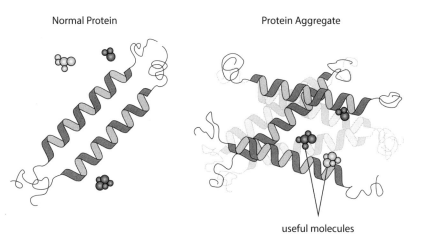

Normal Protein   Protein Aggregate

useful molecules

Figure 22.2. Protein aggregate

disruption of autophagy causes these amyloid beta protein aggregates to accumulate, thus causing Alzheimer's disease, and that activation of autophagy prevents amyloid beta deposition and buildup, thus blocking the progression of neurodegenerative disease.[2]

The takeaway message from these and many similar studies is that autophagy enhancement strategies can play a dramatic role in slowing and reversing cognitive decline.

Autophagy Blocks Aging and Neurodegeneration

From a molecular biological perspective, autophagy is an incredibly complex and medically important undertaking that affects a vast array of cellular functions and disease processes. An intense scientific effort to better understand it has been underway for the past couple of decades, generating thousands of research papers, but there is still a long way to go.

A daily twelve-hour fast turns on autophagy in our cells. Once activated, autophagy blocks—and even reverses—virtually every known major mechanism of cellular aging: protein aggregate buildup, stem cell loss, epigenetic gene silencing, telomere shortening, and oxidative damage to proteins, lipids, and DNA.

Autophagy is like a muscle. If unused, it will weaken. Exercising it, however (by following the protocol below) will keep it strong and support its ability to continue protecting the brain. Your body's cells will heartily welcome your efforts to shore up their autophagic efforts, and will reward you by helping you feel—and think—better.

HOW TO PRACTICE AUTOPHAGY

Food suppresses autophagy; fasting and caloric restriction stimulate it.

While your body's cells are still processing that last meal, they can't initiate autophagy. After eight hours, autophagy will gradually turn back on and will stay on until you eat again. Fasting twelve hours every day will therefore net you about four hours of autophagy.

While you are fasting, it's okay to consume calorie-free liquids. These include water, black coffee, tea, and unsweetened soda. Lemon or lime juice is fine also. All alcoholic beverages are out because ethanol is a high-carbohydrate food.

The most convenient time for autophagy is before or after sleep (since you will be fasting anyway when you are asleep). You can get in your twelve-hour fast by skipping either dinner or breakfast. It doesn't matter which; choose whichever is easier or more comfortable for you.

So, for example, you can fast from 9:00 p.m. to 9:00 a.m. and have breakfast. Or you can have a bedtime snack, sleep, skip breakfast, and have lunch around noon. I personally allow twelve to sixteen hours for autophagy and find it easier to fast in the morning, so I put off my first meal as long as is comfortable. I have a light fruit snack around 9:00 or 10:00 p.m. and usually end my overnight fast between noon and 2:30 p.m. Sometimes I get hungry earlier, like 11:00 a.m. or noon, and sometimes I don't get hungry until 2:00 or 3:00 p.m.

Give your body some time to adjust to this program. At first I found it difficult, and fasting for even just twelve hours was difficult, but as I worked my way into it, it gradually became easier. As my body adjusted, I noticed that my hunger diminished and I actually felt better when I put off the first meal. You may experience a similar transition. On the other hand, starving yourself isn't beneficial; you're just setting the stage for rebound overeating down the road. If I feel significant hunger, I'll eat, and I recommend you do the same.

FOOD CHOICES THAT BOOST AUTOPHAGY

A high-fat, very low-carb, moderate-to-low-protein diet is necessary to achieve autophagy. This is the ketogenic diet discussed in chapter 21.

Sixty to 75 percent of your overall calories should come from healthy fats. Protein—at 15 to 30 percent—should pick up as much of the difference as possible. Just 5 to 10 percent of your calories should come from carbohydrates, with zero sugars or other sweeteners. Avoid all processed grains, pasta, bread, cookies, and sweetened sodas; these are pretty much 100 percent carbs.

For fats, avoid pro-inflammatory omega-6 fats, such as those in processed and polyunsaturated vegetable oils (soy, corn, canola, sunflower, safflower, and cottonseed). Replace them with healthy fats found in real, unprocessed foods such as coconut oil, extra virgin olive oil, palm oil, flaxseed oil, and nuts. (All nuts are good. Omega-3-rich walnuts are especially good.) Also healthy are seeds, flaxseeds, omega-3-fortified eggs, olives, and avocado. As long as your intake of omega-3s and MCT oils is high and omega-6 oils is low, a small amount of saturated fat, like that found in fresh meats and butter, is okay.

AFTER AUTOPHAGY

Knowing I have provided my cells with an opportunity to do some housekeeping, I break my daily twelve- to sixteen-hour fast by easing gently back into eating. I enjoy a small "break-fast" snack: blueberries or a slice of melon and a couple of handfuls of nuts. In another couple of hours (or whenever hunger returns) I'll eat a very low-carb, medium-protein, high-fat meal, usually a couple of eggs cooked in two tablespoons of MCT-rich virgin coconut oil and a cup of blueberries or perhaps a salad and some cooked vegetables. Leftover cooked meat and vegetables from last night's dinner often fill the bill.

I might also blend a fruit smoothie using blueberries, cherries, strawberries, half a banana, 1–2 tablespoons of flaxseed oil, and almond milk. Using this as a starting point, I can be creative. I'll throw in some chia seeds, ground flaxseeds, hemp seeds, walnuts, a little yogurt and maybe a raw egg.

Sometimes I will make a vegetable smoothie with lettuce, romaine, spinach, or other greens, broccoli, kale, tomato, carrot, pepper—whatever vegetables are in the fridge. I add almond milk. I might throw in a couple of handfuls of walnuts and a squirt of flaxseed oil, lemon juice, vinegar, and sometimes salsa or a sauce, favorite spices, and perhaps some high omega-3 salad dressing for flavor.

Give autophagy a chance and I think you will experience some remarkable changes in your body and mind!

CHAPTER 23

Coconut Oil and MCTs: Brain Food

Coconut oil is a superfood for the brain that tastes great, protects you from a slew of diseases, and can reverse dementia. Coconut is the richest source of medium chain triglycerides, which are naturally occurring fatty acids that have been shown to protect and improve brain function in people with mild to moderate cognitive impairment. MCTs do this by providing an alternative energy source for the brain. Coconut oil contains 60 percent MCTs. Butter, cheese, and palm oil also contain significant amounts.

Almost 90 percent of the fatty acids in coconut oil are saturated. But what does this mean, and why is it important?

Saturation has to do with the number of hydrogen atoms and double bonds in a fatty acid molecule. Hydrogenation involves removing double bonds and replacing them with two hydrogen atoms and a single bond. Saturated fatty acids (all animal fats and coconut oil) have no double bonds: their double bonds have all been "saturated" with hydrogen atoms. Unsaturated fats have one or more double bonds. (Monounsaturated fatty acids have one double bond and polyunsaturated fatty acids have two or more double bonds.)

A LITTLE SATURATED FAT IS OKAY

Coconut oil was demonized for decades because it contains so much saturated fat. We have been programmed to shy away from high-saturated-fat foods, but you may be surprised to discover that the latest research has exonerated saturated fats such as those found in meats, butter, cheese, and coconut oil. Studies that scrutinized the dietary habits of hundreds of thousands of people for several decades showed that saturated fats, in modest quantities (especially when accompanied by a high intake of omega-3 oils and a low intake of omega-6 oils), don't cause heart attacks.[1] The real culprit, all along, has been too many sugars and carbs.

A HIGH-CARB DIET CAUSES INSULIN RESISTANCE, WHICH LEADS TO DEMENTIA

Your brain is your most metabolically active organ, accounting for 20 percent of your body's energy consumption but only 2 percent of your body's mass. To power that activity, your brain needs lots of fuel. In the typical American diet, that fuel comes from carbs, which damage the brain and constitute a powerful driving force behind Alzheimer's disease.

Chronic carb overloading causes insulin resistance, a disease of carbohydrate metabolic mismanagement in which receptors on the surface of liver and muscle cells lose their ability to respond to insulin. This prevents the cells from taking in the glucose that is readily available in the bloodstream. Varying degrees of insulin resistance can be found in most people over fifty. The most common signs of insulin resistance include blood sugar elevation, a roll of fat around one's middle, elevated blood lipids (triglycerides, LDL, and cholesterol), and high blood pressure. Unfortunately, these early signs are often dismissed by doctors. When this insulin resistance progresses, we diagnose it as metabolic syndrome or type 2 diabetes. For the sake of brain health and Alzheimer's prevention, addressing this condition early and aggressively is strongly recommended.

Most people with MCI or Alzheimer's disease have insulin resistance that affects their cognitive abilities. In the brain, neurons are unable to extract glucose from the bloodstream and are unable to use it as a source of energy. Sugar levels build up in the bloodstream; levels over 90 mg/dL are a sure sign that the body is having difficulty managing its sugar supply and that insulin receptors on cells' surfaces are damaged and can no longer facilitate the transfer of glucose into cells. The pantry door is locked. Unable to use the ample sugar supply that sits literally next door in the bloodstream, brain cells are being starved in the midst of plenty.

Coconut oil to the rescue! Its medium chain triglycerides and ketones can reverse brain-eroding damage (insulin resistance, high blood sugar, metabolic syndrome, and type 2 diabetes) done by carbohydrates.

COCONUT OIL: "CLEAN BURNING" ALTERNATIVE BRAIN FUEL

The key to understanding why coconut oil supercharges cognition is knowing how the brain's energy needs are supplied. Think of coconut MCT-derived ketones as a "clean green" energy supply for the brain, like solar or wind energy, whereas using sugar for fuel is like burning carbon-based coal or oil that generates pollutants.

Your body uses coconut MCT fats as a backup source of brain fuel to replace the carbs and bypass the insulin resistance problem. That fuel is ketones, which are generated in your brain from the MCTs in coconut oil and from other fats. A high-fat diet is called ketogenic because it generates a lot of brain-protecting ketones.

Diets high in coconut MCTs benefit a long list of neurological diseases, including all forms of dementia, Parkinson's, ALS, epilepsy, stroke, and traumatic brain injury.[2]

MCTs' neurological effects are rapid. Research studies in adults with MCI have demonstrated measurable improvement in memory recall within ninety minutes of a single dose of MCT oil.[3]

COCONUT OIL PREVENTS AND REMOVES
AMYLOID BETA PLAQUE

Amyloid beta—the protein spotted by Dr. Alzheimer and now deeply implicated as a causative agent in dementia—damages nerve cells. A clever group of researchers wondered whether pretreating nerve cells with coconut oil might protect those cells from the neurodegenerative effects of amyloid beta. Sure enough, it did,[4] which strongly suggests that pretreating your own brain cells by consuming coconut oil MCTs will do the same for you. The researchers also showed that coconut pretreatment protects nerve cells from mitochondrial damage.

The take-home message is this: we can pretreat our brains' neurons and protect our hippocampi by consuming 2–4 tablespoons of coconut oil daily while on a ketogenic diet.

USING COCONUT OIL

Many coconut oil products are available. Quality varies. Look for the words pure, organic, and virgin on the label. When you see the words virgin or extra virgin (there is no difference), you can be sure you are getting unprocessed, high-MCT coconut oil. Avoid hydrogenated coconut oil.

Coconut oil tolerates high heat, so you can use it as you would any cooking oil with vegetables, sauces, sautés, and stir-fries. You can cook meat and vegetables in it, stir it into soups, bake with it, and put it in your fruit or vegetable smoothie. Use it to replace those unhealthy oils you may currently be using—such as canola, sunflower, soy, and safflower oils. I cook my morning eggs with coconut oil—the results are delicious!

Coconut oil's melting point is just a tad above room temperature, so in warmer weather, it becomes a liquid.

As a preventive measure against neurodegenerative disease, I recommend 2–4 tablespoons of coconut oil a day. This will supply 20–40 grams of MCT. For an established case of MCI, Alzheimer's, or other dementia, a daily therapeutic dose would be 4–8 tablespoons (40–80 grams) spread out into two or three divided doses.

Most people tolerate coconut oil without any problem, but it has been known to occasionally cause mild GI symptoms in individuals who, in their excitement about the amazing benefits, start taking too much too soon. Your body metabolizes MCTs a little differently, so give it some time to shift gears. You'll have no problem if you start at 1–2 teaspoons per meal and build up gradually over a few days to the full dose.

CHAPTER 24

Polyphenols: Miracle-Gro for Your Brain

Polyphenols are a class of naturally occurring micronutrient compounds. Though present in a variety of foods, they are found in highest concentrations in vegetables, fruit, and herbs. Polyphenols are often the molecules that give a plant its unique color, including yellow, orange, red, blue, and purple pigments.

Polyphenols exhibit a wide range of properties, depending on their particular structures. They are known for their antioxidative, neuroprotective, and cognition-enhancing properties. They promote an impressive array of parameters, including improved overall brain health, better brain metabolism, and improved cerebral blood circulation. Polyphenols also enhance the functionality of the dentate gyrus, that part of the brain that contains the hippocampus and is most involved in memory. Polyphenols have been shown to increase synaptoplasticity, enhance hippocampal functioning, enhance learning and memory, and reduce the risk of developing age-related neurodegenerative diseases.[1]

Polyphenols accomplish this via a combination of mechanisms, the most important of which may be stimulating the release of BDNF, a powerful neurohormone that triggers production of new brain cells and strengthens existing ones. BDNF flips on the switch for a series of genes that grow new brain cells. High BDNF rewires your brain so that you age slower, learn faster, and remember better. BDNF also stimulates neuroplasticity, which protects stressed-out or damaged nerve cells and helps them heal faster.[2] This cornucopia of polyphenol benefits includes another huge bonus: polyphenols block the deposition of amyloid beta in the hippocampus.

More than eight thousand naturally occurring polyphenols have been identified. High-polyphenol foods are listed below and in appendix 2.

Virtually all fruit and vegetables contain some polyphenols. Berries (especially blueberries), grapes, broccoli, eggplant, onions, spinach, cherries, cocoa, green tea, coffee, nuts, and curcumin (turmeric/curry) are particularly good sources.

WHAT POLYPHENOLS CAN DO

Polyphenols exert powerful medicinal effects. They effectively address the diseases of aging that account for most human deaths: cancer, cardiovascular disease, neurodegenerative disease, inflammation, type 2 diabetes, and metabolic syndrome.

Polyphenols have especially attracted the attention of neuroscience researchers because, compared to other molecules, they provide extreme degrees of neuroprotection. In other words, they protect against neurodegenerative diseases like Alzheimer's.[3] Though research efforts have focused for several decades on the molecular mechanisms that explain the health benefits of polyphenols, answers have proved elusive.[4]

Early research efforts focused on polyphenols' potent antioxidant and free-radical-scavenging effects. Oxidative stress (an abundance of free radicals) causes inflammatory disease, and polyphenols such as curcumin and quercetin were able to block the inflammation by scavenging free radicals.[5]

Polyphenols have long been known to be powerful antioxidants, so the assumption for decades has been that the secret to their phenomenal health benefits lay in their great antioxidant powers. That seemed to be a good enough explanation for how they could potentiate the immune system, fight cancer, protect the heart, reverse diabetes, slow the aging process, and protect the nervous system. Recent studies, however, have revealed that polyphenols are active at much deeper, more complex levels in human metabolism.[6] We now know they act as signaling molecules (in a very complex language using chemical messengers that enable cells to talk to one another).[7] They also modulate the expression of genes (epigenetics), which means that you can alter your genetic destiny simply by consuming more high-polyphenol foods.[8] Polyphenols go one step further: they protect and repair damaged DNA.[9]

Perhaps the most remarkable effect of all, however, is their ability to enhance the production of BDNF and, with it, the ability to stimulate new nerve cell growth.[10] This means brain renewal.

Dietary choices exert profound effects on the amount of BDNF generated in the hippocampus. Polyphenols are at the top of the beneficial foods list. Blueberries are perhaps the single richest source of BDNF-generating polyphenols, but many other foods also contain these wonderful compounds.

Published studies have examined the connection between BDNF levels and dietary flavonoid (polyphenol) intake.[11] Diets high in fruit and vegetables increase BDNF, which fosters global improvements in cognitive performance. This correlation is even higher when the diet is high in polyphenols (blueberries, green tea, cocoa, grapes, curcumin/turmeric, etc.), DHA, and coconut oil. A diet rich in these molecules will thwart cognitive decline and reverse neurodegeneration.

Adam M. Brickman, an associate professor of neuropsychology at Columbia University, uses advanced neuroimaging techniques to understand cognitive aging and dementia. Brickman and associates used functional MRI (fMRI) technology to map the precise brain location in the dentate gyrus where dysfunction would occur and then showed that a high-polyphenol food given to a group of healthy fifty to sixty-nine-year-old subjects enhanced cognitive function in that precise anatomical area.[12]

THE MOST IMPORTANT POLYPHENOLS

Some notable examples of powerful polyphenols include resveratrol (from grapes), epigallocatechin gallate (green tea), tannic acid (black tea), quercetin (citrus, onion, apple), curcumin (turmeric, curry), and pterostilbene (blueberries).

Though it's best to consume a broad variety of polyphenol-rich foods, certain ones have been so carefully studied and have shown such powerful neuroprotective, cognition-enhancing, antidementia effects, that I recommend including them in your diet every day as food or as supplements: blueberries, cocoa, curcumin, and green tea. I devote an entire chapter to each one of these.

Here's how I load up on polyphenol-rich foods.

I enjoy a cup of organic blueberries every morning—fresh, or frozen if out of season. Green tea (chapter 30) is a delicious beverage you can have anytime; on the days I don't have a couple of cups, I take two to three green tea capsules.

For curcumin, I might have a curry dish that is cooked using turmeric; if not, I'll take four to eight 500 mg turmeric capsules. The herb must be specially processed to make it absorbable. Turmeric that has not been cooked in oil (or processed with heat and oil) is very poorly absorbed, so don't waste your money on capsules containing unprocessed turmeric. Look for Meriva or Longvida on the label—or cook your own by putting equal parts of oil (olive, coconut, or avocado) along with fresh ground organic turmeric in a frying pan. Stir vigorously on medium heat for a few minutes. (For more about curcumin, see chapter 29.)

POLYPHENOL-RICH FOODS

Here is a list of the foods highest in polyphenols. Cram as many as possible of these into your daily diet! An exhaustive list can be found in appendix 2.

Highest polyphenol content

- Berries (all, but especially blueberries)
- Chocolate (cocoa powder, dark chocolate, hot chocolate made with dark chocolate)
- Coffee
- Cranberries
- Curcumin (curries)
- Green tea
- Pure pomegranate juice

Fruit

- Apricots
- Blackberries
- Blueberries
- Cherries
- Grapes (red or purple)
- Lemon juice
- Marionberries
- Nectarines
- Peaches
- Plums and prunes (dried plums)
- Pomegranates
- Raspberries
- Strawberries

Vegetables

- Broccoli
- Cabbage (red)
- Eggplant
- Garlic
- Greens (dark, leafy—e.g., kale, turnip)
- Lettuce (red)
- Onions (all)

- Olives (black)
- Shallots
- Spinach
- Tomatoes

Beans
- Black beans
- Chickpeas (garbanzo beans)
- Red kidney beans

Nuts
- Hazelnuts
- Pecans
- Walnuts (also high in ALA)

Herbs, spices, and seasonings
- Basil
- Curry

Now that you've got the basics of high-polyphenol eating, let's look at the food that is the single richest source of polyphenols.

CHAPTER 25

Blueberries: Brain-Boosting Bonanza

I f you are looking for ways to increase your intelligence, improve your memory, be better at sports, do better on exams, outwit your opponents, get ahead of the competition, and expand the size of your brain, you need to put blueberries at the top of your list. These are all research-proven blueberry effects. Before I explain how blueberries work, however, let me tell you a fascinating story.

ELIZABETH COLEMAN WHITE AND THE STORY OF BLUEBERRIES

Almost all the plants we eat came from wild ancestors, ancient cultures, and foreign lands—so we usually don't know a plant's pedigree. Not so for blueberries. We know exactly where they came from: they were born and bred in the United States in the vast 1.1-million-acre wilderness of the Pine Barrens of southern New Jersey—now an International Biosphere Reserve bigger than Yosemite and the Grand Canyon National Parks.

Native Americans appreciated the health benefits and versatility of wild blueberries and used them both as a natural flavoring and for medicinal purposes. In the early twentieth century—around the same time that Alois Alzheimer was publishing his dementia studies—Elizabeth Coleman White, daughter of a cranberry farmer in Whitesbog, New Jersey, became fascinated with the wild blueberries growing like weeds on the family farm. Elizabeth was determined to cultivate them for a commercial market, a feat that had been heretofore considered impossible because they were small and the flavor left something to be desired.

Meanwhile, in Washington, DC, Frederick Vernon Coville, chief botanist of the USDA and first director of the United States National Arboretum, also became interested in blueberries. He collected seeds and in 1906 began germination trials. In 1908 Coville identified an outstanding bush in a pasture of his neighbor, Fred Brooks, for whom its berry was named. This fortunate find produced larger berries (over 0.5 inch in diameter) that were, for a change, really tasty.

Between 1906 and 1910, Coville studied blueberries intensely and determined that they require moist but not wet soil, a low soil pH, specific nutrients, and winter chilling. He developed propagation techniques and breeding procedures. He published this information in "Experiments in Blueberry Culture" (USDA Bulletin 193, November 15, 1910). Within weeks, White had read Coville's paper. Excited by the possibility that her family land might be the perfect spot to grow blueberries, she wrote him, offering land and assistance. In early 1911, Coville responded positively to her offer, and they teamed up to identify and cultivate the most desirable wild blueberry bushes.

White and Coville's collaboration continued for twenty-six years until Coville's death in 1937. This was a labor of love and mutual respect, in which they crossbred thousands of varieties to finally create a vibrant new blueberry that was both large and tasty. White later described this work as a "joyous memory" and wrote that "encouraging developments came thick and fast. Dr. Coville and I gloated over them together, the enthusiasm of each fanning to brighter flame that of the other."[1]

In 1916 (one year after Alzheimer died), after five years of research, Coville and White sold their first commercial crop of blueberries out of Whitesbog. Together they had tamed the wild blueberry and given birth to a new delicious business that has—because just about everybody loves blueberries—evolved into a global phenomenon.

POWERFUL EFFECTS

Just as Dr. Alois Alzheimer couldn't have anticipated the profound and lasting significance of his dementia work, White and Coville, in simply developing a marketable blueberry product, couldn't have imagined the spectrum of powerful effects these little blue dynamos can exert on our brains: They had no way of knowing that blueberries would be shown to help people improve verbal learning and memory, improve academic and athletic performance, outwit opponents, get ahead of competition, and even, remarkably, reverse cerebral atrophy. Blueberries also alleviate inflammation, fight cancer, support digestion, promote heart health, and assist in weight loss.

Blueberries are flowering plants of the genus *Vaccinium*. The dark purple berries contain anthocyanins, nature's most potent antioxidants. A study that compared the antioxidant capacity of blueberries, blackberries, and strawberries found that blueberries not only contained the highest total antioxidant capacity, but also contained more different types of antioxidants.

It was long thought that blueberries deliver their multitude of benefits solely through the antioxidant effects of the polyphenols that neutralize free radicals. Now we know that blueberries act at multiple molecular levels to enhance nerve cell function. Blueberry polyphenols exert powerful epigenetic effects, actually reprogramming genetic expression in your brain, switching off genes that increase inflammation or exert other deleterious effects, while switching on an array of neuroprotective neuroplasticity genes like those programmed to make BDNF (brain-derived neurotrophic factor, the neurohormone that triggers neurogenesis, the production of new brain cells).

PTEROSTILBENE MULTITASKING

Blueberries are rich in a type of plant polyphenol known as anthocyanins that give blueberries their deep blue color and powerful antioxidant properties. The principal anthocyanin in blueberries is pterostilbene (trans-3,5-dimethoxy-4-hydroxystilbene), a purple phytonutrient with a tongue-twisting name. Because it exerts beneficial effects on a multiplicity of antidementia mechanisms, a great deal of research has focused on this blueberry molecule.

The pterostilbene in your bowl of blueberries crosses through the blood-brain barrier and goes directly to the brain, where it enhances memory and cognition and improves motor skills and spatial learning abilities.

Pterostilbene blocks age-related memory decline while enhancing hippocampal plasticity and increasing levels of various important chemicals (IGF-1, IGF-2, and ERK) known to encourage the passage of information between brain cells.

This powerful blueberry polyphenol also boosts brain blood flow, fights inflammation, accelerates psychomotor performance, increases intelligence, strengthens bones, enhances cellular defenses, fights cancer, and prevents vascular and neurological disease. Pass the blueberries!

The chemical structure of pterostilbene is remarkably similar to that of its better-known cousin, resveratrol, the antioxidant, anti-aging nutrient in grapes and wine. In fact the only difference is two methyl (CH3) groups. (For more about methyl groups, see chapter 13.)

Resveratrol is especially famous because the wine industry has invested heavily in creating the impression that the resveratrol in wine is good for you—though a glass of pure grape juice or a cup of blueberries will deliver many times more antioxidant power (and a host of other antidementia chemicals) without the sugar and empty calories of the fermented version, and without the well-known adverse effects of ethanol on the brain and liver.

ENHANCING NEUROGENESIS

Blueberries stimulate production of BDNF, the neurohormone that promotes that miracle of new nerve cell growth: neurogenesis. Blueberry-derived BDNF also enhances neuroregeneration (nerve cell healing). These effects are concentrated in the hippocampus, our memory center, where they play significant roles in the prevention of cognitive impairment.

Also, through their action on BDNF, blueberries reverse age-related degenerative decline in nerve cell signal transmission throughout the brain by increasing the number of young, healthy nerve cells, and thus the ability to carry brisker messages. In the process, blueberries enable increased neuroplasticity, so we learn faster and adjust to changes better. Bottom line: thinking, memory, and reflexes remain younger longer. (See chapter 8 on neurogenesis.)

The enhanced BDNF production that comes from eating blueberries every day isn't limited to your hippocampus; it occurs throughout the brain, improving cognitive functioning everywhere.

BREAKTHROUGH RESEARCH SHOWS BLUEBERRIES DIRECTLY ENHANCE COGNITION

A great many studies have shown that blueberries enhance learning, memory, and cognition. All along, the logical assumption had been that blueberries exerted their effects directly on the areas of the brain involved in these activities—but until 2017, no one had actually shown that this was true. The possibility remained that blueberries' brain effects were due to some secondary/indirect phenomenon.

Enter Joanna L. Bowtell and colleagues at the University of Exeter, who used functional MRI (fMRI) imaging techniques to determine whether blueberry supplementation would improve brain blood flow, enhance task-related cerebral activation, and improve cognitive function in healthy older adults. fMRIs were performed on subjects before and after twelve weeks of blueberry supplementation (or placebo). The researchers looked not just for blueberry-induced changes but also pinned down their actual locations in the brain. What they saw was remarkable. The group that got the blueberries learned faster, remembered more, and displayed cognitive superiority. And the MRI patterns reflected increased blood flow to the specific areas of the brain involved in these activities. In other words, the MRI images showed, for the first time, that blueberry-enhanced blood flow to specific areas of the brain was responsible for the cognitive enhancement. The exact brain locations targeted by blueberries lit up on the MRI images, and these were the same areas of the brain that are responsible for thinking, learning, and memory.[2]

IMPROVED SPATIAL AND NAVIGATIONAL MEMORY

The abundant flavonoid compounds found in blueberries target specific molecules in the hippocampus to enhance several different kinds of memory.

As we navigate the world, we store information about our surroundings in our hippocampus in order to form a cohesive spatial representation of our environment. This is spatial and navigational memory: processing and storing information about your location and orientation in space. Examples include remembering the positions of items, geographical layouts (e.g., your hometown or the inside of a friend's house), remembering where you have been, and how to get home. (Of course, we now have Siri and Google Maps, so that part is covered.)

The extremely complicated basic neural processes involved in spatial and navigational memory were elucidated by British American neuroscientist John O'Keefe and Norwegian neuroscientists May-Britt Moser and Edvard I. Moser; the three shared the 2014 Nobel Prize for Physiology or Medicine for these discoveries.

Navigational memory is what enables lab rats to get through a maze or remember how to go back to where the cheese was. In Alzheimer's, this system starts breaking down. Older animals lose the ability to find their way around a maze; cognitively compromised humans, because they can't fully access and retrieve information stored in their hippocampus, can lose track of where they are in space or have difficulty finding their way in a once-familiar setting.

Catarina Rendeiro and her colleagues enhanced spatial/navigational memory and rate of learning by feeding lab rats a blueberry-rich diet for seven weeks. The animals ran their mazes more efficiently and their hippocampal BDNF levels skyrocketed.[3]

Navigational memory is complicated stuff, and I don't need to go into more detail here except to say that blueberries give us an incredibly powerful (and tasty) tool to improve many different types and aspects of memory—as well as across-the-board brain function.

POWERFUL EFFECTS ON THE VASCULAR SYSTEM

The brain's blood vessels have sole responsibility for feeding its neurons. Compromised blood vessels will obstruct the free flow of blood, causing nerve damage, cognitive decline, and, eventually, dementia.

In chapters 1 and 7, I described the distinction between the two main types of dementia, vascular dementia (VaD) and Alzheimer's disease (AD). VaD is caused by damage to the blood vessels that supply the brain, which in turn causes the direct damage to nerve cells we call AD.

Both types are equally important. VaD and AD can't be clinically teased apart and diagnosed separately. Blueberries protect against both. This is a big deal given that the two types coexist in about 90 percent of dementia patients. (See chapter 7.)

Diminished blood flow to the brain is responsible for ischemic strokes, cognitive impairment, VaD, and neurodegenerative disorders in general. Eating blueberries not only lessens the probability of just about every molecular metabolic mechanism that leads to a stroke and vascular dementia, it also dramatically reduces the probability of damage if a stroke does occur.

Acting on multiple targets, blueberry polyphenols enhance blood flow in cerebral vessels to protect against the strokes that lead to vascular dementia. Multiple mechanisms are involved, including antioxidant activity, reducing cholesterol, lowering blood pressure, improving blood sugar control, preventing atherosclerosis, and blocking the causes of the metabolic syndrome and type 2 diabetes. Blueberries also work hard to lower low-density lipoprotein (LDL) oxidation, reduce clotting (platelet aggregation), and maintain healthy endothelial function. [4] (The endothelium is the inner lining of blood vessels—metabolically speaking, a very busy place.)

Keeping the blood vessels in the brain healthy is necessary to protect the hippocampus. Blueberries protect hippocampal memory centers. In research studies, stroke-prone rats given blueberry extract prior to a stroke sustained one-third as much hippocampal damage as those that had strokes with no blueberry.

BLUEBERRY PRODUCTS

Here are a few tips about buying blueberries. The only acceptable blueberry product is fresh or frozen whole unprocessed berries. Buy only certified organic berries. Nonorganic blueberry growers usually use glyphosate (found in Roundup products) to control the weeds that grow near their ("unsprayed" or "sustainable") crop, and you definitely do not want to expose yourself to this nasty endocrine-disrupting human carcinogen.

A lot of processed products contain blueberries in various forms. By the time these get to you, they may still be blue in color, but most of the fragile polyphenols have been destroyed.

Blueberry extracts, freeze-dried berries, syrups, and tinctures are sometimes recommended to cut costs, but processing of the fresh berries (except flash-freezing) destroys much of the flavonoid content. Avoid blueberry products that contain sugar or any other additive.

The notion that fresh blueberries are the ideal has been challenged by folks in the frozen blueberry packaging industry, and they have some good arguments. They claim that flash-frozen berries contain higher polyphenol levels than fresh because fifteen to twenty days may go by as the fresh berries are transported to distributors, stored a while, and then transported again to grocery stores, where they may sit on a shelf for another week before being purchased. As time passes, valuable polyphenols are damaged that would have been instantly preserved in the flash freezing process that is done within an hour or two of picking. Frozen blueberries also usually costs less. (Make sure they are organic.)

I recommend using frozen berries in the off-season when fresh organic blueberries are not available. (The most cost-effective product I've found is at Costco.) You can always find an open bag in my home freezer for my daily smoothie. To obtain maximum brain and blood vessel benefits, I try to consume at least a cup every day. Most days I succeed.

CHAPTER 26

Cocoa and Chocolate: Memory-Boosting Superfoods

S ome very exciting recent research shows that cocoa—and special chocolates made from it—improves cognitive functioning and prevents the changes that lead to dementia. Cocoa and chocolate contain a staggering array of health-promoting chemical molecules that also have been shown to lower blood sugar, blood pressure, and cholesterol. Foremost among these compounds are polyphenols. The cocoa bean is chock-full of flavonoids, the largest family of polyphenol compounds.

Humans have been in love with chocolate for a long time. The Latin name for the cacao tree, *Theobroma cacao*, appropriately summarizes the essence of chocolate: it translates as "food of the gods." Etymologists trace the origin of the word *chocolate* to the Aztec word *xocoatl*, which referred to a bitter drink brewed from cacao beans.

The Aztecs and Mayans attributed magical and divine properties to the cacao bean and used it in sacred rituals of birth, marriage, and death. The Aztecs may have been the first to believe in the connection between chocolate and amorous feelings. Montezuma is said to have consumed large amounts to enhance his romantic forays—and later on Casanova reportedly imbibed preseduction as well.

I can't think of a more flavorful prescription for improving cognitive function than fine chocolate. I speak here of dark, minimally sweetened chocolate bars and hot cocoa.

But hold on. We have a *huge* problem. Despite all of chocolate's goodness, and despite the fact that we all love it, I can't recommend ingesting many kinds of chocolate bars, candy, and cocoa powders. The problem is that many of them—especially the very dark ones, even if they're organic—are contaminated with cadmium, a neurotoxic element that causes dementia. High levels of lead are also found in many of the products. The amounts vary, but every major brand has a significant problem.

These nasty heavy metals get into the cacao plant from the soil in which it is grown, and this makes removal difficult (but not impossible). My guess is that it won't be long before an enterprising chocolate company sees the huge profit potential in advertising and supplying "cadmium- and lead-free chocolate." Then everyone else will have to follow suit. When cadmium-and lead-free chocolates become available, all those wonderful benefits will be too—but that's down the road. Meanwhile, choose carefully from products listed on the As You Sow website.[1]

THE HEAVY METAL PROBLEM

Cadmium is a heavy metal that the human body has no way to remove. It therefore accumulates and damages the kidneys, lungs, bones, and brain. It is a human carcinogen and a potent neurotoxin, as discussed in chapter 18.

The World Health Organization suggests a maximum of 0.3 mcg of cadmium per gram of chocolate. California's Proposition 65, the Safe Drinking Water and Toxic Enforcement Act, requires a warning label on products that have 4.1 mcg of cadmium per daily serving for any single product.[2] Testing commissioned by consumer health watchdog As You Sow in 2014 to 2018, conducted at independent laboratories, revealed that most brands and products, including all the brands considered above reproach, exceed these levels.[3] The chocolate companies are exposing consumers to toxic levels of cadmium and then breaking California law by not providing a legally required label warning that their products contain high levels of a carcinogen and a chemical that causes reproductive toxicity.

These label warnings are important: "As underscored by the Flint disaster . . . we must do everything in our power to protect ourselves and our children, who are the most vulnerable of us, from every possible exposure," said Sean Palfrey, MD, a pediatrician and professor of pediatrics and public health at Boston University School of Medicine.[4] But anyone who has a brain and wants to avoid dementia is also at risk of the severe damage cadmium can inflict.

Cadmium is a well-known neurotoxin that undermines memory, thinking, and vocabulary. Fetuses and children are especially vulnerable to this heavy metal because their brains are in critical growth and development stages. Even at very low levels, exposure causes neurological impairment, learning disabilities, and decreased IQ.

WHY ISN'T THE LAW BEING ENFORCED?

As You Sow petitioned the chocolate industry to fix this problem—to get the lead and cadmium out—or at least warn consumers (many are parents and children) by complying with the law and labeling their chocolates.[5] After years of waiting, an industry response was not forthcoming, so in 2017 As You Sow filed suit against more than twenty chocolate manufacturers—including Whole Foods, Trader Joe's, Hershey's, Green and Black's, Lindt, Kroger, Godiva, See's Candies, Mars, Theo Chocolate, Mondelēz, Chocolove, Equal Exchange, Ghirardelli, and Earth Circle Organics—for failing to provide the legally required warning to consumers that their chocolate products contain cadmium or lead and sometimes both.

In February 2018, a California Superior Court judge approved a settlement "resolving claims" that levels of lead and cadmium in chocolate require warnings under California's stringent Proposition 65 law. The settlement requires a joint study to investigate and report on the main sources of lead and cadmium in chocolate and to publish findings in a public report. The settlement agreement also sets thresholds for determining when Proposition 65 warnings will be required for chocolate products based on their percentage of cacao content and their levels of lead and cadmium. The skeptical consumer might regard this "settlement" as a hand slap that allows continued delays, since the breach in labeling law remains unenforced and no specific plan was put in place to remove the toxic products.

This ruling is an outrage. The only agreement was to "study the problem." It is an insult to the rule of law and to good public health practices. It does nothing to alert consumers of a serious danger. It temporarily takes a toxic industry off the hook while sanctioning the continued widespread brain and fetal damage caused by its products. As a direct consequence of this ruling, many more people will become demented. Most of the companies sued did not even feel compelled to sign on to this agreement. A proper ruling would have been to suspend sales of the offending products until their producers could show they are safe to consume. But the ball stays in the consumer's court: *caveat emptor.* Until this problem is fixed and certified cadmium- and lead-free chocolate products find their way onto the market, As You Sow's list will have to serve as your best guide to safe chocolates.[6] For more about the neurotoxic effects of lead and cadmium, see chapter 18.

GREAT FOR YOUR BRAIN!

Polyphenols protect plants from oxidative injury, environmental toxins, infection, parasites, and harsh climatic conditions. They also help plants repair damage. When ingested by humans, polyphenols exhibit similar properties: they shield our neurons from assaults that cause neurodegeneration.

In general, the darker the chocolate, the higher the polyphenol content. Cocoa's polyphenol bonanza delivers specific biological and medicinal actions that thwart disease and restore good health by exerting powerful effects on brain blood circulation, neuronal health, memory, and cognition.[7] Alzheimer's disease, vascular dementia, and other neurodegenerative diseases have been shown to respond—sometimes dramatically—to cocoa polyphenols. These polyphenols lower the risk for developing Alzheimer's disease, protect against the strokes that lead to vascular dementia, lower blood pressure, preserve cognitive abilities during aging, and even reverse established vascular dementia.[8]

The protection provided by cocoa polyphenols begins at the earliest stages of neurodegenerative disease and follows through at virtually every stage of dementia. In a 2014 study published in *Nature Neuroscience*, Adam Brickman and colleagues gave high- and low-cocoa-flavonoid diets to healthy fifty- to sixty-nine-year-olds for three months and then compared cognitive function in the dentate gyrus, the part of the brain's hippocampus involved in age-related memory decline. The high-cocoa-flavonoid group showed enhanced dentate gyrus function, as measured by fMRI and cognitive testing.[9] This study—and several others like it— tells us that ingestion of high-polyphenol cocoa improves memory and cognition in healthy older people.

As we go through chocolate's amazing array of benefits, keep in mind that only very dark, cocoa-rich, minimally processed versions contain the high percentage of polyphenols necessary to prevent cognitive decline and reverse brain disease. Typical milk chocolate bars and most other chocolate candies do not qualify. In fact, because they are typically loaded with sugar, these low-polyphenol products will do more harm than good.

Here is a list of the amazing things cocoa polyphenols do:

- Improve cognitive functioning
- Enhance memory
- Lower the risk of Alzheimer's disease
- Enhance cerebral blood flow
- Decrease the risk of stroke (a major cause of dementia)
- Preserve cognitive abilities during aging
- Prevent and reverse the neurodegenerative changes that lead to dementia
- Improve insulin resistance
- Lower blood pressure

- Remove amyloid beta
- Change the shape and structure of neurons, especially in regions of the brain involved in learning, memory, and cognition
- Stimulate neurogenesis
- Enhance neuronal survival while inhibiting neuronal death induced by neurotoxic substances such as oxygen free radicals
- Improve synaptoplasticity
- Enhance angiogenesis (growth of new blood vessels) in the brain
- Boost neural function in the dentate gyrus of the hippocampus
- Provide powerful antioxidant protection
- Generate positive mood effects

HOW COCOA PREVENTS AND REVERSES DEMENTIA

When the polyphenols and antioxidants in cocoa first enter the brain, they begin their work by telling the endothelium (the inner lining of the blood vessels) to produce and release nitric oxide. This causes vasodilation: the brain blood vessels open wide, allowing a dramatically increased flow of blood to the entire brain, bringing with it a surge of healing nutrients and oxygen. Expanded vessels also allow faster removal of waste material.

The cocoa polyphenols and flavonoids then induce the growth of new blood vessels (angiogenesis) and new nerves (neurogenesis). These crafty cocoa chemicals also induce beneficial changes in the shape and structure of neurons—especially the ones residing in regions of the brain most involved with learning, memory, and cognition: the hippocampus, dentate gyrus, and cortex.

Neurotoxic substances such as oxygen free radicals damage and kill neurons. Cocoa polyphenols promote neuronal survival by reducing the oxidative damage to nerve pathways in Alzheimer's patients' brains. Nerve impulses carrying memories are free to flow unfettered. And cocoa starts doing this long before cognitive dysfunction has progressed to the point that overt symptoms appear. In other words, cocoa functions as a fabulous preventive.

Cocoa polyphenols also stimulate the production of BDNF, the remarkable protein that supports the survival of existing neurons while encouraging the growth and differentiation of new neurons and synapses. In the brain, BNDF is very active in the hippocampus, cortex, and other areas vital to learning, memory, and higher thinking. Increasing BDNF levels by administering cocoa polyphenols has been shown to stimulate neurogenesis and reverse the neurodegenerative changes seen in Alzheimer's disease. Through BDNF, cocoa also promotes synaptoplasticity, the ability of brain cells to grow, change, adapt, and respond to changing conditions.[10]

Amyloid beta, as you know, is deeply involved in brain inflammation and the loss of cognitive function. In dementia patients, sticky clumps of amyloid beta build up in the synapses, clogging memory circuits and disrupting the ability to pass messages to the next nerve cell.

Cocoa's anti-amyloid effects are truly exciting. Cocoa polyphenols have been shown to reverse amyloid beta accumulation by modifying its physical structure such that it no longer accumulates in the hippocampus. No amyloid beta, no sticky clumps, no interference with synapses: voila!—enhanced cognition.

Amyloid beta also triggers immune inflammatory reactions that summon a rush of chemicals and cells to the area. These are meant to destroy the amyloid invaders but may instead cause further nerve cell damage.

Studies had strongly suggested that cocoa polyphenols prevent degenerative diseases of the brain, but neuroscientist Giulio Pasinetti and his colleagues wanted to know why, so he designed a study using genetically engineered Alzheimer's-prone mice to show that ingesting high-polyphenol cocoa extract blocks dementia. The cocoa polyphenols prevented amyloid beta from forming the sticky clumps that gum up the synapses, damage the nerve pathways, and eventually cause Alzheimer's disease. This work was published in the June 2014 edition of the *Journal of Alzheimer's Disease*.[11]

According to lead investigator Giulio Maria Pasinetti, MD, PhD, Saunders Family Chair and professor of neurology at the Icahn School of Medicine at New York's Mount Sinai Hospital, "Evidence in the current study is the first to suggest that specific cocoa polyphenols in the diet over time may prevent the glomming together of Aβ into oligomers that damage the brain, as a means to prevent Alzheimer's disease." He adds, "Given that cognitive decline in Alzheimer's disease is thought to start decades before symptoms appear, we believe our results have broad implications for the prevention of Alzheimer's disease and dementia."[12]

ALL CHOCOLATE IS NOT CREATED EQUAL

Please think twice before you start devouring chocolate candy bars and handfuls of M&M's and guzzling chocolate milk and hot cocoa in the belief that this will help cognition. It won't. The mere presence of chocolate in a product does not mean it will bolster your brain. To reap the magnificent benefits of cocoa and chocolate, you must pay very close attention to the source of your chocolate and its sugar content.

The amount of polyphenol in chocolate products varies dramatically. The chocolate used in the Mount Sinai study was chosen for its high polyphenol content. Most commercially available chocolate products are too low in polyphenols to benefit cognition and have a high sugar content as well.

Polyphenols are dark and bitter. Since polyphenols are what give chocolate its brain benefits, the darkest, bitterest chocolates work best.

Sugar is often used to hide the bitterness. The average American eats half a pound of chocolate every month, virtually all of which is blended into or coated with sugar. An average three-ounce bar of milk chocolate has 420 calories, and most of these calories come from the added sugars.

Processing (fermentation, alkalizing, roasting, and Dutching) removes the bitter polyphenols but also removes the brain benefits, so the more the chocolate has been processed, the less good it is for the brain. By the time you get down to your typical milk chocolate or even dark chocolate candy bar, the polyphenol benefits are gone, replaced by a lot of vascular-damaging sugar.

I might have a bite of chocolate here and there, but I'm holding back on major gorging until the industry gets its act together and generates a safe product. It is a real shame to not be able to fully indulge because chocolate offers so many remarkable brain health benefits.

Nutritional Supplements That Reverse Alzheimer's

Part 4 contains information about eight amazing nutritional medicines that prevent and reverse dementia. These are the nutritional medicines I believe would make the most useful addition to any anti-Alzheimer's program. I explain what each one is, why it is important, how it works in the body, and how to use it.

The following notes are a few tasty nibbles from a massive smorgasbord of powerful cognitive effects:

- *Low-dose lithium*—Lithium reverses Alzheimer's disease. It also protects the brain from neurodegenerative disease, prevents and reverses age-related cerebral atrophy, improves memory, protects against brain trauma, and reduces both stroke risk and stroke damage. Lithium is just plain amazing!

- *DHA and flaxseed oil*—These omega-3 EFAs increase brain levels of BDNF, the extensively studied remarkable neurohormone that keeps the brain young by stimulating new neuron growth, enhancing neuroplasticity, and guarding against neurodegeneration and cognitive decline.

- *Curcumin*—Curcumin enhances cognitive functioning and reverses dementia by blocking the synthesis of several key pro-inflammatory chemicals. It also suppresses inflammatory triggers for Alzheimer's disease and reverses amyloid beta plaque deposition.

- *Green tea*—Consumption of green tea has been associated with a dramatic reduction of Alzheimer's risk.

- *Citicoline*—Citicoline provides potent stroke protection, boosts cognition, enhances brain blood circulation and overall brain function, and accelerates synaptic growth.

- *Bacopa*—*Bacopa monnieri*, an herb used widely in ancient Indian Ayurvedic medicine, accelerates learning rate and memory and reverses neurodegenerative brain disease.

- *Phosphatidylserine*—This nutrient renews aging brain cells, bolsters memory, enhances alertness and overall mental performance, and rejuvenates just about every function controlled by the central nervous system. It helps regenerate stressed-out or damaged nerve cells, reversing defects in nerve cell message transmission.
- *Berberine*—Berberine has been shown to reverse the loss of spatial memory in Alzheimer's disease and enhance the health and functionality of the brain's memory centers. It also protects against strokes by normalizing blood sugar and reversing metabolic syndrome.

The following chapters present lots more about what these compounds can do and how they work.

CHAPTER 27

Low-Dose Lithium Reverses Dementia

To understand lithium, you must understand the distinction between high-dose lithium and low-dose lithium. There is a world of difference.

High-dose lithium is a powerful and potentially toxic pharmaceutical used to treat severe mental illness. Typical doses used in the treatment of bipolar disorder and mania range from 500 to 2,000 mg a day.

Low-dose (or microdose) lithium, on the other hand, is an essential nutrient (like zinc, calcium, and magnesium), necessary for our survival. Low-dose lithium is taken in much smaller amounts, typically from 20 to 80 mg a day.

Low-dose lithium protects the brain from neurodegenerative disease, blocks the progression of cognitive decline, and reverses Alzheimer's disease. It has been shown to enhance the size of the brain, optimize cognitive health, and boost overall brain function. And remarkably, this harmless miracle mineral also prevents and reverses age-related cerebral atrophy.

My Lithium Story

In 2003, an MRI scan of my brain showed cerebral atrophy. This wasn't a surprising finding; most sixty-year-olds have some brain shrinkage as a "normal" feature of aging. A few months later I read a research article in *Lancet* showing that low-dose lithium reversed cerebral atrophy,[1] so I added 20 mg a day of lithium orotate to my supplement program.

A couple of years ago, a repeat MRI revealed, to my surprise, that the atrophy was completely gone! Recent research has unveiled the mechanism: lithium triggers BDNF production that stimulates the growth of stem cells, leading to neuroregeneration. Nothing else is known to reverse brain atrophy, so I assume it was the lithium. What a gift!

THE "CINDERELLA" ELEMENT

In terms of generating new neurons, lithium is by far the most powerful brain nutrient. Nevertheless, it continues to be viewed by many people as a dangerous and scary drug rather than an essential nutrient that protects and heals the brain. In a 2014 *New York Times* article entitled "Should We All Take a Bit of Lithium?" psychiatrist Anna Fels characterizes the metal this way: "Lithium is the Cinderella of psychotropic medications, neglected and ill-used."[2]

For most, the word lithium suggests a pharmaceutical drug for bipolar disease and conjures up images of mental illness, lobotomies, and Jack Nicholson's character ranting at Nurse Ratched in *One Flew Over the Cuckoo's Nest*. If you are younger, lithium may have become indelibly burned into your consciousnesses as a type of battery most famous for catching fire on airplanes. I want you to start thinking of lithium as a gentle but potent natural medicine that—at extremely low doses—will improve memory, enhance cognition, prevent and reverse dementia, protect against brain trauma, and reduce both stroke risk and stroke damage.

For me, lithium triggers warm, fuzzy feelings of appreciation and amazement—because it reversed age-related shrinkage of my brain. And because it has the remarkable potential to reverse Alzheimer's disease. And because it holds the promise of slowing or even stopping the epidemic of our time.

AN ESSENTIAL NUTRIENT EFFECTIVE IN MICRODOSES

Lithium at high "pharmacologic" doses (typically 500 to 2,000 mg a day), one of the best-known and most effective psychotropic drug medicines ever, has been prescribed since the 1960s for bipolar disease (mania and depression). Lithium at these doses can cause side effects and adverse reactions, so blood levels in high-dose patients must be monitored closely.

But this chapter is about *low-dose* (or microdose) lithium, which—at 20 to 80 mg a day—is free of side effects and adverse reactions. In fact, many scientists believe lithium at these levels is an essential mineral, necessary for human survival. I agree with this assessment. Lithium has been officially added to the World Health Organization's list of nutritionally essential trace elements alongside zinc, iron, selenium, chromium, iodine, and a handful of others.

Low-dose lithium is an over-the-counter nutritional supplement. The published evidence is unequivocal: lithium protects the brain from degenerative disease without causing any side effects, adverse reactions, or toxicity.

Lithium is found naturally in food and water. Grains and vegetables serve as the primary sources of lithium in a standard diet; animal foods such as eggs and milk provide the rest.

THE DISCOVERY THAT LITHIUM PREVENTS AND REVERSES ALZHEIMER'S DISEASE

Several studies done from the 1970s to the '90s revealed that folks drinking water that contained lithium experienced multiple health benefits. Further studies showed that patients taking lithium for depression were apparently immune to dementia. Then a stunning series of discoveries over the past two decades led to the revolutionary finding that low-dose lithium prevents and reverses Alzheimer's disease.[3]

In 2007, Paula Nunes and her research group showed that depressed patients receiving lithium for bipolar disease were far less likely to get Alzheimer's than similar patients who were not taking lithium.[4] Then in 2008, Dr. Lars Kessing and colleagues surveyed the records of over twenty-one thousand depressed patients who had received high-dose lithium treatment. This study confirmed that lithium therapy decreased levels of both Alzheimer's and all dementias.[5]

Their interest piqued, researchers wondered whether low-dose lithium would work as well as the high-dose version to prevent Alzheimer's and would it work in nondepressed patients. The answer was a resounding yes. In 2013, M. A. Nunes and colleagues showed that microdose lithium, given to Alzheimer's patients for fifteen months, prevented decline in cognitive function, while the control group (without lithium) continued declining.[6]

In 2011, a group led by Orestes Forlenza wondered whether lithium could prevent Alzheimer's disease in high-risk individuals. Forty-five participants with MCI, a precursor to Alzheimer's, were randomized to receive lithium or a placebo. At the conclusion of the twelve-month study, researchers discovered that in the patients receiving lithium, levels of destructive tau proteins had declined. This finding was in stark contrast to the tau levels of the placebo group, which had gone up. What's more, the group taking lithium showed significantly improved cognitive performance as measured on multiple cognitive scales. The researchers concluded that lithium prevents dementia and Alzheimer's disease best when initiated early.[7]

To summarize, in just the past few years research has unearthed a harmless way to slow or stop the Alzheimer's epidemic. Lithium blocks the onset of Alzheimer's and reverses the disease once it has begun. Low-dose lithium should be seriously considered as a primary preventive and treatment for cognitive decline and Alzheimer's.

HOW LITHIUM PROTECTS AND HEALS THE BRAIN AND REVERSES DEMENTIA

Low-dose lithium provides a beneficial and safe neuroprotective therapy that goes beyond dramatic dementia risk reduction. Starting at the most fundamental level, that of genetic expression, lithium modifies key cascades of biochemical reactions to increase neuronal viability and resilience. It repairs the damaged biochemical reactions that whip up a metabolic recipe for dementia.

Convincing proof of lithium's effectiveness in blocking and reversing Alzheimer's and healing the brain is seen when we look at how long-term, microdose lithium therapy gradually reorganizes and normalizes a broad spectrum of disturbed metabolic pathways. Lithium inhibits damaging enzymes and stimulates the release of protective neurotrophic factors while removing the plaques and tangles so intimately associated with cognitive decline.

Brains on lithium grow, heal, and function better. Confirmation of these changes can be seen on multiple levels, from cognitive and IQ performance testing to macroscopic anatomy and MRIs to microscopic intracellular signaling, and—even deeper—to submicroscopic molecular enhancements.

Lithium accomplishes these changes through a smorgasbord of effects and a multiplicity of mechanisms. It enhances the synthesis of neurotrophic neuroprotective factors, such as BDNF, that promote the formation of new brain cells. It inhibits cell death (apoptosis), enhances autophagy (cellular cleanup), improves mitochondrial cellular energy production, enhances neurotransmission, inhibits cellular oxidative stress, increases gray matter density and cerebral cortex size, and enlarges the hippocampus.[8]

Prevents Cerebral Atrophy

Cerebral atrophy happens in just about everybody. It can be a "normal" effect of aging in the brain, but when severe, it is a hallmark of Alzheimer's. One of the most remarkable of lithium's many remarkable effects is that it reverses cerebral atrophy. Over time, it literally increases the amount of gray matter and gradually restores the brain to its original size. The size—and functionality—of the memory areas (anterior cingulate cortex, ventral prefrontal cortex, hippocampus, and amygdala) also increases.[9]

Prevents and Reverses Traumatic Brain Injury

Lithium has recently been evaluated in preventing and treating traumatic brain injury, and the mineral appears to protect the nerve cells in the brain from just about everything known to damage them.

Researchers devised a variety of challenges in testing situations. Preadministration with lithium has been shown to protect against them all, including trauma, free radicals, toxins (the kinds of pollutants we all encounter every day from food, air, water, and the environment), chronic depression, excitotoxic neurotransmitters such as glutamate, and even stroke and traumatic brain injury.[10]

Improves Cell Signaling

Cells communicate by continuously sending and receiving chemical signals. The ability of cells to perceive and correctly respond to their microenvironment is the basis of all development, tissue repair, immunity, and normal tissue homeostasis. This communication, known as cell signaling, governs the basic activities of all cells and coordinates cell actions. Metabolic errors that disrupt this signaling are responsible for many diseases, including cancer, autoimmune diseases, diabetes, and Alzheimer's disease.

Lithium exerts a powerful beneficial influence on cell signaling molecules, controlling a number of important ones. In effect, lithium uses the language of cell signaling to explain to neurodegenerating nerve cells exactly how to go back to functioning efficiently.[11]

Triggers Release of BDNF

Lithium induces hippocampal production of BDNF, and higher levels are associated with enhanced neurogenesis and improved cognition.[12]

Inhibits Oxidative Stress

Oxidative stress in neurons damages their membranes, proteins, mitochondria, and genes. This undermines plasticity, signal transmission, and cellular resilience. Numerous studies have examined lithium's powerful antioxidant action in the brain that prevents or reverses DNA damage, membrane disruption, free-radical formation, and lipid peroxidation.

START EARLY

Because the dangerous plaques and tangles involved in Alzheimer's disease begin to accumulate up to forty years before symptoms appear, it is important to take steps to protect your brain at a much younger age. When started early, low-dose lithium may be the single most valuable intervention to prevent cognitive decline.

HOW TO USE LOW-DOSE LITHIUM

Lithium orotate is the most commonly used dietary supplement version of low-dose lithium. It is made and sold by companies that specialize in nutritional medicine and does not require a prescription. Take 20–80 mg per day, all at once or in divided doses.

Do not confuse microdose lithium orotate with pharmaceutical-dose lithium carbonate or lithium chloride. Megadoses of these chemicals bludgeon the brain into submission. These potencies are available only in drugs prescribed for long-term control of bipolar disorder at doses usually ranging from 500 to 2,000 mg per day. High-dose lithium therapy is associated with serious and potentially debilitating side effects, and blood lithium levels must be monitored. Low-dose lithium, on the other hand, is available over-the-counter as a food-grade nutritional supplement. Optimal dosing at microdose levels is an attempt to emulate the physiological lithium levels present in a normal young, healthy brain. These doses have not been associated with side effects or adverse reactions.

CHAPTER 28

DHA and Flaxseed Oil:
The Omega-3 Brain Power Oils

Your brain is about 60 percent fat. The fats you choose to put into your body have a powerful effect on whether healthy fats end up in your brain. The wrong combination of oils will quickly undermine healthy cognition and dramatically increase the risk of dementia.

In this chapter I will show you why taking both supplemental FSO (flaxseed oil) and DHA (docosahexaenoic acid) provides all the omega-3s you need and why this is a crucial step toward achieving peak brain performance and maximum Alzheimer's protection. We'll zero in on the two omega-3 essential fatty acids:

- *DHA*—Fish have lots of DHA, but, because they are contaminated with mercury, fish and seafood are not good sources of DHA. It is therefore necessary to take a DHA supplement; the one you want is derived from algae.

- *ALA* (alpha-linolenic acid)—Getting enough ALA is a different kind of problem. No single food, except flaxseeds, contains more than a small amount of ALA. Flaxseeds don't fit into most diets very well; the best way to get your ALA is to use liquid flaxseed oil every day.

These EFAs target and correct defects in the metabolic pathways that cause Alzheimer's. You'll need to supplement with both DHA and FSO for dementia protection and optimum brain health.

ABOUT ESSENTIAL FATTY ACIDS

All fats can be divided into two groups: essential and nonessential. (*Essential* means that you must have it but your body can't make it out of other oils, so you need to get it from diet or supplements.)

EFAs can be further subdivided into two categories: omega-3 and omega-6. These are the only two kinds of EFAs. All other fats and oils are nonessential.

Omega-3s are extremely important for brain health, but it's hard to get enough of them. Omega-6 oils are the opposite: they're very easy to come by, and consuming more than a little of them causes inflammation and undermines brain health.

Even though, technically, omega-6 oils are "essential," no one ever worries about an omega-6 deficiency; the real challenge with omega-6 oils is limiting our intake. We tend to overconsume them because they are everywhere: soy, canola, corn, safflower, sunflower, peanut, and cottonseed oils are all rich omega-6 sources and should, for the most part, be avoided.

On the other hand, we can get small amounts of omega-3 oils derived from fruit, vegetables, and nuts (see the lists below), but we need supplements to get enough. The two supplemental sources you can rely on are DHA (in capsules) from algae (*not from fish*) and ALA from liquid flaxseed oil.

DHA IMPROVES COGNITION AND REDUCES ALZHEIMER'S RISK

Age-related cognitive decline (ARCD), the earliest sign of possible onset of Alzheimer's, manifests as forgetfulness, decreased ability to stay focused, and decreased problem-solving capacity. MCI (mild cognitive impairment) is a slightly more advanced stage of the disease in which the cognitive impairment has been documented by testing. Left unchecked, symptoms of ARCD or MCI may progress to dementia and Alzheimer's. Karin Yurko-Mauro and colleagues showed, in a double-blind trial, that

DHA reverses ARCD. The investigators identified 485 individuals with ARCD and divided them into two groups. The research group received DHA while the control group received a placebo. The researchers concluded, "Twenty-four-week supplementation with 900 mg/day DHA improved learning and memory function in ARCD and is a beneficial supplement that supports cognitive health with aging."[1]

Researchers with the world-famous Framingham Heart Study have sung the praises of DHA. In a 2006 article published in the *Archives of Neurology*, they compared DHA levels in the bloodstream of subjects with and without Alzheimer's. They discovered that the risk of dementia and Alzheimer's disease in people with the highest levels of DHA was cut in half.[2]

Shouldn't we all be getting brain-protective amounts of DHA into our bodies?

WHAT OMEGA-3 EFAS DO AND WHY THEY ARE IMPORTANT

Omega-3 fatty acids support a broad range of functions in the brain and vascular system and represent a powerful resource for protection against—and even reversal of—cognitive decline. DHA and ALA are hardworking, versatile molecules that display a spectrum of neural support activities. They're kind of like a utility fielder who plays multiple positions on a baseball team—except they can play all the positions at once.

Omega-3 fatty acids serve two main purposes in the body: as building blocks for nerve cell walls and as precursors for neurotransmitters and inflammation-fighting chemicals called prostaglandins.

In the heart and cardiovascular system, omega-3s from DHA and FSO increase blood flow to the brain, reduce heart disease, and protect against vascular dementia by lowering LDL (bad) cholesterol while increasing HDL (good) cholesterol. They thin the blood (reducing clotting risk), prevent inflammation, lower blood pressure, and slow plaque buildup in the arteries.

In the immune system, omega-3s help block autoimmune inflammatory diseases like lupus, Sjögren's syndrome, psoriasis, ankylosing spondylitis, rheumatoid arthritis, fibromyalgia, Graves' disease, Hashimoto's thyroiditis, scleroderma, Addison's disease, celiac disease, and Crohn's disease.

In the brain, DHA and ALA stimulate BDNF, which spurs the growth of new dendritic spines, the projections from dendrites that "reach out" to connect with nearby neurons and grow the brain. DHA and ALA are thus deeply involved in the synaptic development and repair that nurture this aspect of brain plasticity.[3]

It is exciting that we have these easily obtained natural compounds—foods, no less—that can do so much to improve brain function. They help us think more clearly, do better on tests, handle stress better, do work more easily, and communicate better.

HOW DHA WORKS TO PREVENT AND REVERSE ALZHEIMER'S

In their extensive and illuminating review article in the *Journal of Nutrition*, Greg M. Cole and Sally A. Frautschy outline four main molecular mechanisms by which DHA slows and reverses AD and vascular dementia:

- First, DHA reduces the production of amyloid beta, the protein that forms the plaques intimately associated with AD.
- Second, DHA helps block the production of tau protein, the main component of neurofibrillary tangles.
- Third, DHA slows neuroinflammation and oxidative damage. It is a potent antioxidant and anti-inflammatory, so it decreases levels of lipid peroxides and reduces oxidative and ischemic damage in neurons, the factors that contribute to loss of synapses, neuronal dysfunction, and dementia.
- Last, but not least, DHA reduces the major pro-inflammatory (omega-6) fatty acid, arachidonic acid, the fatty acid that is converted into pro-inflammatory prostaglandins that promote AD.[4]

EFAS WORK HARD TO PREVENT AND
REVERSE ALZHEIMER'S

Probably the most important thing you need to know about DHA and ALA is that they increase brain levels of BDNF.

DHA levels in the body are highly negatively correlated with dementia risk; in other words, people with higher DHA levels are less likely to become demented.[5] When consumed in the early stages of a neurodegenerative disorder, DHA will slow and reverse the cognitive decline and block the progression to dementia.[6]

When neuropathologists aim their microscopes at the brains of people who have consumed a diet rich in omega-3 EFAs, they see more nerve cell connections and fewer amyloid beta plaques. Brains from people with low levels of omega-3 EFAs in their blood and brain, on the other hand, have fewer connections between nerve cells, more plaque, and more cognitive impairment.

Researchers have shown that both exercise and DHA, separately, will enhance BDNF and neuroplasticity, improve cognitive function, promote neuroplasticity, and protect against neurodegenerative disease. But are these separate effects (and therefore not additive) or two different causes for the same effect (additive)? To get the answer, Aiguo Wu and his team at UCLA studied rats that were getting exercise; they gave DHA to some of them and none to a control group. The researchers stated the problem this way: "In this study, we investigated a possible synergistic action between DHA dietary supplementation and voluntary exercise on modulating synaptic plasticity and cognition." Maybe they were wondering if they could get their brain enhancement effect from DHA supplementation and slack off on their exercise program. The results showed a clear additive effect: the DHA-enriched diet enhanced the effects of exercise on cognition and BDNF-related synaptoplasticity, learning, and memory.[7] (I am going to assume the researchers didn't quit their gym memberships.) Bottom line: do both.

DHA from Seafood: Not Recommended

Fish are the best-known and most readily available source of the all-important DHA. Unfortunately, consuming seafood, even in small amounts, is not at all a good idea because sea animals spend their entire lives soaking in a vast methylmercury bathtub (a.k.a. the world's oceans). Their tissues are thoroughly saturated with one of the most neurotoxic substances known to science. Because our bodies are unable to remove mercury, it bioaccumulates. It is toxic at the level of a single atom. A safe level of methylmercury has never been established, and there is no scientific reason to believe a safe level exists. Zero is the only safe level.

Beyond mercury, seafood often contains brain-damaging levels of dioxin, PCBs (polychlorinated biphenyls), and other toxins.

My personal diet does not contain any seafood. I recommend you follow my example for the sake of your brain—and if you're a pregnant woman, for the sake of your unborn child's brain.

Winds and water currents mix the seas well, so the mercury is evenly distributed. The notion that some area of the sea has been spared is ludicrous. Nonetheless, creative marketers have conjured slick labels suggesting otherwise: "Arctic," "wild," "North Sea," "Alaskan," and "Nordic" are misleading and meaningless hogwash. Don't be fooled. Some fish are more toxic than others, but none is mercury-free. I don't want a little poison. I want none at all.

The "Arctic" moniker is particularly troubling. Recent research has shown that global weather currents have turned the earth into a kind of mercury distillery, concentrating mercury in the Arctic such that over 2.2 billion pounds (a million cubic meters of pure liquid mercury) has been sequestered in the Arctic ice cap permafrost. According to research published in the journal *Geophysical Research Letters*, the amount of mercury bound up in this way is about ten times greater than all the mercury humans have pumped into the atmosphere from coal burning and other pollution sources over the last thirty years.[8] Global warming is melting this vast mercury reservoir, dumping enormous quantities into the earth's oceans.

You will have no trouble finding platoons of doctors who recommend eating fish and feel the benefits of the DHA content outweigh the adverse effects of the mercury. Unfortunately, they are dead wrong; they haven't examined the evidence and thought it through. Mercury, like ionizing radiation, is toxic at the atomic level—orders of magnitude more toxic than substances such as the pesticides and BPA that we now routinely avoid.

Here is how mercury sabotages the formation of nerve cells, leaving neurofibrillary tangles (NFTs) in its wake. In the synthesis of tubulin (the protein that links together to form the support structure for our nerve cells), just *one mercury atom* can abort the DNA-programmed synthesis of tau protein molecules, thus preventing tubulin proteins from linking together in a linear sequence to form the tubular structure. The tubular structure disintegrates into free tubulin molecules, which then reassemble in a scrambled manner, forming the NFTs so intimately associated with neurodegenerative conditions such as AD.

In fetuses of mothers consuming mercury, this metabolic nightmare provides a springboard for developmental brain defects, spina bifida, ADHD, and autism. Because the fetal brain is assembling microtubules at an incredible rate, the toxic effects of mercury are magnified, so it is especially important that pregnant moms steer clear of fish.

All the studies of the adverse effects of mercury have been short term, but humans live a long time, and extended exposure has never been examined. Also, the effects of mercury on the human microbiome have not been studied, but it is safe to assume that those effects are substantial and that mercury would favor the growth of pathogens over the health-promoting probiotic species.

For more information about mercury and other neurotoxic metals, please see chapter 18.

OPTIMIZING YOUR OMEGA-3S

Use the lists provided below to enrich your diet with the highest possible omega-3 content.

Flaxseeds, walnuts, chia seeds, and hemp seeds are great sources of omega-3s. Leafy green vegetables and cruciferous vegetables have a surprising amount of omega-3s: cauliflower, broccoli, Brussels sprouts, cabbage, arugula, bok choy, Chinese cabbage, collard greens, radish, daikon radish, horseradish, kale, kohlrabi, and mustard greens are all good choices.

All berries are a good source of omega-3 EFAs, as are mangos and honeydew melons.

Beans, seeds, and nuts are great choices when you're trying to consume more omega-3s.

Winter squash is a surprisingly good source of omega-3s.

Virtually all common herbs and spices contain significant amounts of EFAs.

HOW TO USE EFA SUPPLEMENTS

Diet alone will not supply optimum amounts of EFAs. ALA and DHA are the two main EFAs you'll need to take as supplements.

The ALA in flaxseed oil is an omega-3 oil from which our cells can manufacture small amounts of DHA. Our genetic program makes an enzyme that converts dietary ALA to DHA (it also converts DHA to EPA). But our body's ability to make this enzyme slowly declines as we age—so in the years when we need DHA the most, we are making very little of it.

Two strategies can get around this obstacle, and because DHA is so important for scaling the heights of cognitive performance and dementia prevention, I recommend both. One is to increase your daily dose of flaxseed oil. You'll find no better source of omega-3s, and your body will convert some of the oil's ALA into DHA. The liquid is easier to take, a tablespoon contains over 7 grams of omega 3s, and it disappears into lots of different foods, such as soups, smoothies, and salad dressings. Take 1–3 tablespoons a day. Flaxseed oil can be taken anytime and can be added to any food. The only proviso is that the ALA in FSO is sensitive to temperatures above the boiling point of water, so you can't fry or bake with it. But you can stir it into or pour it on foods that have been cooked and are cooling.

Flaxseed oil will get you only part of the way to optimum DHA levels, so you will need to supplement with algae-derived (and therefore mercury-free) DHA in capsules. The high-quality product I use is Neuromins (Cardiovascular Research); one capsule contains 100 mg

DHA. The daily dose for people with a good memory who want to keep it that way is 800–1,500 mg/day. For individuals who have mild to moderate cognitive impairment, the dose needs to be higher, 1,500–2,000 mg daily.

CHAPTER 29

Curcumin: The Secret to India's Low Alzheimer's Rate?

ndia has a spectacularly low incidence of Alzheimer's disease. Indians are about one-tenth as likely as Americans to get the disease.

What's their secret?

Many believe it is the curcumin in the turmeric used in curries and other spicy Indian dishes. It's omnipresent in India, a staple in the Indian curry-based diet.

Turmeric (*Curcuma longa*), a plant of the ginger family, is the most popular spice in Indian cooking. In addition to being used in large quantities in daily cuisine, turmeric is also used as a preservative, coloring agent, and medicine. Curcumin is the phytonutrient molecule in turmeric that gives the root its distinctive orange-yellow hue.

Curcumin is a polyphenol (see chapter 24) that shares antioxidant, anti-inflammatory, and antidementia properties with similar compounds in grapes (resveratrol), green tea (catechins), chocolate (cocoa), blueberries (pterostilbene), strawberries, and pomegranates. Considered a "cleanser of the body," curcumin has been used for centuries in Ayurvedic medicine to reduce pain and inflammation. Modern science has embraced curcumin's molecular biological medicinal effects. Curcumin is one of the most thoroughly researched botanicals in the biomedical literature, the focus of more than fourteen thousand journal articles to date. Many of the studies strongly support its role in the prevention and reversal of Alzheimer's, Parkinson's, and other neuro-degenerative diseases.[1]

In addition, curcumin has demonstrated effectiveness in treating the following disorders:

- Arthritis (all types)
- Cardiovascular disease
- Indigestion or dyspepsia
- High cholesterol and LDL
- Cancer, including prostate, breast, skin, and colon cancer
- Bloating and gas
- Ulcerative colitis
- Bacterial and viral infections
- Uveitis

CURCUMIN BLOCKS INFLAMMATION

Curcumin may be helpful in any medical situation where inflammation is part of the problem. That's a big deal, because inflammation causes or contributes to just about every major chronic disease, including cardiovascular disease, diabetes, cancer, depression, autoimmune diseases, arthritis, and, of course, dementia.

Curcumin suppresses inflammatory triggers for Alzheimer's disease, in effect acting as a master switch that turns inflammation off by blocking the biosynthesis of several key pro-inflammatory chemicals.

The chemistry of chronic inflammation is very complex. To oversimplify, a signaling protein called tumor necrosis factor alpha (TNFα) plays a huge role in driving most inflammation. Pharmaceutical drugs that block or inhibit TNFα are used to treat autoimmune disease, inflammatory bowel disease, psoriasis, rheumatoid arthritis, ankylosing spondylitis, and many other inflammatory diseases. Because these drugs cause serious side effects and toxicity, the price of using them is high. Curcumin lowers TNFα without the side effects or adverse reactions caused by these drugs.

CURCUMIN PREVENTS AND REVERSES DEMENTIA

Curcumin enhances cognitive functioning, learning, and memory.

In animal studies, curcumin supplements given even after the onset of Alzheimer's-like symptoms result in improved performance on mazes and reduction of mistakes on memory-dependent tasks. When the brains of these animals were examined, they demonstrated significantly reduced cell death in hippocampal (memory-processing) areas. No drug has these kinds of effects.

Curcumin prevents and reverses dementia through several mechanisms. First, it enhances neurogenesis, the repair of damaged nerve cells and the growth of new ones from stem cells.[2] Inflammation plays a key role in causing and perpetuating Alzheimer's and other neurodegenerative disorders. Curcumin exerts powerful anti-inflammatory effects that have been shown to reverse Alzheimer's.[3]

Next, curcumin removes amyloid beta plaque. Not everyone is afforded the unique opportunity of working with demented mice— expensive rodents that have been genetically engineered to develop early Alzheimer's. Their brains become loaded with amyloid beta plaque, just like that of a human with advanced Alzheimer's disease. These mice come in handy as an experimental model to study dementia.

One research group did enjoy this option, however, and they designed a study in which they gave curcumin to these so-called amyloid precursor protein (APP) mice. After just one week, the researchers observed plaque size reduction.[4] Numerous research studies have corroborated this effect and have shown it works in humans as well. (Researchers used doses that were the human equivalent of 4–8 grams a day. These doses in human patients are safe and produce no toxic effects.)

Curcumin demonstrates activity at several stages in the development of amyloid beta plaque. APPs aggregate to form oligomers, which quickly coalesce into amyloid fibrils and are then incorporated into amyloid plaque. Curcumin passes through the blood-brain barrier into the brain, where it gets busy preventing the formation of oligomers and amyloid beta fibrils. It also binds to and destroys preexisting amyloid beta plaques and dissolves any free amyloid protein molecules (prior to forming plaques) in the brain.[5] This remarkable combination of effects, especially active in the hippocampus, reverses the Alzheimer's disease process throughout the brain. Then curcumin takes one final, fabulous step: it rescues nerve cells from further toxic damage by commanding local macrophages (your body's natural cleanup cells) to increase their rate of phagocytosis (eating unwanted junk) to quickly chew up the broken pieces of amyloid beta plaque before they can be reassembled into plaque.

These three properties—removal, cleanup, and prevention—push curcumin to the top of the dementia protection and treatment program list. In animal studies, curcumin increased cognitive function and decreased amyloid deposits by around 40 percent.

Mitochondria are the tiny power plants in every cell that provide the energy necessary for that cell to do its job. Internal oxidation can damage and destroy mitochondria, setting the stage for neurodegenerative disease. Curcumin, a powerful antioxidant, scavenges dangerous oxygen free radicals inside mitochondria, protecting them from damage.[6]

Curcumin's antioxidant and free radical scavenging properties are estimated to be more powerful than those of vitamin E. Curcumin inhibits lipid peroxidation better than vitamin E and therefore is able to protect against neurotoxic and genotoxic agents that promote dementia.

Curcumin also protects against vascular dementia by improving the bioavailability of nitric oxide, a molecule required for healthy functioning of blood vessels.

CURCUMIN BIOAVAILABILITY ISSUES

Moving curcumin from the spice jar and into your brain tissues is a dicey proposition for several reasons. Curcumin is rapidly metabolized and rapidly eliminated by the body. Curcumin is not soluble in water and is poorly absorbed from the gut unless it is delivered with a fat. Traditionally, this absorption problem was solved when turmeric was cooked in ghee, coconut oil, or some other fat as a part of a curry.

This creates a liposomal delivery system in which the curcumin molecule is bundled inside a fat globule, a form in which curcumin can be easily absorbed through the intestinal wall.

For centuries, people had no idea they were automatically creating a liposomal delivery system when they dumped turmeric, with some oil, into their stir-fries. To be able to put an absorbable form of curcumin into a capsule, scientists have tackled the issue by developing advanced liposomal formulations to improve curcumin's bioavailability.

Avoid curcumin products that are simply powdered curcumin or turmeric powder stuffed into a capsule. Regardless of product claims, these are not going to be successfully absorbed. For the same reason, it is futile to sprinkle turmeric on food. The herb will not be absorbed unless it has been heated with an oil. This requires cooking with it or purchasing a product that has processed the curcumin before encapsulation.

NEW PRODUCTS AND CREATIVE DELIVERY SYSTEMS

The bioavailability problem has generated numerous attempts to enhance curcumin delivery. Proprietary "liposomal delivery system" products have been developed in which the curcumin has been pre-cooked in oil and then put into capsules. Meriva is one such product. This is curcumin complexed with soy phosphatidylcholine (a fat) that optimizes absorption and delivers curcumin's anti-inflammatory effects directly into body tissues.

But Meriva is not pure curcumin; it is a downstream metabolite, and some researchers maintain that only pure curcumin is able to pass through the blood-brain barrier and get to the brain to work against Alzheimer's disease. Others maintain curcumin is a pleitrophic molecule, which means it is medicinally effective in several molecular forms, including downstream metabolites.

A new product, Longvida, was developed to solve the possible problem of brain bioavailability. (I say "possible" because Indians, experimental animals, and others had been benefitting from curcumin cooked in oil long before Longvida or Meriva arrived on the scene.) Longvida encapsulates the curcumin to protect it from hydrolyzing enzymes in the upper digestive system, thus maintaining its original chemical structure and preventing transformation into downstream metabolites. It's supposedly the only product shown in research studies to deliver pure curcumin directly to the brain and therefore to be effective for the prevention and treatment of Alzheimer's. However, no one has done a study comparing Longvida to Meriva or other forms of curcumin in terms of ability to cross the blood-brain barrier.

Meriva, Longvida, and cooked curcumin all work. If you can fit it into your busy schedule, I think getting some of your curcumin the old-fashioned way, by cooking it with coconut oil and some pepper (the piperidine in pepper enhances absorption) is a very good idea.

HOW I GET MY CURCUMIN

Most mornings, I fry up two eggs in 1–2 tablespoons of coconut oil. I sprinkle a teaspoon of turmeric powder and black pepper into the hot oil before adding the eggs. This makes a delicious ketogenic dish. I also usually cook up some vegetables in a separate frying pan (with a little butter or more coconut oil) to eat along with my "eggs curcumin."

To increase my curcumin intake, I sometimes add powdered turmeric when cooking meat and vegetable stir-fries. Our family also frequently enjoys Indian curry dishes. If I don't get enough of the herb in my cooked food, I will make sure to take Meriva or Longvida curcumin supplements that day.

HOW TO USE CURCUMIN

Like most Alzheimer's treatments, curcumin is most likely to succeed if started early in the disease process because the brain begins to deteriorate years or even decades before full-blown dementia occurs.

Optimum curcumin dosing depends on where one is on the cognitive decline spectrum. To prevent cognitive decline before it has begun, I recommend at least 1,000–2,000 mg of curcumin a day. For established dementia, the safe, reasonable, and therapeutically effective dose range is 2–8 grams of curcumin a day. No side effects or adverse reactions have been observed at these doses. You can achieve your target dose using any combination of fresh cooked (in coconut or olive oil) and commercial versions (Meriva, Longvida).

CHAPTER 30

Green Tea: Jack-of-All-Trades

If you were looking for a health food that is a jack-of-all-trades, my vote would go to green tea, a flavorful drink consumed by billions. Green tea is the second most consumed beverage in the world (after water). Depending on how you look at it, green tea is simultaneously a simple ancient drink, a cultural tradition, and a phytochemical-rich nutritional medicinal bonanza that protects the aging brain and reduces the incidence of all dementia, including Alzheimer's and Parkinson's.[1]

Research tells us that green tea can fix just about anything. It reverses cardiovascular disease, lowers blood pressure and cholesterol, defends against insulin resistance and stabilizes blood sugar levels, blocks cancer, and fights obesity. It even blocks autoimmune diseases. So it shouldn't come as a great surprise that green tea consumption has been associated with dramatic reductions in the risk of developing cognitive decline.[2]

Green tea is prepared from dried leaves of *Camellia sinensis*, a small perennial evergreen shrub grown mainly in China, Japan, and Southeast Asia. Green tea contains several compounds beneficial to brain health, including caffeine, various catechins (polyphenols), and L-theanine (an amino acid derivative), but EGCG (epigallocatechin gallate) is the major catechin constituent, accounting for more than 10 percent of the dry weight.

HOW GREEN TEA IMPROVES COGNITION

High levels of EGCG are responsible for much of green tea's anti-Alzheimer's effects. EGCG is the most prominent polyphenol in green tea. It's a profound antioxidant that can also be found in cocoa, blackberries, raspberries, cherries, purple grapes, and beans. EGCG increases brain blood flow, lowers blood pressure, and reduces the risk of cardiovascular disease, cancer, obesity, and periodontal disease.

Black and oolong teas, though they also originate from the leaves of *Camellia sinensis*, exert a much weaker effect, probably because they contain much smaller amounts of EGCG.

EGCG protects neurons by simultaneously manipulating multiple brain targets.[3] EGCG physically blocks the assembly of amyloid beta proteins, preventing them from clumping together to form those nasty plaques so intimately associated with the impairment and death of brain cells in Alzheimer's disease. If some amyloid plaque has already been deposited in the brain, EGCG can break it down and remove it.[4]

EGCG is a busy little chemical. It upregulates the antioxidant defense system by binding to transcription factors, chemicals that play a large role in the epigenetic regulation of genes. EGCG also blocks the action of NF-kB, a chemical known to cause production of pro-inflammatory chemicals. EGCG scavenges neuroinflammation-causing oxygen free radicals, chelates metals, improves communication between cells, turns on cell survival genes, and enhances mitochondrial function.[5]

That's quite a bag of tricks—all especially useful for preventing and reversing Alzheimer's.

HOW TO USE GREEN TEA

Green tea is available loose or in bags. A typical cup of brewed green tea (200 mL) contains 40–60 mg of caffeine (decaf is okay too), 8–25 mg of L-theanine, and 25–200 mg of catechins.

Green tea supplements are available in pills, capsules, liquid, and powder. I take the capsules on the days I'm not guzzling tea.

For more about polyphenols and their powerful antidementia effects, see chapter 24.

CHAPTER 31

Citicoline: Potent Stroke Protection

Citicoline (cytidine 5'-diphosphocholine, also known as CDP-choline) is a safe, effective, bioidentical food-derived brain-function enhancer with extensive research support and clinical experience. Citicoline is about as natural as it gets. It is derived from a B-complex vitamin, choline. Most of us don't get enough choline in our diet, but even minor deficiencies can lead to mental impairment.

Your brain makes citicoline, the immediate biochemical precursor of your brain's main neurotransmitter, acetylcholine (ACh). Taking supplemental citicoline increases levels of ACh, dopamine, and norepinephrine throughout the central nervous system. This may explain why many users report that citicoline lowers their overall stress levels and generates a feeling of general well-being.

Citicoline serves dual functions in nerve cells. First, it provides the raw material from which nerve cells build (or repair) their cell walls. Second, and equally important, citicoline can be converted directly into several of the brain's neurotransmitters (the chemicals that transmit messages from one nerve to the next by jumping across the synapse, the gap between nerve cells) as shown in figure 31.1. As a measure of how important these two functions are, it is safe to say that all brain function—including memory, cognition, and even consciousness—would come to a screeching halt if we suddenly became unable to make nerve cell walls and ACh.

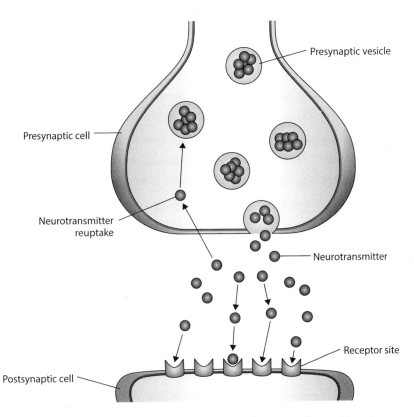

Figure 31.1 Neurons synthesizing acetylcholine from citicoline. ACh is then released from the presynaptic cell axon and travels across the synapse to stimulate receptors on dendrites of the postsynaptic cell.

Citicoline has a long track record of safely and successfully enhancing memory, learning, logical reasoning, and ability to focus. With the improved bioavailability of ACh made possible by citicoline, anyone's brain will perform more efficiently.

Supplemental citicoline not only accelerates the synthesis of ACh but also boosts production of three other important brain phospholipids: phosphatidylcholine, phosphatidylethanolamine, and phosphatidylserine. These also act as both cell membrane material and as neurotransmitter precursors.

Acetylcholine, the neurotransmitter of memory and cognition, protects those areas of the brain most vulnerable to dementia: the hippocampus, cingulate gyrus, and cortex. Increased ACh also improves synaptoplasticity—the ability of synapses to strengthen or weaken over time in response to increases or decreases in their activity. This supercharges the speed of memory, recall, and learning.

In this chapter, we are going to focus on the extensive use of citicoline in the treatment of neurodegenerative disorders associated with head trauma, stroke, brain aging, cerebrovascular pathology, and Alzheimer's disease.

CITICOLINE TO THE RESCUE

We've all known people who have an uncanny ability to quickly spot what needs to be done next and then just jump in and do it. My buddy Paul is one of those people. He would identify high-risk situations— such as accidents about to happen—that needed quick intervention long before anyone else would notice. He'd quickly step in and apply the appropriate remedy. He wouldn't stop to ask questions; he immediately knew what needed to be done—and he'd go ahead and do it. Then, just as abruptly, expecting no praise, compliment, or reward, he'd slip back into the background, having headed off a disaster.

Citicoline is like a mini-Paul inside of us—always on the lookout for problems, identifying and locating neurons that need repair. When it spots them, it quickly moves in and rebuilds, revamps, renovates, and repairs the broken part or renews the damaged structural component.

Citicoline is the raw material used for making much of the outer membrane that covers nerve cells, including the ends of the axons called synaptic vesicles that make and release acetylcholine neurotransmitter molecules. And, as you know, citicoline is also just one step away from becoming ACh. When it finishes rebuilding a broken nerve cell, fixing a defective synapse, or beefing up dendritic spine production (this happens in microseconds), citicoline, like Paul, fades into the background, ready for more action whenever and wherever needed.

On a cellular level, these repair situations arise at rates that stagger the imagination. Millions of times a second or more, neurons are damaged and quickly restored by citicoline.

CITICOLINE ENHANCES NEUROTRANSMITTER PRODUCTION

Our bodies make their own citicoline, but dementia patients—and even individuals experiencing mild memory problems and early cognitive decline—can't make acetylcholine and other related brain phospholipids fast enough to supply optimum requirements. Creative nutritional biochemists figured out a way to speed up production: giving ACh's immediate precursor, citicoline, dramatically accelerates the body's rate of ACh synthesis. This provides a quick, effective, sustained increase in ACh production.

Alzheimer's disease and age-related cognitive decline are characterized by a widespread loss of acetylcholine in the brain. Billions of dollars have been spent on research to find a patentable drug that will help reverse some of the symptoms of the disease by restoring ACh availability at receptor sites. Several such drugs have been developed, but every one of them—besides being completely unnatural and toxic—has failed to work.

But wait: citicoline—a natural medication that restores ACh availability—already exists. Why not use that? The answer is that because the human body makes citicoline, it fits the definition of *natural*, and natural is not patentable and therefore not profitable.

CITICOLINE IMPROVES MENTAL ENERGY

Individuals who take supplemental citicoline often report that their overall brain function seems enhanced. Users note improved mental energy—an increase in attention span, focus, and concentration as well as greater motivation and vitality. This makes sense because increased ACh not only increases neurotransmitter production (especially norepinephrine and dopamine), but also enhances brain blood circulation (cerebral perfusion), which increases oxygen uptake and glucose metabolism. Together, these translate into improved communication between neurons, lowered stress levels, and a general feeling of well-being. My patients remark, "It's as if my brain is communicating better with itself." I tell them that's because with citicoline, it actually is.

Improved mental energy is nice, and feeling good is great, but the vascular benefits of citicoline go far deeper. Citicoline repairs and enhances blood flow to the small vessels of the brain, the ones most likely to be blocked in a stroke.

TIMELY CITICOLINE ADMINISTRATION REDUCES STROKE SIZE, HEALING TIME, AND RESIDUAL DAMAGE

Stroke increases the probability of dementia. Citicoline has proven its value in prevention and treatment of stroke.[1] In fact, citicoline is the only substance ever shown to have a significant neuroprotective effect in patients who have suffered mild to moderate strokes. Taking citicoline after a stroke reduces the size of the stroke lesions as seen on MRIs. Patients experience a decrease of neurologic deficits and improvement in learning, memory, and behavioral performance. The sooner after a stroke the citicoline is begun, the more effective it is.

Here's a fact that all cardiologists and neurologists should be aware of and implement in their clinical practice: stroke patients given citicoline, 500–2,000 mg/day orally within twenty-four hours of acute ischemic stroke, are more likely to have a complete recovery within three months compared to patients given a placebo.[2]

Also, intravenous citicoline, 500 mg within twelve hours of the appearance of ischemic stroke symptoms and then daily for seven days thereafter, improves symptoms, speeds healing, and reduces the risk of subsequent dementia when compared to a group not treated with citicoline.[3]

Overall, patients who receive citicoline have significantly reduced rates of death and disability following an ischemic stroke. Citicoline accomplishes this by intervening with a multiplicity of mechanisms at several stages. It enhances neurotransmitter production by repairing the outer nerve cell wall and protecting the membranes that surround its organelles (mitochondria, nucleus, lysosomes, Golgi apparatus, etc.).[4]

When strokes happen, much of the damage is caused by the loss of blood supply to local nerve cell tissues. We call this *ischemic* damage. Citicoline intervenes and protects the injured tissue against early and delayed mechanisms responsible for ischemic brain injury. Citicoline also enhances the circulation of blood to the entire brain, and—as a potent free radical scavenger—protects against the oxidative stress that would slow healing.[5]

Citicoline has one final trick up its sleeve for strokes. It accelerates neurorepair by enhancing synaptic outgrowth and dendritic spine density. This promotes neuroplasticity in stroke-damaged tissues.[6] For all the above reasons, citicoline for stroke patients decreases residual neurologic deficits (loss of arm or tongue or eye control, for example) and improves poststroke behavioral performance, learning, and memory.[7]

Why aren't all doctors who treat stroke (family physicians, internists, cardiologists, neurologists) using citicoline for their stroke patients? Their counterparts in Europe and Asia certainly find it effective.

CITICOLINE BLOCKS STROKE RECURRENCE

Beyond speeding up healing and reducing residual stroke damage, citicoline blocks ischemic strokes, thus reducing the likelihood of a recurrence.[8] I certainly wish I had known about citicoline's stroke-protective effects prior to December 2012 when I had a small stroke (see chapter 7). When I first learned about citicoline in 2014 (while conducting research for this book), I started taking it immediately and have taken it ever since.

Citicoline might have prevented my stroke because it actually locates and identifies defects in neurons and neurotransmitters—and then it repairs them!

Paul would approve.

PRODUCTS AND DOSE

Citicoline is marketed as a supplement in over seventy countries under a variety of brand names: Cognizin, Ceraxon, NeurAxon, Somazina, and Synapsine.

Citicoline is usually sold as 250 mg capsules. Typical dosing would be 500–2,000 mg (two to eight 250 mg capsules) per day of citicoline (CDP-choline).

HOW TO USE CITICOLINE

Citicoline occurs naturally in the human body and has an extremely low-toxicity profile.

Pregnant and breast-feeding women should avoid taking this supplement because we do not have enough information at this point to determine its safety for this group.

Oral citicoline is generally well-tolerated with no known interactions with herbs, supplements, drugs, or foods. Adverse reactions and side effects are virtually absent when used at the recommended dose range of 500–2,000 mg a day.

CHAPTER 32

Bacopa: Botanical Brain Booster

What do Vedic scholars, Australian researchers, and Dr. Mehmet Oz have in common? They all believe that *Bacopa monnieri* enhances memory, attention, and cognition.

Bacopa monnieri (also known as water hyssop) is a creeping perennial with small oblong leaves and purple flowers native to the warm wetlands of Australia and India. It is commonly found as a weed in rice fields and grows throughout East Asia and the United States.

Bacopa monnieri is an herb used widely in Ayurveda, the ancient Indian system of medicine, to rejuvenate intellect and heighten memory. Indian texts dating as far back as the sixth century classify it as *medhya rasayana*, medicinal plants that support and enhance cognitive health.[1]

Known then as Brahmi (after Brahma, the Hindu god of creation), Bacopa was recommended to "sharpen the intellect and attenuate mental deficits." Ancient Vedic scholars used it to facilitate the memorization of lengthy sacred hymns and scriptures.[2] Bacopa is frequently found in traditional Ayurvedic preparations prescribed for cognitive dysfunction, where it is often combined with other intellect-sharpening herbs such as *Centella asiatica* (gotu kola).

BACOPA ENHANCES SYNAPTOPLASTICITY

Bacopa has been extensively researched and shown to exert a diverse array of antidementia effects. In an extensive 2017 review of

Bacopa's remarkable neurocognitive effects published in the *Annals of Neurosciences*, K. S. Chaudhari and colleagues outline its multiple neuroprotective effects and discuss the molecular biological mechanisms behind its antidementia effect. Bacopa reduces amyloid beta deposition in the hippocampus and shields it from oxidation and stress-induced damage, thus improving memory and providing powerful protection against Alzheimer's disease.[3]

Venkata Ramana Vollala of the Department of Anatomy at the Rajiv Gandhi Institute of Medical Sciences in India and colleagues gave Bacopa to lab rats for six weeks. The herb significantly bolstered spatial learning and memory retention. Microscopic examination of the memory areas of the neurons in the Bacopa-treated rats revealed impressive increases in the number, length, and complexity of dendritic branching points. The researchers concluded that constituents in *Bacopa monnieri* extract "have neuronal dendritic growth-stimulating properties."[4] In other words, the herb enhances synaptoplacticity.

RESEARCH-PROVEN MEMORY AND COGNITION ENHANCEMENT

Traditionally used for a variety of ailments, Bacopa is best known as a neural tonic that improves just about every aspect of brain function. Several randomized, double-blind, placebo-controlled trials have substantiated the herb's value as a nootropic (memory and cognition enhancement) agent in humans. In these studies, people who consumed Bacopa over periods of months demonstrated multiple cognitive benefits, including a reduction in the rate of forgetting newly learned information and an enhanced ability to retain new information.[5] The herb also improved mood and reduced depression and anxiety.[6]

Research evidence strongly suggests the herb's potential for protection from dementia, Parkinson's disease, and epilepsy. One Australian research group examined Bacopa's effect on cognitive function in healthy humans. In a double-blind, placebo-controlled study, subjects were randomly allocated to one of two groups. Group A received *Bacopa monnieri* (as KeenMind, 300 mg daily). Group B received a placebo. The Bacopa group demonstrated a significantly improved speed of visual information processing, learning rate, and memory compared to the placebo group, with maximal effects evident after twelve weeks. The researchers concluded that "*B. monnieri* may improve higher order cognitive processes that are critically dependent on the input of information from our environment such as learning and memory."[7]

Of possible interest to individuals with ADHD, Bacopa enhanced subjects' ability to ignore irrelevant information and increased their attention time. Other studies have shown that Bacopa improves cortisol responses, prevents synaptic decline, eases anxiety, and helps people focus better in stressful situations.[8]

HOW DOES IT WORK?

Bacopa exhibits tranquilizing and antioxidant properties.

A standardized Bacopa extract contains about thirty different chemicals that support learning, cognition, and memory by promoting neuronal health and efficient nerve impulse transmission. Bacopa exerts both short- and long-term beneficial cognitive effects using multiple neuromolecular metabolic mechanisms, including antioxidant neuroprotection, neurotransmitter modulation, reduction in the production of amyloid beta, and an increase in blood flow to the brain.[9]

In terms of short-term changes that prevent and reverse Alzheimer's, Bacopa inhibits acetylcholinesterase (that is, it blocks the breakdown of acetylcholine), activates choline acetyltransferase (this increases the synthesis of acetylcholine), reduces amyloid beta, increases cerebral blood flow, and regulates the activity of several neurotransmitters (acetylcholine, 5-hydroxytryptamine, and dopamine).[10]

Bacopa's longer-term effects have to do with enhanced synaptic remodeling, prevention of synaptic decline, and enhanced hippocampal memory center function. These cognitive benefits require more time because new dendrites must grow, and this takes six to twelve weeks.[11]

In 2013, researchers Sebastian Aguiar and Thomas Borowski published a neuropharmacological review and extensive analysis of the molecular biological mechanisms at work in the cognitive-enhancing action of *Bacopa monnieri*. Aguiar and Borowski summarize their findings by stating,

> BM [*Bacopa monnieri*] demonstrates immense potential in the amelioration of cognitive disorders, as well as prophylactic reduction of oxidative damage, [NT neurotransmitter] modulation, and cognitive enhancement in healthy people. . . . The social implications of cognition-enhancing drugs are promising but must be appropriately tempered with ethical consideration as researchers enter the brave new world of neural enhancement.[12]

All this, and no toxicity.

HOW TO USE BACOPA

A typical dosage is 300–1,000 mg per day.

As an important piece of my personal brain protection program, I take 600 mg of Bacopa every day.

CHAPTER 33

Phosphatidylserine: Guarding against Cognitive Decline

Phosphatidylserine (PS) is a fatty acid made by our brains that plays key roles in neuronal health and brain energy production. Taking a soy-derived PS supplement is a powerful way for all of us to put the kibosh on ARCD, the gradual erosion that occurs in an aging brain. In effect, PS switches on a light bulb in your brain. It renews aging brain cells and rejuvenates memory, alertness, and overall mental performance.

The discovery of PS is an exciting development in the study of dementia. Clinical PS studies have shown that supplementation not only prevents but also reverses age-related memory loss and Alzheimer's disease.[1] That's a bold claim, but a ton of research backs it up.

A youthful brain makes plenty of PS, but production declines with advancing age, and the aging brain is particularly sensitive to low levels. An older person with impaired mental function and depression almost certainly has a PS deficiency, and this is associated with common age-related conditions. Supplementing PS reverses the symptoms.

As Elizabeth Somer explains in her book *Food & Mood*, "PS supplements restock brain cell membranes, boosting nerve chemical activity such as dopamine and serotonin, stimulating nerve cell growth, lowering levels of the stress hormones, generating new connections between cells, and stirring activity in all brain centers, especially higher brain centers such as the cortex, hypothalamus, and pituitary gland."[2]

Research focusing on PS has yielded results that are nothing short of astonishing. This nutrient rejuvenates just about every function controlled by the central nervous system. PS supplementation helps regenerate stressed-out or damaged nerve cells, actually reversing defects in nerve cell message transmission.

Phosphatidylserine expert and author Professor Parris Kidd, who reviewed more than three thousand peer-reviewed research papers on PS, calls it "the single best means for conserving memory and other higher brain functions as we age."[3]

HOW PS WORKS

PS is a naturally occurring "good fat." Technically, it's a phospholipid—a fat with a phosphate group attached, derived from essential fatty acids. Membranes, the work surfaces of our cells, are composed of a double layer of phospholipid molecules. Vital phospholipids such as PS can be found in the membranes of all cells, but PS is especially concentrated in the membranes of the brain's nerve cells, where its primary role is to facilitate the transmission of chemical messages from one brain cell to other nearby brain cells.

PS also plays a major role in determining the integrity and fluidity of brain cell membranes. As part of the membrane, PS works to eliminate waste and improve intercellular communications, cellular movement, and ion transport.

In young people the brain can manufacture sufficient levels of PS, but as we get older, or if we have a deficiency of B-complex vitamins (such as folic acid and B12) or of essential fatty acids, the brain may not be able to make sufficient PS.

PREVENTION OF AGE-RELATED COGNITIVE DECLINE

PS benefits those brain functions that tend to decline with age: memory, learning, vocabulary skills, concentration, mood, alertness, and sociability. PS has also been shown to improve adrenal functioning and stress tolerance. Clinical research indicates that PS is a premier candidate for inclusion in any program aimed at supporting cognitive function and preventing cognitive decline. Students, professionals, seniors—practically anyone interested in maintaining and maximizing their mental abilities, and improving stress tolerance, can benefit from taking PS.[4] An essential building block of nerve cell membranes, PS stimulates membrane repair and drives brain cell growth and communication. These are the mechanisms by which it slows, halts, or even reverses structural damage in our brains.

For many years, doctors experienced in nutrition and anti-aging medicine have prescribed PS to keep brains young and healthy by blocking ARCD.[5]

Several clinical trials involving thousands of subjects have demonstrated that PS fine-tunes the brain's biochemical environment, effectively halting and even reversing the progressive cognitive degeneration that results in ARCD, senility, and dementia. In a comprehensive report that summarizes twenty-seven double-blind studies—over fifteen years of research—in the use of PS in the treatment of memory loss, cognitive decline, and the brain deterioration of early Alzheimer's disease, Georges Ramalanjaona examined the best current evidence on the role of PS in the treatment of Alzheimer's disease, depressive states, and age-related memory loss involving more than one thousand patients. Ramalanjaona focused specifically on typical age-associated memory loss commonly seen in individuals age fifty and older. Here is how he summarizes his analysis:

> The results show statistically significant improvements in the PS-treated group (P < 0.05) compared to placebo both in terms of behavioral and cognitive parameters. This finding is clinically significant because these patients are representative of the typical geriatric population seen in clinical practice. These results are in agreement with smaller randomized, double-blind, placebo-controlled trials of more than 500 patients with Alzheimer's or other age-related dementia followed over a short period of time. These studies consistently show lasting and statistically significant

improvement in cognitive tests and brain function behavior in PS-treated dementia and Alzheimer's patients vs. placebo.[6]

In one US study, volunteers between the ages of fifty and seventy-five with ARCD took 100 mg of PS three times a day for three months. The nutrient reversed the decline in name-face recognition skills (pairing a face with the correct name) by a statistical twelve years! In other words, the average scores attained by sixty-four-year-olds rose to match the average scores attained by fifty-two-year-olds. The people taking PS showed significant overall reductions in memory impairment, with those who had the worst memory lapses improving the most.[7]

Depression in older people and depressive mood changes during the fall and winter months (seasonal affective disorder) are particularly responsive to PS therapy.

SYNERGISTIC BENEFITS

Despite the phenomenal ability of PS to enhance stress tolerance and boost learning rate, concentration, and memory, this nutritional medicine produces even stronger, synergistic benefits when combined with other neuronutrients for the treatment and prevention of dementia: citicoline, acetyl-L-carnitine, DHA, and MCT. You can also enhance the anti-Alzheimer's effects of PS by taking vitamin B12 (as methylcobalamine, 1,000–5,000 mcg daily), vitamin C (1,000–5,000 mg daily), folic acid (as methylfolate, 1,000–5,000 mcg daily), and alpha-linolenic acid (from flaxseed oil, 2,000–10,000 mg daily).

HOW TO USE PHOSPHATIDYLSERINE

I recommend taking 300 to 500 mg of PS per day.

PS is a friendly molecule. Your body makes its own, and the supplemental form is bioidentical—derived from a natural source: soybean phospholipids. Research has shown PS to be a remarkably safe nutritional supplement with no side effects of any kind.[8]

Because it's a food product, PS is compatible with all other foods and supplements. No drug interactions have been observed. It does work best when used as part of a comprehensive anti-aging program that also includes proper diet, regular exercise, and supplementation with other brain nutrients.

Can you get PS directly from eating soy foods? Unfortunately, no. The amount of PS in soy is so small that you'd never be able to consume enough to reach beneficial levels.

When you start taking PS supplements, give them a chance to work. After all, rebuilding brain cells takes time. You won't turn into Einstein overnight; PS requires about a month to improve memory and several months to achieve peak results. (Let's hope that during the wait you won't forget why you're taking it.)

LASTING BENEFITS

If you stop taking PS, the memory enhancement it generated will gradually fade after several months. This does not mean it didn't work; it means that to continue getting the benefits, one must continue taking the supplement.

Several studies have noted that the benefits of PS supplementation persist for up to three months after people discontinue it. Your brain knows a good thing when it sees it, so when PS comes down the pike, your brain latches onto it, stores it, and recycles it. That's why its effects linger even after supplementation has been discontinued. Of course, continuing it is preferable.

CHAPTER 34

Berberine: Protection against Vascular Dementia

've long admired those perky California poppies that burst forth from the soil around our ranch every spring. I recently learned that they get their bright golden-orange color from berberine. Berberine is the color of the sun, and to me these poppies, my state flower, suggest sunlight and energy. I find it somehow good and proper that this effusion of volunteers that bless our gardens contains copious quantities of berberine, an herbal powerhouse that has the potential to block cognitive decline and slam the door on Alzheimer's disease.

As you will see, the golden herbal medicine in these flowers is—like the sun—very directly involved with the burning of fuel to generate warmth and energy. The berberine in poppies demonstrates a kind of grace and elegance and beauty in the way it tweaks our metabolic molecular reactions to benefit our brains.

BERBERINE HAS BEEN AROUND FOR A LONG TIME

Berberine is a single chemical compound—a powerful, versatile, naturally occurring phytochemical medicine that can be extracted from the roots, rhizomes, stems, and bark of several plants, including barberry (*Berberis vulgaris*), tree turmeric (*Berberis aristata*), Oregon grape (*Mahonia aquifolium*), goldenseal (*Hydrastis canadensis*), yellowroot (*Xanthorhiza simplicissima*), Chinese goldthread (*Coptis chinensis*),

Amur cork tree (*Phellodendron amurense*), and the Californian poppy (*Eschscholzia californica*).

Berberine is a natural plant alkaloid revered for centuries by herbalists practicing both Ayurvedic and traditional Chinese Medicine. The earliest known mention of berberine's medicinal properties dates back to the *Ben Cao Jing*, a Chinese book on agriculture and medicinal plants written about two thousand years ago. Berberine was used mainly for its antibiotic, antiprotozoal, and antidiarrheal activity. Science has verified its antimicrobial activity against a variety of organisms, including bacteria, viruses, fungi, protozoans, helminths, and chlamydia.

BIG-TIME PROTECTION

Berberine is an anti-inflammatory and antioxidant polyphenol that plays multiple roles in protection from—and reversal of—dementia. It reduces plaque formation in the brain (by inhibiting beta-secretase, the enzyme that converts amyloid beta precursor protein to amyloid beta protein).

By blocking the development of neurofibrillary tangles, berberine has been shown to reverse the loss of spatial memory in animal models of Alzheimer's disease and enhance the health and functionality of the brain's memory centers.[1]

Berberine retards the breakdown of our main neurotransmitter, acetylcholine, which in turn enhances nerve message transmission. The herb also promotes intestinal health and protects intestinal mucosal integrity. Berberine discourages the bad (pathogenic) bugs that disrupt the small intestines and damage the inner surface of the intestinal tract, thus protecting the body from undesirable material (wheat, dairy, partially digested food, and other foodborne allergens) that would leak into the bloodstream, setting the stage for autoimmune diseases such as lupus, rheumatoid arthritis, and ankylosing spondylitis, as well as neurodegenerative diseases. (See chapter 16.) Berberine also helps the damaged gut wall heal, which reduces mucosal barrier permeability.[2]

BERBERINE PREVENTS VASCULAR DEMENTIA

As if this extraordinary smorgasbord of beneficial effects wasn't sufficient, berberine's most impressive effects actually lie in the breathtaking power with which it enhances so many different aspects of cardiovascular health—including every major metabolic factor involved in causing vascular dementia. (See chapter 7.) This is extremely important because significant arterial damage is present in over 90 percent of patients with cognitive decline or dementia.

If you wanted to develop a drug that addresses all the metabolic derangements that cause vascular dementia—and does a far better job than currently available drugs (which don't do it at all)—berberine would fill the bill. You may recall that almost all patients diagnosed with Alzheimer's actually have a mixture of AD and VaD and that VaD is caused by damage to the systems that regulate blood sugar, cholesterol, and blood pressure. Berberine lowers the level of all three. It reduces blood sugar better than the most-used pharmaceutical, metformin. It lowers cholesterol—not as dramatically as statin drugs, but it can be added to a statin regimen to get just as much cholesterol-lowering with less drug. And it reverses insulin resistance and type 2 diabetes. Because it multitasks so well, berberine is the perfect natural medicine for treating atherosclerotic cardiovascular, heart, and brain disease—and metabolic syndrome.[3] (See chapters 10, 11, and 12.)

If you have even minimally elevated fasting blood sugar (FBS above 90 mg/dL), you should be taking berberine. It is normoglycemic, which means it reduces blood sugar only if it is elevated.[4]

Berberine also reduces inflammation in the endothelium (the inner lining of all blood vessels), an important effect because such inflammation is the first step in the pathophysiological cascade of atherosclerotic changes that lead directly to vascular dementia. In other words, berberine protects against vascular dementia.

In numerous randomized, placebo-controlled trials, patients diagnosed with diabetes and blood lipid abnormalities who took berberine had significantly lower blood sugar, triglycerides, LDL cholesterol, and total cholesterol. Furthermore, groups taking berberine had lower blood pressure accompanied by loss of weight and abdominal fat.[5]

BERBERINE REVERSES ARTERIAL BLOCKAGE

In 2017, Mahila Aski and colleagues did a mouse study in which they demonstrated the neuroprotective effect of berberine for stroke and vascular dementia. They first surgically induced carotid arterial narrowing, which reduced blood supply to the brain, in effect surgically generating in the mice the equivalent of a human stroke. They then documented the resulting hippocampal damage and cognitive impairment caused by the blocked blood vessels. Next, they fed berberine to the mice. (The mouse dose was equivalent to 4,000 mg/day—eight 500 mg capsules in a 150-pound human.) The berberine reversed the hippocampal damage and cognitive deficits caused by stroke and blood vessel occlusion, strongly reinforcing the theme that winds its way through hundreds of other berberine studies: the herb prevents and reverses vascular disease, including stroke damage, and is therefore a valuable tool for preventing and treating vascular dementia.[6]

HOW DOES BERBERINE DO IT?

Possibly the most important of berberine's multiplicity of molecular actions has to do with its ability to regulate the enzyme AMPK (adenosine monophosphate–activated protein kinase), your body's master regulator of cellular energy production. AMPK—found in all plants and animals and a fundamental (ancient) activator of metabolism—regulates the energy supply to all our metabolic processes.

Here is a little bit about how it works. Our cells burn nutrients (from the food we eat) in oxygen (from the air we breathe) to generate the energy that makes life possible. This energy is released in the form of a free electron that must be grabbed (because otherwise it would turn into a damaging free radical). AMP (adenosine monophosphate) is the molecule that grabs the freed-up electron and passes it on to our storage systems to be used later as a source of energy. AMPK is the enzyme that generates AMP.

When berberine activates AMPK, it delivers an increase in the energy our cells use to drive our complicated biochemical machinery. AMPK controls all metabolism involved in managing fuel and energy storage and utilization in skeletal muscle, liver cells, fat tissues, and pancreatic beta cells (the ones that secrete the insulin that regulates cellular glucose utilization). This includes blood-sugar-regulating systems and other aspects of the synthesis of important lipids and proteins involved in blood sugar regulation. By activating AMPK, berberine benefits insulin resistance, metabolic syndrome, and type 2 diabetes and provides a diversity of other cardiovascular benefits.

For people with blood-sugar-regulation problems, berberine-driven AMPK activation stimulates the uptake of glucose into the cells, lowers insulin and improves insulin sensitivity, reduces glucose production in the liver, slows the release of free fatty acids (which lowers lipid levels and prevents harmful fat deposition), boosts fat burning in the mitochondria, stimulates the release of nitric oxide (a signaling molecule that relaxes the arteries), increases blood flow, lowers blood pressure, reverses diabetic neuropathy, and protects against atherosclerosis.

BETTER THAN METFORMIN

In my clinical practice over the years, I've seen how effective berberine is at lowering my patients' elevated blood sugar levels. Research studies have done head-to-head comparisons with metformin (the go-to mainstream type 2 diabetes sugar-lowering drug), and berberine is the clear winner.

Though widely used, metformin is not a fun drug. The body does not want it. It has a long list of side effects. It very often makes people sick, causing nausea and diarrhea and other symptoms as the body fights hard to expel it. Metformin interferes with thyroid function, reduces testosterone, lowers energy levels, depletes vital nutrients such as B12 and folate, and elevates homocysteine, which is very bad for the brain. (See chapter 13.)

In a 2008 clinical study published in *Metabolism*, people with newly diagnosed type 2 diabetes were randomly divided into groups and assigned to take either metformin or berberine. Improvements were noted the very first week, and by the end of the study, the average blood sugar and hemoglobin A1C levels significantly decreased in both groups. Remarkably, berberine helped fight diabetes every bit as effectively as metformin. The researchers concluded that the two had "an identical effect in the regulation of glucose metabolism." But that was where the similarities ended. When it came to lipid metabolism (cholesterol, triglycerides, LDL, and HDL), berberine was the clear champ: "By week 13, triglycerides and total cholesterol in the berberine group had decreased and were significantly lower than in the metformin group."[7]

In a significant recent development, Chinese researchers explained how berberine reverses diabetic neuropathy and increases the expression of BDNF. Berberine was shown to reverse diabetic neuropathic pain while lowering cholesterol, triglycerides, insulin, and blood sugar.[8]

POTENTIAL DRUG INTERACTIONS

As noted, berberine reduces blood sugar only if it is elevated. Berberine will reduce or even eliminate the need for other blood-sugar-lowering medications.

Berberine is known to interact with liver enzymes that metabolize specific drugs. Berberine may, for example, inhibit the enzyme systems CYP2D6, CYP2C9, and CYP3A4, and this may slow down the removal of macrolide antibiotics such as azithromycin and clarithromycin.

HOW TO USE BERBERINE

The usual dose of berberine is one or two 500 mg capsules taken twice daily, for a total of 1,000–2,000 mg/day.

Epigenetics and the Future of Alzheimer's Research

Thanks to the emergence of epigenetics, you now have an opportunity to make changes that will send you down a different metabolic path that leads to a keen dementia-free mind and a vibrant body.

These are special times for us humans. After learning and growing and evolving for over 5 million years, our species has, just in the past few years, arrived at a momentous milestone: we have achieved the power to manipulate our own genes. The recent discovery of epigenetics has enabled us to make conscious lifestyle choices that change—and enhance—the way our genes will be expressed. For the first time ever, genetic events inside your body and brain are under your conscious control. Applying the principles of epigenetics empowers you to change your genetic and cognitive destiny. Thanks to this new science, whether you have a healthy, dementia-resistant brain is completely up to you.

Allow me to explain what epigenetics is and how it works.

ABOUT EPIGENETICS

Epigenetics is the science of understanding what controls the expression of our genes.

We have known about our DNA genetic blueprint since the 1950s and '60s. Our genome has been carefully studied and completely mapped. We have long known that it consists of twenty-three pairs of chromosomes, twenty-two thousand genes, and about 3 billion base pairs. It's an incredibly complex language that uses rearrangements of just four different letters.

But a huge piece of the puzzle was missing. For several decades after the discovery of DNA—from the 1950s until just a few years ago—scientists had no idea what controlled genetic expression. What tells a gene to express itself? What turns it on? What turns it off? How are the choices made as to which genes are expressed and which are not? What controls the timing of expression of a sequence of genes? Why does a specific gene express itself while others nearby remain dormant? Until epigenetics arrived on the scene, scientists were unable to answer these questions. Now, with the help of epigenetics, they can.[1]

Our understanding of epigenetics enables us to tinker with our DNA and make decisions that change how and when it is expressed. We can now turn genes off and on at will. A lot more work is needed to fully understand the complexities of this, but the age of epigenetics has arrived.

The genes in our DNA molecules bathe in a watery soup in a huge cellular bathtub that surrounds and engulfs them. Transcription factor protein molecules floating in this bath with the genes tell them whether or not to express themselves. Together, thousands of different transcription factors form a complex system that guides and controls expression of the genome.[2]

If the transcription factors control the expression of the genes, what controls the transcription factors? You! Choices you make directly determine which transcription factors are in the soup. The foods you eat, the supplements you take, the exercise you do, whether you practice autophagy and low-carb ketogenic eating—these all exert powerful influences on the composition of the soup and the expression of the genes. By altering the types and amounts of transcription factors in this fluid, we can directly influence genetic expression.[3]

This knowledge arms you with a mighty tool for making conscious and deliberate decisions determining how your DNA blueprint performs and whether or not you get Alzheimer's. Every brain health recommendation I make in this book directly facilitates optimum transcription factors that generate optimum gene transcription. When you incorporate these ideas into your lifestyle, you are decisively upregulating a broad range of neuroprotective and neuroregenerative gene functions, including neurogenesis and synaptoplasticity. It's a smart thing to do that makes you smarter![4]

Now you can understand the molecular benefits of scarfing down the specific foods and supplements I've covered. This is why I have recommended low-dose lithium, high-polyphenol foods, omega-3 essential fatty acids such as DHA and flaxseed oil, coconut oil and MCTs, vitamin D, B-complex vitamins, blueberries, curcumin, green tea, Bacopa, berberine, phosphatidylserine, and citicoline. These *endogenous regulators* of gene transcription enhance multiple aspects of brain health and reverse Alzheimer's disease.[5]

We can further enhance these epigenetic effects to benefit our brains by utilizing the *exogenous modulators* of gene transcription—physical activity, caloric restriction, a ketogenic diet, healthy fat choices, and low-carb dieting—to further amplify cognition and brain health.[6]

Suppose, for example, you wish to improve your memory by epigenetically enhancing neurogenesis in your hippocampus. A malfunctioning hippocampus and compromised neurogenesis are the principal pathologic features of Alzheimer's. Because the brain is not replacing lost neurons fast enough, compromised neurogenesis leads to a decline of neurons and subsequent cognitive and motor disabilities.[7]

BDNF reverses this decline by stimulating neurogenesis: the growth of new nerve cells and the repair of damaged nerve cells. You can increase BDNF levels by turning on the expression of the BDNF genes in your brain. When you choose to eat blueberries or take low-dose lithium—or when you indulge in any of the other BDNF-enhancing foods, supplements, and behaviors (see the list in chapter 8)—you are instantaneously epigenetically upregulating your neurogenesis genes—the genes that make BDNF, grow new brain cells, enhance neuroplasticity, and heal the brain.

These principles work in reverse as well. Whether we do it intentionally or accidentally, we are continually influencing the composition of this bath our genes are floating in. If we make haphazard dietary choices that end up surrounding our genes in a fluid that is toxic, there will be adverse outcomes. When you choose to eat a diet high in sugars, bad fats, or methylmercury from seafood, you are epigenetically encouraging the expression of multiple genes associated with dysfunctional transcription factors and encouraging dementia. Conversely, when you choose to avoid carbs, bad fats, fish, and so on you are downregulating the expression of dysfunctional, disease-inducing genes.[8]

Every single food, supplement, lifestyle, and exercise recommendation I make in this book is designed to encourage a healthy balance of transcription factors. We want to epigenetically upregulate the genes that protect you from Alzheimer's and downregulate those that encourage it. (Not coincidentally, these same choices also upregulate anti-inflammatory, anti-aging mechanisms that enable you to live a longer, healthier life.) You are literally the first, the leading edge of future generations able to exercise what I call the epigenetic option—to consciously and intelligently choose to redirect the way you want your genes to be expressed to change your health, control your cognition, and optimize your genetic destiny.

As you get older, you want to maintain and maximize cognitive function—the ability to remember accurately, plan rationally, and think clearly. With epigenetics, you can take control of your body in ways that were never before possible! Teaching you how to harness this information, engage yourself in the practical application of epigenetics, and make optimum epigenetic choices has been my job.[9]

Start gradually and work toward doing everything: get all the recommended tests and fix every biomarker that is outside the optimum range. Incorporate autophagy, ketogenesis, and low-carb eating into your everyday lifestyle. Load up on blueberries, coconut oil, flaxseed oil, and high-polyphenol foods. (See chapter 24 and appendix 2.) Seek out healthy fats and dump the bad ones. Remember that low-dose lithium acts directly on the epigenome to promote the expression of more than fifty genes.[10] *Bacopa monniera* upregulates learning and memory genes.[11] Vitamin D, flaxseed oil, DHA, berberine, green tea, citicoline, phosphatidylserine, and curcumin have been shown to exert similar broad-spectrum epigenetic effects.[12] Daily exercise enhances your brain's epigenomic outlook.[13]

YOU CAN DO THIS

The recommendations made in this book—every single one—will enhance the epigenetics of gene expression. The cumulative effect will be to renew and invigorate your body and mind.[14]

I can't overemphasize the importance of early preventive action. About a third of all people reading this book will end up demented, and it is a sad fact that most of these cases could be prevented. The metabolic changes that lead to dementia start decades before symptoms appear. The earlier you start, the sooner you can begin to protect yourself. Whether you just want to maintain good brain health or you already have some memory loss and wish to reverse it, the time to start is right now! Yes, the program is challenging, but the rewards are phenomenal. Yes, this'll require giving up some old habits, but in terms of longevity and (more importantly) quality of life, you'll be way ahead. You can do it!

Laboratory Test Order

Lee Jones, MD
123 Grand Avenue, #610
Anytown, CA 98765
Phone: (555) 555-1234
Fax: (555) 555-2345
Email: drleejones@mywebsite.com

Laboratory Test Order

Date _____

Name _____

Address _____

Phone _____

Email address _____

Date of Birth _____

Blood Tests (with ICD-10 diagnosis codes)

☐ Comprehensive Metabolic Panel (includes Fasting Blood Sugar) E88.81

☐ Lipid Panel E78.0

☐ Homocysteine, plasma E72.10

☐ TSH E03.9

☐ Free T3 E03.9

☐ Free T4 E03.9

(Continued)

☐ Antithyroid Antibody Panel E03.9

☐ 25-Hydroxy Vitamin D E55.9

☐ DHEA-S E27.9

☐ Ferritin Serum E83.119

☐ Testosterone, serum, Free and Total E29.1

☐ Estradiol, serum E28.9

☐ Progesterone, serum E28.9

Other Tests:

☐ Comprehensive Stool Analysis—Genova Diagnostics GI Effects Microbial Ecology Profile: https://www.gdx.net/product /gi-effects-comprehensive-stool-test

☐ Polysomnogram—Physician referral to a sleep lab required; home tests are now available

☐ Hair Mineral Analysis—Doctor's Data "Toxic and Essential Elements" Hair Mineral Analysis (https://www.doctorsdata.com /hair-elements)

High-Polyphenol Foods

Here is a list of foods high in polyphenols. The ones with very high polyphenol content are marked with an asterisk.

Highest polyphenol content
- Berries (all)*
- Black tea
- Chocolate (dark chocolate* and hot chocolate made with dark chocolate*)
- Cocoa powder (minimally processed) and very dark chocolate*
- Coffee*
- Curcumin (curries)*
- Green tea*
- Pure pomegranate juice*

Fruit
- Apples
- Apple butter or applesauce
- Apple cider and juice
- Apricots*
- Blackberries*
- Blueberries*
- Cherries*

- Citrus: blood oranges, navel oranges, tangelos, tangerines, etc. (The white spongy pith is flavonoid-rich.)
- Cranberries*
- Currants (black or red)
- Dates
- Elderberries
- Gooseberries
- Grapes (red or purple)*
- Hazelnuts
- Kiwis
- Lemon juice*
- Limes
- Mangos
- Marionberries*
- Nectarines*
- Peaches*
- Pears
- Plums and prunes (dried plums)*
- Pomegranates*
- Quinces
- Raisins
- Raspberries*
- Rhubarb
- Strawberries*

Vegetables
- Artichoke
- Broccoli*
- Cabbage (red)*
- Celery
- Eggplant*
- Fennel
- Garlic*

- Greens (dark, leafy—e.g., kale, turnip)*
- Kohlrabi
- Leeks
- Lettuce (red)
- Lovage
- Onions (all)*
- Olives (black)*
- Peppers (small, hot)
- Parsnips
- Peas (green or English)
- Red lettuce*
- Rutabagas
- Scallions
- Shallots*
- Spinach*
- Sweet potatoes
- Tomatoes*
- Watercress

Nuts and Seeds

- Almonds
- Cashews
- Flaxseeds and flaxseed meal
- Hazelnuts*
- Nut butters
- Peanuts
- Pecans*
- Pistachios
- Pumpkin seeds
- Sunflower seeds
- Walnuts (high in ALA)*

Beans

- Black-eyed peas
- Chickpeas (garbanzo beans)*
- Fava beans
- Lentils
- Red kidney beans*
- Snap peas

Herbs, Spices, and Seasonings

- Basil*
- Capers (red or green)
- Chives
- Cinnamon
- Curry*
- Dill weed
- Horseradish
- Ketchup
- Oregano
- Parsley
- Rosemary
- Sage
- Tarragon
- Thyme
- Turmeric
- Vinegar

Notes

Chapter 1

1. Alzheimer's Association, *2019 Alzheimer's Disease Facts and Figures* (Washington, DC: Alzheimer's Association, 2019), https://www.alz.org/media /documents/alzheimers-facts-and-figures-2019-r.pdf.
2. Alzheimer's Association, *Alzheimer's Disease Facts.*
3. "10 Facts on Dementia," World Health Organization, updated September 2019, https://www.who.int/features/factfiles/dementia/en.
4. Alzheimer's Association, *Alzheimer's Disease Facts.*
5. B. D. James et al., "Contribution of Alzheimer Disease to Mortality in the United States," *Neurology* 82, no. 12 (March 5, 2014): 1045–50, http://doi.org/10.1212 /WNL.0000000000000240.
6. J. Weuve et al., "Deaths in the United States among Persons with Alzheimer's Disease (2010-2050)," *Alzheimer's & Dementia* 10, no. 2 (2014): e40–46, https:// www.ncbi.nlm.nih.gov/pubmed/24698031.
7. Alzheimer's Association, *Alzheimer's Disease Facts.*
8. Andrew E. Budson and Neil W. Kowall, eds., *The Handbook of Alzheimer's Disease and Other Dementias* (West Sussex, UK: Wiley-Blackwell, 2011).
9. Wikipedia, s.v. "Mini–Mental State Examination," last modified December 4, 2019, https://en.wikipedia.org/wiki/Mini–Mental_State_Examination#Test_features.
10. Mini-Cog, https://mini-cog.com/.

Chapter 3

1. Feng-Juan Zhuang et al., "Prevalence of White Matter Hyperintensities Increases with Age," *Neural Regeneration Research* 13, no. 12 (2018): 2141–46, http://doi .org/10.4103/1673-5374.241465.
2. A. Kapasi, C. DeCarli, and J. A. Schneider, "Impact of Multiple Pathologies on the Threshold for Clinically Overt Dementia," *Acta Neuropathologica* 134, no. 2 (August 2017): 171–86, http://doi.org/10.1007/s00401-017-1717-7. See also Johannes Attems, "The Multi-Morbid Old Brain," *Acta Neuropathologica* 134, no. 2 (August 2017): 169–70, http://doi.org/10.1007/s00401-017-1723-9.
3. Alina Solomon et al., "Midlife Serum Cholesterol and Increased Risk of Alzheimer's and Vascular Dementia Three Decades Later," *Dementia and Geriatric Cognitive Disorders* 28, no. 1 (2009): 75–80, http://doi.org/10.1159/000231980.

4. Robert Clarke et al., "Folate, Vitamin B12, and Serum Total Homocysteine Levels in Confirmed Alzheimer Disease," *Archives Neurology* 55, no. 11 (November 1998): 1449–55, http://doi.org/10.1001/archneur.55.11.1449. See also Sudha Seshadri et al., "Plasma Homocysteine as a Risk Factor for Dementia and Alzheimer's Disease," *New England Journal of Medicine* 346, no. 7 (February 14, 2002): 476–83, http://doi.org/10.1056/NEJMoa011613; and Katherine L. Tucker et al., "High Homocysteine and Low B Vitamins Predict Cognitive Decline in Aging Men: The Veterans Affairs Normative Aging Study," *American Journal of Clinical Nutrition* 82, no. 3 (September 2005): 627–35, http://doi.org/10.1093/ajcn/82.3.627.

5. A. David Smith et al., "Homocysteine-Lowering by B Vitamins Slows the Rate of Accelerated Brain Atrophy in Mild Cognitive Impairment: A Randomized Controlled Trial," *PLOS ONE* 5, no. 9 (September 8, 2010), http://doi.org/10.1371/journal.pone.0012244.

6. Gwenaëlle Douaud et al., "Preventing Alzheimer's Disease-Related Gray Matter Atrophy by B-Vitamin Treatment," *PNAS* 110, no. 23 (2013): 9523–28, http://doi.org/10.1073/pnas.1301816110.

7. Cédric Annweiler et al., "Higher Vitamin D Dietary Intake Is Associated with Lower Risk of Alzheimer's Disease: A 7-Year Follow-up," *Journals of Gerontology: Series A* 67, no. 11 (November 2012): 1205–11, http://doi.org/10.1093/gerona/gls107.

8. Thomas J. Littlejohns et al., "Vitamin D and the Risk of Dementia and Alzheimer Disease," *Neurology* 83, no. 10 (August 6, 2014): 920–28, http://doi.org/10.1212/WNL.0000000000000755.

9. Syrjyadipta Bhattacharjee and Walter J. Lukiw, "Alzheimer's Disease and the Microbiome," *Frontiers in Cellular Neuroscience* 7 (September 2013): 153, http://doi.org/10.3389/fncel.2013.00153.

10. Julian R. Marchesi et al., "The Gut Microbiota and Host Health: A New Clinical Frontier," *British Medical Journals: Gut* 65, no. 2 (February 2016): 330–39, http://doi.org/10.1136/gutjnl-2015-309990.

11. A. Benjafield et al., "Global Prevalence of Obstructive Sleep Apnea in Adults: Estimation Using Currently Available Data," *American Journal of Respiratory and Critical Care Medicine* 197 (2018): A3962.

12. Terry Young et al., "The Occurrence of Sleep-Disordered Breathing among Middle-Aged Adults," *New England Journal of Medicine* 328 (April 29, 1993): 1230–35, http://doi.org/10.1056/NEJM199304293281704.

13. Vishesh Kapur et al., "Underdiagnosis of Sleep Apnea Syndrome in U.S. Communities," *Sleep and Breathing* 6 (2002): 49–54, http://doi.org/10.1007/s11325-002-0049-5.

14. Paul E. Peppard et al., "Increased Prevalence of Sleep-Disordered Breathing in Adults," *American Journal of Epidemiology* 177, no. 9 (April 14, 2013): 1006–14, http://doi.org/10.1093/aje/kws342.

15. "General Information Press Room," American Thyroid Association, https://www.thyroid.org/media-main/press-room/.

16. Broda O. Barnes, *Hypothyroidism: The Unsuspected Illness* (New York: Harper, 1976).

Chapter 4

All the references below were used to gather and arrange information about the history of Alois Alzheimer, Auguste Deter, and the emergence of the disease that came to be referred to as "Alzheimer's."

1. Hanns Hippius and Gabriele Neundorfer, "The Discovery of Alzheimer's Disease," *Dialogues in Clinical Neuroscience* 5, no. 1 (March 2003): 101–8.
2. J. M. S. Pearce, "Historical Note: Alzheimer's Disease," *Journal of Neurology, Neurosurgery, and Psychiatry* 68 (March 2000): 348, http://dx.doi.org/10.1136 /jnnp.68.3.348.
3. Hippius and Neundorfer, "Discovery of Alzheimer's," 101–8.
4. Konrad Maurer, Stephan Volk, and Hector Gerbaldo, "Auguste D and Alzheimer's Disease," *Lancet* 349, no. 9064 (May 24, 1997): 1546–49, http://doi.org/10.1016/S0140-6736(96)10203-8.
5. Alois Alzheimer, "Über eine eigenartige Erkrankung der Hirnrinde," *Allgemeine Zeitschrift fur Psychiatrie und Psychisch-gerichtliche Medizin* 64 (1907): 146–48.
6. M. B. Graeber et al., "Histopathology and APOE Genotype of the First Alzheimer Disease Patient, Auguste D.," *Neurogenetics* 1, no. 3 (March 1998): 223–28. See also M. B. Graeber and Parviz Mehraein, "Reanalysis of the First Case of Alzheimer's Disease," *European Archives of Psychiatry and Clinical Neuroscience* 249 (1999): S10–S13, http://doi.org/10.1007/PL00014167.

Chapter 5

1. Dale E. Bredesen, "Reversal of Cognitive Decline: A Novel Therapeutic Program," *Aging* 6, no. 9 (September 27, 2014): 707–17, http://doi.org/10.18632 /aging.100690.
2. Suzana Herculano-Houzel, "The Human Brain in Numbers: A Linearly Scaled-Up Primate Brain," *Frontiers in Human Neuroscience* 3, no. 31 (November 9, 2009), http://doi.org/10.3389/neuro.09.031.2009.
3. Syrjyadipta Bhattacharjee and Walter J. Lukiw, "Alzheimer's Disease and the Microbiome," *Frontiers in Cellular Neuroscience* 7 (September 2013): 153, http://doi.org/10.3389/fncel.2013.00153. See also Julian R. Marchesi et al. "The Gut Microbiota and Host Health: A New Clinical Frontier," *British Medical Journals: Gut* 65, no. 2 (February 2016): 330–39, http://doi.org/10.1136 /gutjnl-2015-309990.

Chapter 6

1. Scott A. Small and Sam Gandy, "Sorting through the Cell Biology of Alzheimer's Disease: Intracellular Pathways to Pathogenesis," *Neuron* 52 (October 5, 2006): 15–31, https://doi.org/10.1016/j.neuron.2006.09.001.
2. Joseph Altman and Gopal Das, "Autoradiographic and Histological Evidence of Postnatal Hippocampal Neurogenesis in Rats," *Journal of Comparative Neurology* 124, no. 3 (June 1965): 319–35, https://doi.org/10.1002/cne.901240303.

3. Daniel A. Berg et al., "A Common Embryonic Origin of Stem Cells Drives Developmental and Adult Neurogenesis," *Cell* 177, no. 3 (March 28, 2019): 654–68, http://doi.org/10.1016/j.cell.2019.02.010.

Chapter 7

1. Zhiyou Cai et al., "Cerebral Small Vessel Disease and Alzheimer's Disease," *Clinical Interventions in Aging* 10 (2015): 1695–704, http://doi.org/10.2147/CIA .S90871.

2. Leslie Kernisan, "The Most Common Aging Brain Problem You've Never Heard Of," Health, *Next Avenue*, May 10, 2017, https://www.nextavenue.org /common-aging-brain-problem. See also F-E. de Leeuw et al., "Prevalence of Cerebral White Matter Lesions in Elderly People: A Population Based Magnetic Resonance Imaging Study. The Rotterdam Scan Study," *Journal of Neurology, Neurosurgery, and Psychiatry* 70, no. 1 (January 2001): 9–14, http://doi.org /10.1136/jnnp.70.1.9.

3. Yuan Wang et al., "White Matter Injury in Ischemic Stroke," *Progress in Neurobiology* 141 (June 2016): 45–60, http://doi.org/10.1016/j.pneurobio .2016.04.005.

4. Jose Álvarez-Sabín and Guistavo C. Román, "Citicoline in Vascular Cognitive Impairment and Vascular Dementia after Stroke," *Stroke* 42, no. 1 (January 2011): S40–S43, http://doi.org/10.1161/STROKEAHA.110.606509.

5. Atte Meretoja et al., "Stroke Thrombolysis: Save a Minute, Save a Day," *Stroke* 45, no. 4 (March 2014): 1053–58, http://doi.org/10.1161/STROKEAHA.113.002910.

6. Atte Meretoja et al., "Endovascular Therapy for Ischemic Stroke: Save a Minute— Save a Week," *Neurology* 88, no. 22 (May 2017): 2123–27, http://doi.org/10.1212 /WNL.0000000000003981.

7. George B. Weiss, "Metabolism and Actions of CDP-Choline as an Endogenous Compound and Administered Exogenously as Citicoline," *Life Sciences* 56, no. 9 (1995): 637–60, https://www.ncbi.nlm.nih.gov/pubmed/7869846.

8. Jeffrey Saver, "Citicoline: Update on a Promising and Widely Available Agent for Neuroprotection and Neurorepair," *Reviews in Neurological Diseases* 5, no. 4 (Fall 2008): 167–77.

Chapter 8

1. Charles H. Hillman, Kirk I. Erickson, and Arthur F. Kramer, "Be Smart, Exercise Your Heart: Exercise Effects on Brain and Cognition," *Nature Reviews Neuroscience* 9 (January 2008): 58–65, http://drlardon.com/wp-content/uploads /2014/06/Perspectives.pdf.

2. Kirk I. Erickson et al., "Exercise Training Increases Size of Hippocampus and Improves Memory," *PNAS* 108, no. 7 (February 15, 2011): 3017–22, http://doi .org/10.1073/pnas.1015950108.

3. Ericksen Mielle Borba et al., "Brain-Derived Neurotrophic Factor Serum Levels and Hippocampal Volume in Mild Cognitive Impairment and Dementia Due to Alzheimer Disease," *Dementia and Geriatric Cognitive Disorders Extra* 6 (2016): 559–67, http://doi.org/10.1159/000450601.

4. Joseph Altman, "Autoradiographic Investigation of Cell Proliferation in the Brains of Rats and Cats," *Anatomical Record* 145, no. 4 (April 1963): 573–91, https://doi.org/10.1002/ar.1091450409.

5. Maura Boldrini et al. "Human Hippocampal Neurogenesis Persists throughout Aging," *Cell Stem Cell* 22, no. 4 (April 5, 2018): 589–99, http://doi.org/10.1016 /j.stem.2018.03.015.

6. Emily Underwood, "New Neurons for Life? Old People Can Still Make Fresh Brain Cells, Study Finds," Brain Behavior, *Science* March 25, 2019, https://www.sciencemag.org/news/2019/03/new-neurons-life-old-people -can-still-make-fresh-brain-cells-study-finds.

7. Éadaoin W. Griffin et al., "Aerobic Exercise Improves Hippocampal Function and Increases BDNF in the Serum of Young Adult Males," *Physiology Behavior* 104, no. 5 (October 24, 2011): 934–41, http://doi.org/10.1016/j.physbeh.2011.06.005.

8. Ioannis Bakoyiannis et al., "Phytochemicals and Cognitive Health: Are Flavonoids Doing the Trick?," *Biomedicine & Pharmacotherapy* 109 (January 2019): 1488–97, https://doi.org/10.1016/j.biopha.2018.10.086.

9. W. J. P. Henneman et al., "Hippocampal Atrophy Rates in Alzheimer Disease," *Neurology* 72, no. 11 (March 17, 2009): 999–1007, http://doi.org/10.1212/01 .wnl.0000344568.09360.31.

10. Erickson et al., "Exercise Training," 3017–22.

11. Erickson et al., "Exercise Training," 3017–22.

12. Khadije Ebrahimi et al., "Physical Activity and Beta-Amyloid Pathology in Alzheimer's Disease: A Sound Mind in a Sound Body," *EXCLI Journal* 16 (2017): 959–72, http://doi.org/10.17179/excli2017-475.

13. Paul J. Lucassen et al., "Regulation of Adult Neurogenesis and Plasticity by (Early) Stress, Glucocorticoids, and Inflammation," *Cold Spring Harbor Perspectives in Biology* 7 (November 2019), http://doi.org/10.1101/cshperspect.a021303.

Chapter 10

1. Endang Susalit et al., "Olive (*Olea europaea*) Leaf Extract Effective in Patients with Stage-1 Hypertension: Comparison with Captopril," *Phytomedicine* 18, no. 4 (February 15, 2011): 251–58. See also Anwar-ul H. Gilani et al., "Blood Pressure Lowering Effect of Olive Is Mediated through Calcium Channel Blockade," *International Journal of Food Science and Nutrition* 56, no. 8 (December 2005): 613–20.

2. Naghmeh Mirhosseini, Hassanali Vatanparast, and Samantha M. Kimbal, "The Association between Serum 25(OH)D Status and Blood Pressure in Participants of a Community-Based Program Taking Vitamin D Supplements," *Nutrients* 9, no. 11 (2017): 1244–59, https://doi.org/10.3390/nu9111244.

3. F. L. Rosenfeldt et al., "Coenzyme Q_{10} in the Treatment of Hypertension: A Meta-Analysis of the Clinical Trials," *Journal of Human Hypertension* 21 (February 8, 2007): 297–306, https://doi.org/10.1038/sj.jhh.1002138.

4. Alexander Medina-Remón et al., "The Effect of Polyphenol Consumption on Blood Pressure," *Mini-Reviews in Medicinal Chemistry* 13, no. 8 (August 2012): 1137–49, http://doi.org/10.2174/1389557511313080002.

5. Naomi D. L. Fisher, "Stress Raising Your Blood Pressure? Take a Deep Breath," *Harvard Health Blog,* Harvard Health Publishing, February 15, 2016, https://www.health.harvard.edu/blog/stress-raising-your-blood-pressure -take-a-deep-breath-201602159168.

6. Gary Craig, "The EFT Basic Recipe by Founder Gary Craig," emofree, YouTube, July 9, 2013, https://www.youtube.com/watch?v=1wG2FA4vfLQ.

Chapter 11

1. University of California, San Francisco, "Chronically High Blood Sugar Linked to Risk of Cognitive Impairment," ScienceDaily, August 9, 2006, https://www .sciencedaily.com/releases/2006/08/060809153824.htm.

2. University of California, "Chronically High Blood Sugar."

3. Nicolas Cherbuin, Perminder Sachdev, and Kaarin J. Anstey, "Higher Normal Fasting Plasma Glucose Is Associated with Hippocampal Atrophy: The PATH Study," *Neurology* 79, no. 10 (September 4, 2012): 1019–26, http://doi .org/10.1212/WNL.0b013e31826846de.

4. Paul K. Crane et al., "Glucose Levels and Risk of Dementia," *New England Journal of Medicine* 369 (August 8, 2013): 540–48, http://doi.org/10.1056 /NEJMoa1215740.

5. Heidi Godman, "Above-Normal Blood Sugar Linked to Dementia," *Harvard Health Blog,* Harvard Health Publishing, August 7, 2013, https://www.health .harvard.edu/blog/above-normal-blood-sugar-linked-to-dementia-201308076596.

6. Lucia Kerti et al., "Higher Glucose Levels Associated with Lower Memory and Reduced Hippocampal Microstructure," *Neurology* 81, no. 20 (November 12, 2013): 1746–52, http://doi.org/10.1212/01.wnl.0000435561.00234.ee.

7. Kerti, "Higher Glucose Levels," 1746–52.

8. Honor Whiteman, "High Blood Sugar Levels Linked to Memory Loss," *Medical News Today*, October 24, 2013, https://www.medicalnewstoday.com /articles/267727.

9. Moyra E. Mortby et al., "High 'Normal' Blood Glucose Is Associated with Decreased Brain Volume and Cognitive Performance in the 60s: The PATH through Life Study," *PLOS ONE* 8, no. 9 (September 4, 2013): e73897, https://doi .org/10.1371/journal.pone.0073697.

10. "Seniors and Diabetes: A Complete Guide," National Council for Aging Care, May 23, 2017, https://www.aging.com/seniors-and-diabetes-a-complete-guide/.

11. "New CDC Report: More Than 100 Million Americans Have Diabetes or Prediabetes," Centers for Disease Control and Prevention, July 18, 2017, https:// www.cdc.gov/media/releases/2017/p0718-diabetes-report.html; and Centers for Disease Control and Prevention, *National Diabetes Statistics Report, 2017: Estimates of Diabetes and Its Burden in the United States*, July 2017, https://www .cdc.gov/diabetes/pdfs/data/statistics/national-diabetes-statistics-report.pdf.

12. David Perlmutter, *Grain Brain: The Surprising Truth about Wheat, Carbs, and Sugar* (New York: Little, Brown, 2013); and David Perlmutter, *Brain Maker: The Power of Gut Microbes to Heal and Protect Your Brain for Life* (New York: Little, Brown, 2015).

13. "Toxic Chocolate," As You Sow, May 25, 2019, https://www.asyousow.org /environmental-health/toxic-enforcement/toxic-chocolate.

Chapter 12

1. M. Sjögren and K. Blennow, "The Link between Cholesterol and Alzheimer's Disease," *World Journal of Biological Psychiatry* 6, no. 2 (2005): 85–97, https://www.ncbi.nlm.nih.gov/pubmed/16156481. See also Christiane Reitz, "Dyslipidemia and Dementia: Current Epidemiology, Genetic Evidence, and Mechanisms behind the Associations," *Journal of Alzheimer's Disease* 30, no. 2 (2012): S127–S145, http://doi.org/10.3233/JAD-2011-110599.

2. Luigi Puglielli, Rudolph E. Tanzi, and Dora M. Kovacs, "Alzheimer's Disease: The Cholesterol Connection," *Nature Neuroscience* 6, no. 4 (April 2003): 345–51, http://doi.org/10.1038/nn0403-345.

3. Bruce Reed et al., "Associations between Serum Cholesterol Levels and Cerebral Amyloidosis," *JAMA Neurology* 71, no. 2 (2014): 195–200, http://doi.org/10.1001 /jamaneurol.2013.5390.

4. Reed et al., "Associations between Serum Cholesterol," 195–200.

5. Catharine Paddock, "Cholesterol levels linked to brain deposits that cause Alzheimer's," *Medical News Today*, December 31, 2013, https://www.medical newstoday.com/articles/270710.

6. Richard Deichmann, Carl Lavie, and Samuel Andrews, "Coenzyme Q10 and Statin-Induced Mitochondrial Dysfunction," *Ochsner Journal* 10, no. 1 (Spring 2010): 16–21, https://www.ncbi.nlm.nih.gov/pmc/articles/PMC3096178/.

Chapter 13

1. Sudha Seshadri et al., "Plasma Homocysteine as a Risk Factor for Dementia and Alzheimer's Disease," *New England Journal of Medicine* 346, no. 7 (February 14, 2002): 476–83, http://doi.org/10.1056/NEJMoa011613. See also Robert Clarke et al., "Folate, Vitamin B12, and Serum Total Homocysteine Levels in Confirmed Alzheimer Disease," *Archives of Neurology* 55, no. 11 (1998): 1449–55, http://doi .org/10.1001/archneur.55.11.1449.

2. A. David Smith et al., "Homocysteine-Lowering by B Vitamins Slows the Rate of Accelerated Brain Atrophy in Mild Cognitive Impairment: A Randomized Controlled Trial," *PLOS ONE* 5, no. 9 (September 8, 2010): e12244, https://doi .org/10.1371/journal.pone.0012244.

3. Gwenaëlle Douaud et al., "Preventing Alzheimer's Disease-Related Gray Matter Atrophy by B-Vitamin Treatment," *PNAS* 110, no. 23 (2013): 9523–28, https:// doi.org/10.1073/pnas.1301816110.

4. Douaud et al., "Preventing Alzheimer's," 9523–28.

5. If you want a more detailed examination, Health Diagnostics and Research Institute offers the Methylation Pathway Parameters test:
   Health Diagnostics and Research Institute
   540 Bordentown Ave., Suite 2300
   South Amboy, NJ 08879

Tel 732-721-1234

Fax 732-525-3288

Email info@hdri-usa.com

For more than you ever wanted to know about B vitamins and methylation, go to Health Diagnostics' website (http://www.hdri-usa.com).

For complex methylation problem situations, you may need to enlist the services of a methylation specialist.

Chapter 14

1. Kimberly Y. Forrest and Wendy L. Stuhldreher, "Prevalence and Correlates of Vitamin D Deficiency in US Adults," *Nutrition Research* 31, no. 1 (January 2011): 48–54, http://doi.org/10.1016/j.nutres.2010.12.001. The majority of adult Americans are deficient in vitamin D.

2. Zahid Naeem, "Vitamin D Deficiency—An Ignored Epidemic," *International Journal of Health Sciences* 4, no. 1 (January 2010): v–vi; and M. F. Holick and T. C. Chen, "Vitamin D Deficiency: A Worldwide Problem with Health Consequences," *American Journal of Clinical Nutrition* 87, no. 4 (April 2008): 1080S–1086S, https://doi.org/10.1093/ajcn/87.4.1080S.

3. Barbara J. Hawgood, "Sir Edward Mellanby (1884–1955) GBE KCB FRCP FRS: Nutrition Scientist and Medical Research Mandarin," *Journal of Medical Biography* 18, no. 3 (August 26, 2010): 150–57, http://doi.org/10.1258/jmb.2010.010020.

4. Anthony W. Norman, "From Vitamin D to Hormone D: Fundamentals of the Vitamin D Endocrine System Essential for Good Health," *American Journal of Clinical Nutrition* 88, no. 2 (August 2008): 491S–499S, https://doi.org/10.1093/ajcn/88.2.491S.

5. Cédric Annweiler et al., "Higher Vitamin D Dietary Intake Is Associated with Lower Risk of Alzheimer's Disease: A 7-Year Follow-up," *Journals of Gerontology: Series A* 67, no. 11 (November 2012): 1205–11, https://doi.org/10.1093/gerona/gls107.

6. Thomas J. Littlejohns et al., "Vitamin D and the Risk of Dementia and Alzheimer Disease," *Neurology* 83, no. 10 (August 6, 2014): 920–28, http://doi.org/10.1212/WNL.0000000000000755.

7. Renee Tessman, "Link between Vitamin D and Dementia Risk Confirmed," *Press Room–American Academy of Neurology,* August 5, 2014, https://www.aan.com/PressRoom/Home/PressRelease/1300.

8. Duygu Gezen-Ak, Selma Yilmazer, and Erding Dursun, "Why Vitamin D in Alzheimer's Disease? The Hypothesis," *Journal of Alzheimer's Disease* 40, no. 2 (March 2014): 257–69, http://doi.org/10.3233/JAD-131970. See also Khanh Vin Quoc Luo'ng and Lan Thi Hoang Nguyen, "The Role of Vitamin D in Alzheimer's Disease: Possible Genetic and Cell Signaling Mechanisms," *American Journal of Alzheimer's Disease & Other Dementias* 28, no. 2 (January 2013): 126–36, https://doi.org/10.1177/1533317512473196.

9. Anindita Banerjee et al., "Vitamin D and Alzheimer's Disease: Neurocognition to Therapeutics," *International Journal of Alzheimer's Disease* 2015 (August 17, 2015), http://doi.org/10.1155/2015/192747.

10. Duygu Gezen-Ak, Erding Dursun, and Selma Yilmazer, "The Effect of Vitamin D Treatment on Nerve Growth Factor (NGF) Release from Hippocampal Neurons," *Archives of Neuropsychiatry* 51, no. 2 (June 2014): 157–62, http://doi.org/10.4274 /npa.y7076.

11. A. Masoumi et al., "1α,25-Dihydroxyvitamin D_3 Interacts with Curcuminoids to Stimulate Amyloid-β Clearance by Macrophages of Alzheimer's Disease Patients," *Journal of Alzheimers Disease* 17 (2009): 703–17, http://doi.org/10.3233/JAD -2009-1080, pmid:19433889.

12. Banerjee et al., "Vitamin D."

13. D. A. Youssef et al., "Antimicrobial Implications of Vitamin D," *Dermatoendocrinology* 3, no. 4 (October–December 2011): 220–24, http://doi .org/10.4161/derm.3.4.15027.

14. Ibrar Anjum et al., "The Role of Vitamin D in Brain Health: A Mini Literature Review," *Cureus* 10, no. 7 (July 2018): e2960, http://doi.org/10.7759/cureus.2960.

Chapter 15

1. Naresh M. Punjabi, "The Epidemiology of Adult Obstructive Sleep Apnea," *Proceedings of the American Thoracic Society* 5, no. 2 (February 15, 2008): 136–43, http://doi.org/10.1513/pats.200709-155MG.

2. R. Budhiraja, S. Parthasarathy, and S. F. Quan, "Endothelial Dysfunction in Obstructive Sleep Apnea," *Journal of Clinical Sleep Medicine* 3, no. 4 (June 2007): 409–15, https://www.ncbi.nlm.nih.gov/pubmed/17694731.

3. N. J. Buchner et al., "Microvascular Endothelial Dysfunction in Obstructive Sleep Apnea Is Caused by Oxidative Stress and Improved by Continuous Positive Airway Pressure Therapy," *Respiration* 82 no. 5 (October 2011): 409–17, http:// doi.org/10.1159/000323266.

4. Terry Young et al., "Sleep Disordered Breathing and Mortality: Eighteen-Year Follow-Up of the Wisconsin Sleep Cohort," *Sleep* 31, no. 8 (August 2008): 1071–78.

5. J. Feng et al., "Hippocampal Impairments Are Associated with Intermittent Hypoxia of Obstructive Sleep Apnea," *Chinese Medical Journal* 125, no. 4 (February 2012): 696–701, https://www.ncbi.nlm.nih.gov/pubmed/22490498.

6. Paul M. Macey, "Is Brain Injury in Obstructive Sleep Apnea Reversible?," *Sleep* 35, no.1 (January 1, 2012): 9–10, http://doi.org/10.5665/sleep.1572.

7. Maria Bonsignore, "Sleep Apnea and Its Role in Transportation Safety," *F1000 Research* 6 (December 2017): 2168, https://doi.org/10.12688/f1000 research.12599.1.

Chapter 16

1. International Human Genome Sequencing Consortium, "Initial Sequencing and Analysis of the Human Genome," *Nature* 409 (February 15, 2001): 860–921, http://doi.org/10.1038/35057062.

2. Peter J. Turnbaugh et al., "The Human Microbiome Project," *Nature* 449 (October 17, 2007): 804–10, http://doi.org/10.1038/nature06244.

3. Gil Sharon et al., "The Central Nervous System and the Gut Microbiome," *Cell* 167, no. 4 (November 3, 2016): 915–32, http://dx.doi.org/10.1016/j.cell.2016.10.027.

4. James M. Hill et al., "Pathogenic Microbes, the Microbiome, and Alzheimer's Disease (AD)," *Frontiers in Aging Neuroscience* 6 (June 2014): 127, http://doi .org/10.3389/fnagi.2014.00127.

5. Andy Coghlan, "Autoimmune Disorders Linked to an Increased Risk of Dementia," Health New Scientist, March 1, 2017, https://www.newscientist.com /article/2123274-autoimmune-disorders-linked-to-an-increased-risk-of-dementia/.

6. "Autoimmune Disease List," American Autoimmune Related Diseases Association, February 13, 2019, https://www.aarda.org/diseaselist.

7. David Perlmutter, *Grain Brain: The Surprising Truth about Wheat, Carbs, and Sugar* (New York: Little, Brown, 2013); and David Perlmutter, *Brain Maker: The Power of Gut Microbes to Heal and Protect Your Brain for Life* (New York: Little, Brown, 2015).

Chapter 17

1. "General Information Press Room," American Thyroid Association, November 13, 2019, https://www.thyroid.org/media-main/press-room.

2. Broda O. Barnes, *Hypothyroidism: The Unsuspected Illness* (New York: Harper, 1976).

3. Gillian E. Cooke et al., "Hippocampal Volume Is Decreased in Adults with Hypothyroidism," *Thyroid* 24, no. 3 (March 7, 2014): 433–40, http://doi.org /10.1089/thy.2013.0058.

4. Sherine M. Abdalla and A. C. Bianco, "Defending Plasma T3 Is a Biological Priority," *Clinical Endocrinology* 81, no. 5 (January 4, 2016): 633–41, http://doi. org/10.1111/cen.12538.

5. Johannes W. Dietrich, John E. M. Midgley, and Rudolf Hoermann, "Editorial: Homeostasis and Allostasis of Thyroid Function," *Frontiers in Endocrinology* 9 (June 5, 2018): 287, https://doi.org/10.3389/fendo.2018.00287.

6. G. S. Kelly, "Peripheral Metabolism of Thyroid Hormones: A Review," *Alternative Medicine Review* 5, no. 4 (August 2000): 306–33.

7. Kent Holtorf, "Peripheral Thyroid Hormone Conversion and Its Impact on TSH and Metabolic Activity," *Journal of Restorative Medicine* 3, no. 1 (April 1, 2014): 30–52.

8. Sarah J. Peterson et al., "An Online Survey of Hypothyroid Patients Demonstrates Prominent Dissatisfaction," *Thyroid* 28, no. 6 (June 1, 2018): 707–21, http://doi .org/10.1089/thy.2017.0681.

9. Chris Kresser, "Three Reasons Why Your Thyroid Medication Isn't Working," March 5, 2019, https://chriskresser.com/three-reasons-why-your-thyroid -medication-isnt-working/comment-page-9/.

10. Order your tests from www.directlabs.com. On Direct Labs' home page, find "Test Categories," select "Thyroid," then locate "Free T's plus TSH" on the menu.

The results will be sent directly to you. (Services are not available in Maryland, New Jersey, New York, and Rhode Island.)

Chapter 18

1. Lin Xu et al., "Circulatory Levels of Toxic Metals (Aluminum, Cadmium, Mercury, Lead) in Patients with Alzheimer's Disease: A Quantitative Meta-Analysis and Systematic Review," *Journal of Alzheimer's Disease* 62, no. 1 (February 6, 2018): 361–72, http://doi.org/10.3233/JAD-170811.

2. Dale W. Jenkins, *Toxic Trace Metals in Mammalian Hair and Nails* (Washington, DC: US Environmental Protection Agency, 1979), https://cfpub.epa.gov/si/si _public_record_Report.cfm?Lab=ORD&dirEntryID=45357.

3. Joachim Mutter et al., "Does Inorganic Mercury Play a Role in Alzheimer's Disease? A Systematic Review and an Integrated Molecular Mechanism," *Journal of Alzheimer's Disease* 22, no. 2 (October 1, 2010): 357–74, http://doi .org/10.3233/JAD-2010-100705.

4. C. Hock et al., "Increased Blood Mercury Levels in Patients with Alzheimer's Disease," *Journal of Neural Transmission* 105, no. 1 (March 1998): 59–68, http://doi.org/10.1007/s007020050038.

5. James C. Pendergrass et al., "Mercury Vapor Inhalation Inhibits Binding of GTP to Tubulin in Rat Brain: Similarity to a Molecular Lesion in Alzheimer Diseased Brain," *Neurotoxicology* 18, no. 2 (1997): 315–24.

6. "How Mercury Causes Brain Neuron Damage – Uni. of Calgary," steffyweffy777, YouTube, May 15, 2007, https://www.youtube.com/watch?v=XU8nSn5Ezd8.

7. Paul F. Schuster et al., "Permafrost Stores a Globally Significant Amount of Mercury," *Geophysical Research Letters* 45, no. 3 (February 5, 2018): 1463–71, http://doi.org/10.1002/2017GL075571.

8. The International Academy of Oral Medicine and Toxicology at https://iaomt.org.

9. Qing Peng et al., "Cadmium and Alzheimer's Disease Mortality in U.S. Adults: Updated Evidence with a Urinary Biomarker and Extended Follow-up Time," *Environmental Research* 157 (August 2017): 44–51, http://doi.org/10.1016/j .envres.2017.05.011.

10. Bo Wang and Yanli Du, "Cadmium and Its Neurotoxic Effects," *Oxidative Medicine and Cellular Longevity* (2013), http://dx.doi.org/10.1155/2013/898034; and Ling-Feng Jiang et al., "Impacts of Cd(II) on the Conformation and Self-Aggregation of Alzheimer's Tau Fragment Corresponding to the Third Repeat of Microtubule-Binding Domain," *Biochimica et Biophysica Acta* 1774, no. 11 (November 2007): 1414–21, https://doi.org/10.1016/j.bbapap.2007.08.014.

11. "Toxic Chocolate," As You Sow, May 25, 2019, https://www.asyousow.org /environmental-health/toxic-enforcement/toxic-chocolate/#chocolate-tables.

12. L. D. White et al., "New and Evolving Concepts in the Neurotoxicology of Lead," *Toxicology and Applied Pharmacology* 225, no. 1 (November 15, 2007): 1–27, http://doi.org/10.1016/j.taap.2007.08.001.

13. Jinfang Wu et al., "Alzheimer's Disease (AD)-Like Pathology in Aged Monkeys after Infantile Exposure to Environmental Metal Lead (Pb): Evidence

for a Developmental Origin and Environmental Link for AD," *Journal of Neuroscience* 28, no. 1 (January 2, 2008): 3–9, http://doi.org/10.1523/J NEUROSCI.4405-07.2008.

14. Tatyana Verina, C. A. Rohde, and T. R. Guilarte, "Environmental Lead Exposure during Early Life Alters Granule Cell Neurogenesis and Morphology in the Hippocampus of Young Adult Rats," *Neuroscience* 145, no. 3 (March 30, 2007): 1037–47, http://doi.org/10.1016/j.neuroscience.2006.12.040.

15. Kirstie H. Stansfield et al., "Dysregulation of BDNF-TrkB Signaling in Developing Hippocampal Neurons by Pb: Implications for an Environmental Basis of Neurodevelopmental Disorders," *Toxicological Sciences* 127, no. 1 (May 2012): 277–95, http://doi.org/10.1093/toxsci/kfs090; Jinfang Wu, Riyaz Basha, and Nasser H. Zawia, "The Environment, Epigenetics and Amyloidogenesis," *Journal of Molecular Neuroscience* 34, no. 1 (January 2008): 1–7, http://doi.org /10.1007/s12031-007-0009-4; and Syed Waseem Bihaqi and Nasser H. Zawia, "Enhanced Taupathy and AD-like Pathology in Aged Primate Brains Decades after Infantile Exposure to Lead (Pb)," *Neurotoxicology* 39 (December 2013): 95–101, http://doi.org/10.1016/j.neuro.2013.07.010.

16. Kim M. Cecil et al., "Decreased Brain Volume in Adults with Childhood Lead Exposure," *PLOS Medicine* 5, no. 5 (May 2008): e112, http://doi.org/10.1371 /journal.pmed.0050112.

17. Cecil et al., "Decreased Brain Volume," e112.

18. Erica P. Raven et al., "Increased Iron Levels and Decreased Tissue Integrity in Hippocampus of Alzheimer's Disease Detected *In Vivo* with Magnetic Resonance Imaging," *Journal of Alzheimer's Disease* 37, no. 1 (2013): 127–36, http://doi.org /10.3233/JAD-130209.

19. George Bartzokis et al., "In Vivo Evaluation of Brain Iron in Alzheimer Disease Using Magnetic Resonance Imaging," *Archives of General Psychiatry* 57, no. 1 (January 2000): 47–53, http://doi.org/10.1001/archpsyc.57.1.47.

20. Raven et al., "Increased Iron Levels," 127–36.

21. George Bartzokis et al., "Brain Ferritin Iron as a Risk Factor for Age at Onset in Neurodegenerative Diseases," *Annals of the New York Academy of Sciences* 1012, no. 1 (March 2004): 224–36, http://doi.org/10.1196/annals.1306.019.

22. Masahiro Kawahara and Midori Kato-Negishi, "Link between Aluminum and the Pathogenesis of Alzheimer's Disease: The Integration of the Aluminum and Amyloid Cascade Hypotheses," *International Journal of Alzheimer's Disease* 2011 (January 5, 2011), http://doi.org/10.4061/2011/276393.

Chapter 19

1. Ann Hathaway, "Women, Estrogen, Cognition and Alzheimer's Disease," *Townsend Letter*, June 2012, https://pdfs.semanticscholar.org/be61/74fdd5419 a1f37f6af1b6ba6919ca6cac7da.pdf.

2. Writing Group for the Women's Health Initiative Investigators, "Risks and Benefits of Estrogen Plus Progestin in Healthy Postmenopausal Women: Principal Results from the Women's Health Initiative Randomized Controlled

Trial," *JAMA* 288, no. 3 (July 17, 2002): 321–33, http://doi.org/10.1001/jama
.288.3.321.

3. Women's Health Initiative, "Risks and Benefits," 321–33.

4. Natalie L. Rasgon et al., "Prospective Randomized Trial to Assess Effects of
   Continuing Hormone Therapy on Cerebral Function in Postmenopausal Women
   at Risk for Dementia," *PLOS One* 9, no. 3 (March 12, 2014): e89095, http://doi.org
   /10.1371/journal.pone.0089095.

5. Bruce Goldman, "Estradiol—but Not Premarin—Prevents Neurodegeneration in
   Women at Heightened Dementia Risk," Scope (blog), *Stanford Medicine*, March
   12, 2014, https://scopeblog.stanford.edu/2014/03/12/estradiol-but-not-premarin
   -prevents-neurodegeneration-in-women-at-heightened-dementia-risk/.

6. Joanna L. Spencer et al., "Uncovering the Mechanisms of Estrogen Effects on
   Hippocampal Function," *Frontiers in Neuroendocrinology* 29, no. 2 (May 2008):
   219–37, http://doi.org/10.1016/j.yfrne.2007.08.006.

7. Maya Yankova, Sharron A. Hart, and Catherine S. Woolley, "Estrogen Increases
   Synaptic Connectivity between Single Presynaptic Inputs and Multiple
   Postsynaptic CA1 Pyramidal Cells: A Serial Electron Microscope Study," *PNAS*
   98, no. 6 (March 2001): 3525–30, http://doi.org/10.1073/pnas.051624598. See
   also Maya Frankfurt and Victoria Luine, "The Evolving Role of Dendritic Spines
   and Memory: Interaction(s) with Estradiol," *Hormones and Behavior* 74 (August
   2015): 28–36, http://doi.org/10.1016/j.yhbeh.2015.05.004.

8. Victoria Luine and Maya Frankfurt, "Interactions between Estradiol, BDNF and
   Dendritic Spines in Promoting Memory," *Neuroscience* 239 (June 3, 2013): 34–45,
   https://doi.org/10.1016/j.neuroscience.2012.10.019.

9. Claudia Barth, Arno Villringer, and Julia Sacher, "Sex Hormones Affect
   Neurotransmitters and Shape the Adult Female Brain During Hormonal
   Transition Periods," *Frontiers in Neuroscience* 9 (2015), http://doi.org/10.3389
   /fnins.2015.00037.

10. Rodrigo A. Loiola et al., "Estrogen Promotes Pro-Resolving Microglial Behavior
    and Phagocytic Cell Clearance through the Actions of Annexin a1," *Frontiers of
    Endocrinology* 10 (June 26, 2019): 420, http://doi.org/10.3389/fendo.2019.00420.

11. Jon Nilsen et al., "Estrogen Protects Neuronal Cells from Amyloid Beta-Induced
    Apoptosis via Regulation of Mitochondrial Proteins and Function," *BMC
    Neuroscience* 7 (November 3, 2006), https://doi.org/10.1186/1471-2202-7-74.

12. Michael E. Mendelsohn and Richard H. Karas, "The Protective Effects of
    Estrogen on the Cardiovascular System," *New England Journal of Medicine* 340
    (June 10, 1999): 1801–11, http://doi.org/10.1056/NEJM199906103402306.

13. Whitney Wharton et al., "Short-Term Hormone Therapy with Transdermal
    Estradiol Improves Cognition for Postmenopausal Women with Alzheimer's
    Disease: Results of a Randomized Controlled Trial," *Journal of Alzheimer's
    Disease* 26, no. 3 (March 13, 2012): 495–505, http://doi.org/10.3233/JAD
    -2011-110341.

14. O. Scheyer et al., "Female Sex and Alzheimer's Risk: The Menopause
    Connection," *Journal of Prevention of Alzheimer's Disease* 5, no. 4 (2018): 225–30,
    http://doi.org/10.14283/jpad.2018.34.

15. Joann T. Tschanz et al., "The Cache County Study on Memory in Aging: Factors Affecting Risk of Alzheimer's Disease and Its Progression after Onset," *International Review of Psychiatry* 25, no. 6 (December 2013): 673–85, http://doi.org/10.3109/09540261.2013.849663.

Chapter 20

1. Sarah J. Spencer et al., "Food for Thought: How Nutrition Impacts Cognition and Emotion," *NPJ Science of Food* 1 (December 6, 2017), https://doi.org/10.1038/s41538-017-0008-y.

2. Rebecca J. Denniss, Lynne A. Barker, and Catherine J. Day, "Improvement in Cognition Following Double-Blind Randomized Micronutrient Interventions in the General Population," *Frontiers in Behavioral Neuroscience* 13 (May 28, 2019), http://doi.org/10.3389/fnbeh.2019.00115.

3. Ralph A. Nixon, "The Role of Autophagy in Neurodegenerative Disease," *Nature Medicine* 19, no. 8 (August 6, 2013): 983–97, http://doi.org/10.1038/nm.3232.

4. Rosebud O. Roberts et al., "Relative Intake of Macronutrients Impacts Risk of Mild Cognitive Impairment or Dementia," *Journal of Alzheimer's Disease* 32, no. 2 (October 9, 2012): 329–39, http://doi.org/10.3233/JAD-2012-120862.

5. James Hamblin, "This Is Your Brain on Gluten," *Atlantic*, December 20, 2013, https://www.theatlantic.com/health/archive/2013/12/this-is-your-brain-on-gluten/282550/.

6. Maciej Gasior, Michael A. Rogawski, and Adam L. Hartman, "Neuroprotective and Disease-Modifying Effects of the Ketogenic Diet," *Behavioral Pharmacology* 17, no. 5–6 (September 2006): 431–39, https://www.ncbi.nlm.nih.gov/pmc/articles/PMC2367001.

7. Regina Wierzejska, "Can Coffee Consumption Lower the Risk of Alzheimer's Disease and Parkinson's Disease? A Literature Review," *Archives of Medical Science* 13, no. 3 (April 1, 2017): 507–14, http://doi.org/10.5114/aoms.2016.63599.

8. Marco Cascella et al., "The Efficacy of Epigallocatechin-3-Gallate (Green Tea) in the Treatment of Alzheimer's Disease: An Overview of Pre-Clinical Studies and Translational Perspectives in Clinical Practice," *Infectious Agents and Cancer* 12 (June 19, 2017), http://doi.org/10.1186/s13027-017-0145-6.

9. M. I. Greenberg and D. Vearrier, "Metal Fume Fever and Polymer Fume Fever," *Clinical Toxicology* 53, no. 4 (May 2015): 195–203, http://doi.org/10.3109/15563650.2015.1013548.

10. H. J. Roberts, "Aspartame and Brain Cancer," *Lancet* 349, no. 9048 (February 1, 1997): 362, https://doi.org/10.1016/S0140-6736(05)62868-1.

11. P. Humphries, E. Pretorius, and H. Naude, "Direct and Indirect Cellular Effects of Aspartame on the Brain," *European Journal of Clinical Nutrition* 62 (April 2008): 451–62, https://doi.org/10.1038/sj.ejcn.1602866.

    See also Kaayla T. Daniel, *The Whole Soy Story: The Dark Side of America's Favorite Health Food* (Washington, DC; New Trends, 2005). In her 2005 book *The Whole Soy Story*, Dr. Kaayla T. Daniel (who did her doctoral research on this topic) covers the health dangers of soy in great depth and presents thousands of studies linking soy to cognitive decline and a host of other health problems, including malnutrition, digestive distress, immune-system breakdown, thyroid dysfunction, cancer, heart disease, and reproductive disorders—including infertility. If you are still thinking that soy is a health food, Dr. Daniels's book is a must read. See also Sally Fallon and Mary G. Enig, "Soy: The Dark Side of America's Favorite 'Health' Food," Weston A. Price Foundation, February 17, 2004, https://www.westonaprice .org/health-topics/soy-alert/soy-the-dark-side-of-americas-favorite-health-food.

Chapter 21

1. "How Much Sugar Do You Eat? You May Be Surprised," New Hampshire Department of Health and Human Services, December 11, 2017, https://www .dhhs.nh.gov/dphs/nhp/documents/sugar.pdf.
2. Rosebud O. Roberts et al., "Relative Intake of Macronutrients Impacts Risk of Mild Cognitive Impairment or Dementia," *Journal of Alzheimer's Disease* 32, no. 2 (October 9, 2012): 329–39, http://doi.org/10.3233/JAD-2012-120862.
3. Roberts, "Relative Intake," 329–39.
4. "Harvesting and Producing Sucrose," Sucrose (blog), December 12, 2016, https:// sucrose-isu-common-and-consumer-chemical.weebly.com/productionharvest-ing-of-sucrose.html.

Chapter 22

1. Per Nilsson et al., "Aβ Secretion and Plaque Formation Depend on Autophagy," *Cell Reports* 5, no. 1 (October 17, 2013): 61–69, http://doi.org/10.1016/j.celrep .2013.08.042.
2. Zoe Mputhia et al., "Autophagy Modulation as a Treatment of Amyloid Diseases, *Molecules* 24, no. 18 (September 2019): 3372, http://doi.org/10.3390 /molecules24183372.

Chapter 23

1. Aseem Malhotra, Rita F. Redberg, and Pascal Meier, "Saturated Fat Does Not Clog the Arteries: Coronary Heart Disease Is a Chronic Inflammatory Condition, the Risk of Which Can Be Effectively Reduced from Healthy Lifestyle Interventions," *British Medical Journal: British Journal of Sports Medicine* 51, no. 15 (April 25, 2017), http://dx.doi.org/10.1136/bjsports-2016-097285.
2. Maciej Gasior, Michael A. Rogawski, and Adam L. Hartman, "Neuroprotective and Disease-Modifying Effects of the Ketogenic Diet," *Behavioral Pharmacology* 17, no. 5–6 (September 2006): 431–39, https://www.ncbi.nlm.nih.gov/pmc /articles/PMC2367001.
3. Mark A. Reger et al., "Effects of β-Hydroxybutyrate on Cognition in Memory-Impaired Adults," *Neurobiology Aging* 25, no. 3 (March 2004): 311–14, http://doi .org/10.1016/S0197-4580(03)00087-3.
4. Firoozeh Nadar and Karen M. Mearow, "Coconut Oil Attenuates the Effects of Amyloid-β on Cortical Neurons In Vitro," *Journal of Alzheimer's Disease* 39, no. 2 (January 24, 2014): 233–37, http://doi.org/10.3233/JAD-131436.

Chapter 24

1. Ines Figueira et al., "Polyphenols beyond Barriers: A Glimpse into the Brain," *Current Neuropharmacology* 15, no. 4 (May 2017): 562–94, http://doi.org/10.2174/1570159X14666161026151545.

2. Giselle P. Dias et al., "The Role of Dietary Polyphenols on Adult Hippocampal Neurogenesis: Molecular Mechanisms and Behavioural Effects on Depression and Anxiety," *Oxidative Medicine and Cellular Longevity* 2012 (2012), http://doi.org/10.1155/2012/541971.

3. Rui F. M. Silva and Lea Pogacnik, "Food, Polyphenols and Neuroprotection," *Neural Regeneration Research* 12, no. 4 (April 2017): 582–83, http://doi.org/10.4103/1673-5374.205096.

4. Véronique Cheynier, "Polyphenols in Food Are More Complex Than Often Thought," *American Journal of Clinical Nutrition* 81, no. 1 (January 1, 2005): 223S–229S, http://doi.org/10.1093/ajcn/81.1.223S.

5. Tarique Hussain et al., "Oxidative Stress and Inflammation: What Polyphenols Can Do for Us?" *Oxidative Medicine and Cellular Longevity* 2016 (2016), http://doi.org/10.1155/2016/7432797.

6. Robert J. Williams, Jeremy P. E. Spencer, and Catherine Rice-Evans, "Flavonoids: Antioxidants or Signalling Molecules?," *Free Radical Biology and Medicine* 36, no. 7 (April 1, 2004): 838–49, http://doi.org/10.1016/j.freeradbiomed.2004.01.001.

7. Helmut M. Hügel and Neale Jackson, "Polyphenols for the Prevention and Treatment of Dementia Diseases," *Neural Regeneration Research* 10, no. 11 (November 2015): 1756–58, http://doi.org/10.4103/1673-5374.169609.

8. Joyce Joven et al., "Polyphenols and the Modulation of Gene Expression Pathways: Can We Eat Our Way out of the Danger of Chronic Disease?," *Critical Reviews in Food Science and Nutrition* 54, no. 8 (2014): 985–1001, http://doi.org/10.1080/10408398.2011.621772.

9. Shin Yen Chong et al., "Green Tea Extract Promotes DNA Repair in a Yeast Model," *Scientific Reports* 9 (March 7, 2019), http://doi.org/10.1038/s41598-019-39082-9.

10. Catarina Rendeiro, Justin S. Rhodes, and Jeremy P. E. Spencer, "The Mechanisms of Action of Flavonoids in the Brain: Direct *versus* Indirect Effects," *Neurochemistry International* 89 (October 2015): 126–39, https://doi.org/10.1016/j.neuint.2015.08.002.

11. Ioannis Bakoyiannis et al., "Phytochemicals and Cognitive Health: Are Flavonoids Doing the Trick?," *Biomedicine & Pharmacotherapy* 109 (January 2019): 1488–97, https://doi.org/10.1016/j.biopha.2018.10.086.

12. Adam M. Brickman et al., "Enhancing Dentate Gyrus Function with Dietary Flavanols Improves Cognition in Older Adults," *Nature Neuroscience* 17, no. 12 (December 2014): 1798–803, http://doi.org/10.1038/nn.3850.

Chapter 25

1. Dan Charles, "How New Jersey Tamed the Wild Blueberry for Global Production," *The Salt* (blog), NPR, August 4, 2015, https://www.npr.org/sections

/thesalt/2015/08/04/428984045/how-new-jersey-tamed-the-wild-blueberrgy
-for-global-production.

2. Joanna L. Bowtell et al., "Enhanced Task-Related Brain Activation and Resting
   Perfusion in Healthy Older Adults after Chronic Blueberry Supplementation,"
   Applied Physiology, Nutrition, and Metabolism 42, no. 7 (March 1, 2017): 773–79,
   http://doi.org/10.1139/apnm-2016-0550.

3. Catarina Rendeiro et al., "Blueberry Supplementation Induces Spatial Memory
   Improvements and Region-Specific Regulation of Hippocampal BDNF mRNA
   Expression in Young Rats," *Psychopharmacology* 223, no. 3 (May 9, 2012):
   319–30, http://doi.org/10.1007/s00213-012-2719-8.

4. Peter J. Curtis et al., "Blueberries Improve Biomarkers of Cardiometabolic
   Function in Participants with Metabolic Syndrome—Results from a 6-Month,
   Double-Blind, Randomized Controlled Trial," *American Journal of Clinical
   Nutrition* 109, no. 6 (June 2019): 1535–45, http://doi.org/10.1093/ajcn/nqy380.

Chapter 26

1. "Toxic Chocolate," As You Sow, July 14, 2018, https://www.asyousow.org
   /environmental-health/toxic-enforcement/toxic-chocolate.

2. "Proposition 65 Law and Regulations," California Office of Environment Health
   Hazard Assessment, November 14, 2016, https://oehha.ca.gov/proposition-65
   /law/proposition-65-law-and-regulations.

3. "Toxic Chocolate," As You Sow.

4. "Toxic Chocolate," As You Sow.

5. "Toxic Chocolate," As You Sow.

6. "Toxic Chocolate," As You Sow.

7. Astrid Nehlig, "The Neuroprotective Effects of Cocoa Flavanol and Its Influence
   on Cognitive Performance," *British Journal of Clinical Pharmacology* 75, no. 3
   (March 2013): 716–27, http://doi.org/10.1111/j.1365-2125.2012.04378.x.

8. Jean-Claude Stoclet et al., "Vascular Protection by Dietary Polyphenols,"
   European Journal of Pharmacology 500, no. 1–3 (October 2004): 299–313, http://
   doi.org/10.1016/j.ejphar.2004.07.034.

9. Adam M. Brickman et al., "Enhancing Dentate Gyrus Function with Dietary
   Flavanols Improves Cognition in Older Adults," *Nature Neuroscience* 17, no. 12
   (December 2014): 1798–803, http://doi.org/10.1038/nn.3850.

10. Annamaria Cimini et al., "Cocoa Powder Triggers Neuroprotective and
    Preventive Effects in a Human Alzheimer's Disease Model by Modulating BDNF
    Signaling Pathway," *Journal of Cellular Biochemistry* 114, no. 10 (October 2013):
    2209–20, http://doi.org/10.1002/jcb.24548.

11. Jun Wang et al., "Cocoa Extracts Reduce Oligomerization of Amyloid-β:
    Implications for Cognitive Improvement in Alzheimer's Disease," *Journal of
    Alzheimer's Disease* 41, no. 2 (June 23, 2014): 643–50, http://doi.org/10.3233
    /JAD-132231.

12. Mount Sinai Medical Center, "Cocoa Extract May Counter Specific Mechanisms
    of Alzheimer's Disease," ScienceDaily, June 23, 2014, http://www.sciencedaily
    .com/releases/2014/06/140623224910.htm.

Chapter 27

1. Gregory J. Moore et al., "Lithium-Induced Increase in Human Brain Grey Matter," *Lancet* 356, no. 9237 (October 7, 2000): 1241–42, http://doi.org/10.1016 /S0140-6736(00)02793-8.

2. Anna Fels, "Should We All Take a Bit of Lithium?," *New York Times*, September 13, 2014, https://www.nytimes.com/2014/09/14/opinion/sunday/should-we-all -take-a-bit-of-lithium.html.

3. Multiple studies published between 1970 and 1990 showed an association between higher levels of lithium in local water and beneficial clinical, behavioral, legal, and medical outcomes. Victor Bluml et al., "Lithium in the Public Water Supply and Suicide Mortality in Texas," *Journal of Psychiatric Research* 47, no. 3 (March 2013): 407–11, http://doi.org/10.1016/j.psychires.2012.12.002. This 2013 study examined data from 226 Texas counties from 1978 to 1987 and found that rates of suicide, homicide, and rape were significantly higher in counties whose drinking water contained little or no lithium. The group whose water had the highest lithium level had almost 40 percent fewer suicides than those with the lowest lithium level.

   See also U. Lewitzka et al., "The Suicide Prevention Effect of Lithium: More Than 20 Years of Evidence—A Narrative Review," *International Journal of Bipolar Disorders* 3 (July 18, 2015), http://doi.org/10.1186/s40345-015-0032-2. This 2015 Japanese study that looked at eighteen municipalities with a total of 1,206,174 individuals over a twenty-year period; lithium in the local water supply exerted a suicide prevention effect. The study also showed lower levels of all-cause mortality in people ingesting more lithium.

   See also Lars Vedel Kessing et al., "Association of Lithium in Drinking Water with the Incidence of Dementia," *JAMA Psychiatry* 74, no. 10 (October 1, 2017): 1005–10, http://doi.org/10.1001/jamapsychiatry.2017.2362. In this 2017 Danish study, Lars Vedel Kessing at the University of Copenhagen scrutinized the water consumed by 73,731 dementia patients compared with 733,653 normal controls. He found that increased lithium exposure in drinking water was associated with a lower incidence of Alzheimer's disease and vascular dementia.

4. Paula V. Nunes, Orestes V. Forlenza, and Wagner F. Gattaz, "Lithium and Risk for Alzheimer's Disease in Elderly Patients with Bipolar Disorder," *British Journal of Psychiatry* 190, no. 4 (April 2007): 359–60, http://doi.org/10.1192/bjp .bp.106.029868.

5. Lars Vedel Kessing et al., "Lithium Treatment and Risk of Dementia," *Archives of General Psychiatry* 65, no. 11 (November 3, 2008): 1331–35, http://doi.org /10.1001/archpsyc.65.11.1331.

6. M. A. Nunes, T. A. Viel, and H. S. Buck, "Microdose Lithium Treatment Stabilized Cognitive Impairment in Patients with Alzheimer's Disease," *Current Alzheimer's Research* 10, no. 1 (January 2013): 104–7, https://www.ncbi.nlm.nih .gov/pubmed/22746245.

7. Orestes V. Forlenza et al., "Disease-Modifying Properties of Long-Term Lithium Treatment for Amnestic Mild Cognitive Impairment: Randomised Controlled Trial," *British Journal of Psychiatry* 198, no. 5 (May 2011): 351–56, http://doi.org /10.1192/bjp.bp.110.080044.

8. James Greenblatt and Kayla Grossman, "Lithium: The Cinderella Story about a Mineral That May Prevent Alzheimer's Disease," *Neuropsychotherapist* (blog), Walden Psychiatric Care, December 2015, https://www.waldenpsychiatric.com /lithium-may-prevent-alzheimers-disease.

9. S. Zung et al., "The Influence of Lithium on Hippocampal Volume in Elderly Bipolar Patients: A Study Using Voxel-Based Morphometry," *Translational Psychiatry* 6 (June 28, 2016): e846, http://doi.org/10.1038/tp.2016.97.

10. Pretreatment with low-dose lithium reduces the severity of injury in cases of brain damage. In a 2014 study Dr. Peter Leeds stated that lithium had "demonstrated robust beneficial effects in experimental models of traumatic brain injury (TBI). These effects include decreases in TBI-induced brain lesion, suppression of neuroinflammation, protection against blood-brain barrier disruption, normalization of behavioral deficits, and improvement of learning and memory." Peter R. Leeds et al., "A New Avenue for Lithium: Intervention in Traumatic Brain Injury," *ACS Chemical Neuroscience* 5, no. 6 (April 3, 2014): 422–33, http://doi.org/10.1021/cn500040g.

11. The signaling molecule GSK-3, an enzyme involved in gene transcription and synaptic plasticity, provides an excellent example of how lithium influences cell signaling to reverse the pathogenesis of Alzheimer's disease (AD). GSK-3 plays pivotal roles in the growth and development of nerves by controlling the synaptic remodeling that drives memory formation in the hippocampus and frontal cortex. Chronic stress damages GSK-3, causing it to become overactive.

    In a 2007 paper published in the *Journal of Neurochemistry*, Claudie Hooper, Richard Killick, and Simon Lovestone proposed the "GSK-3 hypothesis of AD," which proposes that damaged, hyperactive GSK-3 redirects normal nerve growth and development down a dead-end street, leading to memory impairment, increased β amyloid production, neurofibrillary tangles, and local inflammatory responses—all of which are hallmark characteristics of AD. Lithium literally puts the GSK-3 train back on the tracks. Lithium repairs the broken cell signaling mechanism by restoring the correct level of activity to the derailed GSK-3. This halts inappropriate amyloid plaque and neurofibrillary tangle production, blocking the decline that would otherwise have led to Alzheimer's. Claudie Hooper, Richard Killick, and Simon Lovestone, "The GSK3 Hypothesis of Alzheimer's Disease," *Journal of Neurochemistry* 104 no. 6 (December 18, 2007): 1433–39, https://doi.org/10.1111/j.1471-4159.2007.05194.x.

12. Thomas Leyhe et al., "Increase of BDNF Serum Concentration in Lithium Treated Patients with Early Alzheimer's Disease," *Journal of Alzheimer's Disease* 16, no. 3 (March 9, 2009): 649–56, http://doi.org/10.3233/JAD-2009-1004.

Chapter 28

1. Karin Yurko-Mauro et al., "Beneficial Effects of Docosahexaenoic Acid on Cognition in Age-Related Cognitive Decline," *Alzheimer's & Dementia* 6, no. 6 (November 2010): 456–64, https://www.ncbi.nlm.nih.gov/pubmed/20434961.

2. Ernst J. Schaefer et al., "Plasma Phosphatidylcholine Docosahexaenoic Acid Content and Risk of Dementia and Alzheimer's Disease: The Framingham Heart Study," *Archives of Neurology* 63, no. 11 (November 2006): 1545–50, http://doi.org/10.1001/archneur.63.11.1545.

3. Dehua Cao et al., "Effects of Docosahexaenoic Acid on the Survival and Neurite Outgrowth of Rat Cortical Neurons in Primary Cultures," *Journal of Nutritional Biochemistry* 16, no. 9 (September 2005): 538–46, http://doi.org/10.1016/j.jnutbio.2005.02.002. See also Mahmoudreza Hadjighassem et al., "Oral Consumption of α-Linolenic Acid Increases Serum BDNF Levels in Healthy Adult Humans," *Nutrition Journal* 14 (February 26, 2015), http://doi.org/10.1186/s12937-015-0012-5.

4. Greg M. Cole and Sally A. Frautschy, "DHA May Prevent Age-Related Dementia," *Journal of Nutrition* 140, no. 4 (February 24, 2010): 869–74, https://doi.org/10.3945/jn.109.113910.

5. Thekkuttuparambil A. Ajith, "A Recent Update on the Effects of Omega-3 Fatty Acids in Alzheimer's Disease," *Current Clinical Pharmacology* 13, no. 4 (2018): 252–60, http://doi.org/10.2174/1574884713666180807145648.

6. J. Thomas et al., "Omega-3 Fatty Acids in Early Prevention of Inflammatory Neurodegenerative Disease: A Focus on Alzheimer's Disease," *BioMed Research International* 2015 (August 2, 2015), http://doi.org/10.1155/2015/172801.

7. Aiguo Wu, Zhengxin Ying, and Fernando Gomez-Pinilla, "Docosahexaenoic Acid Dietary Supplementation Enhances the Effects of Exercise on Synaptic Plasticity and Cognition," *Neuroscience* 155, no. 3 (August 26, 2008): 751–59, http://doi.org/10.1016/j.neuroscience.2008.05.061.

8. Paul F. Schuster et al., "Permafrost Stores a Globally Significant Amount of Mercury," *Geophysical Research Letters* 45, no. 3 (February 5, 2018), http://doi.org/10.1002/2017GL075571.

Chapter 29

1. S. Mishra and P. Kalpana, "The Effect of Curcumin (Turmeric) on Alzheimer's Disease: An Overview," *Annals of Indian Academy of Neurology* 11, no. 1 (January 2008): 13–9, http://doi.org/10.4103/0972-2327.40220.

2. Suzhen Dong et al., "Curcumin Enhances Neurogenesis and Cognition in Aged Rats: Implications for Transcriptional Interactions Related to Growth and Synaptic Plasticity," *PLOS* 7, no. 2 (February 16, 2012): e31211, https://doi.org/10.1371/journal.pone.0031211.

3. Meiling Jin et al., "Anti-Neuroinflammatory Effect of Curcumin on Pam3CSK4-Stimulated Microglial Cells," *International Journal of Molecular Medicine* 41 (October 27, 2017): 521–30, https://doi.org/10.3892/ijmm.2017.3217.

4. Fusheng Yang et al., "Curcumin Inhibits Formation of Amyloid β Oligomers and Fibrils, Binds Plaques, and Reduces Amyloid *in Vivo*," *Journal of Biological Chemistry* 280, no. 7 (December 7, 2004): 589–901, http://doi.org/10.1074/jbc.M404751200.

5. Yang, "Curcumin Inhibits Formation," 589–901.

6. A. Barzegar and A. A. Moosavi-Movahedi, "Intracellular ROS Protection Efficiency and Free Radical-Scavenging Activity of Curcumin," *PLOS One* 6, no. 10 (October 10, 2011): e26012, http://doi.org/10.1371/journal.pone.0026012.

Chapter 30

1. Moeko Noguchi-Shinohara et al., "Consumption of Green Tea, but Not Black Tea or Coffee, Is Associated with Reduced Risk of Cognitive Decline," *PLoS ONE* 9, no. 5 (May 14, 2014): e96013, https://doi.org/10.1371/journal.pone.0096013.

2. Yasutake Tomata et al., "Green Tea Consumption and the Risk of Incident Dementia in Elderly Japanese: The Ohsaki Cohort 2006 Study," *American Journal of Geriatric Psychiatry* 24, no. 10 (October 2016): 881–89, http://doi.org/10.1016/j.jagp.2016.07.009.

3. Silvia A. Mandel et al., "Molecular Mechanisms of the Neuroprotective/Neurorescue Action of Multi-Target Green Tea Polyphenols," *Frontiers in Bioscience* 4, no. 2 (January 1, 2012): 581–98.

4. Rashik Ahmed et al., "Molecular Mechanism for the (–)-Epigallocatechin Gallate-Induced Toxic to Nontoxic Remodeling of Aβ Oligomers," *Journal of the American Chemical Society* 139, no. 39 (August 25, 2017): 13720–34, https://doi.org/10.1021/jacs.7b05012. See also Curt Anthoy Polito et al., "Association of Tea Consumption with Risk of Alzheimer's Disease and Anti-Beta-Amyloid Effects of Tea," *Nutrients* 10, no. 5 (May 22, 2018): 655, http://doi.org/10.3390/nu10050655.

5. Jose M. Rubio-Perez et al., "Effects of an Antioxidant Beverage on Biomarkers of Oxidative Stress in Alzheimer's Patients," *European Journal of Nutrition* 55, no. 6 (September 2016): 2105–16, http://doi.org/10.1007/s00394-015-1024-9. See also Ide Kazuki et al., "Effects of Tea Catechins on Alzheimer's Disease: Recent Updates and Perspectives," *Molecules* 23, no. 9 (September 2018): 2357, http://doi.org/10.3390/molecules23092357; and Marco Cascella et al., "The Efficacy of Epigallocatechin-3-Gallate (Green Tea) in the Treatment of Alzheimer's Disease: An Overview of Pre-Clinical Studies and Translational Perspectives in Clinical Practice," *Infectious Agents and Cancer* 12 (June 19, 2017), http://doi.org/10.1186/s13027-017-0145-6.

Chapter 31

1. M. Martynov and E. Gusev, "Current Knowledge on the Neuroprotective and Neuroregenerative Properties of Citicoline in Acute Ischemic Stroke," *Journal of Experimental Pharmacology* 7 (October 1, 2015): 17–28, http://doi.org/10.2147/JEP.S63544.

2. Antoni Davalos et al., "Oral Citicoline in Acute Ischemic Stroke: An Individual Patient Data Pooling Analysis of Clinical Trials," *Stroke* 33, no. 12 (October 24, 2002): 2850–57, https://doi.org/10.1161/01.STR.0000038691.03334.71.

3. Jose Álvarez-Sabín and Gustavo C. Román, "The Role of Citicoline in Neuroprotection and Neurorepair in Ischemic Stroke," *Brain Science* 3, no. 3 (September 23, 2013): 1395–414, http://doi.org/10.3390/brainsci3031395.
4. Álvarez-Sabín and Román, "The Role of Citicoline," 1395–414.
5. Jeffrey L. Saver, "Citicoline: Update on a Promising and Widely Available Agent for Neuroprotection and Neurorepair," *Reviews in Neurological Diseases* 5, no. 4 (Fall 2008): 167–77.
6. O. Hurtado et al., "A Chronic Treatment with CDP-Choline Improves Functional Recovery and Increases Neuronal Plasticity after Experimental Stroke," *Neurobiology of Disease* 26, no. 1 (April 2007): 105–11, http://doi.org/10.1016/j.nbd.2006.12.005.
7. Álvarez-Sabín and Román, "The Role of Citicoline," 1395–414.
8. Álvarez-Sabín and Román, "The Role of Citicoline," 1395–414.

Chapter 32

1. Reena Kulkarni, K. J. Girish, and Abhimanyu Kumar, "Nootropic Herbs (*Medhya Rasayana*) in Ayurveda: An Update," *Phamacognosy Reviews* 6, no. 12 (July 2012): 147–53, http://doi.org/10.4103/0973-7847.99949, https://www.researchgate.net/publication/232232232_Nootropic_herbs_Medhya_Rasayana_in_Ayurveda_An_update.
2. Sebastian Aguiar and Thomas Borowski, "Neuropharmacological Review of the Nootropic Herb *Bacopa monnieri*," *Rejuvenation Research* 16, no. 4 (August 14, 2013): 313–26, http://doi.org/10.1089/rej.2013.1431.
3. K. S. Chaudhari et al., "Neurocognitive Effect of Nootropic Drug Brahmi (*Bacopa monnieri*) in Alzheimer's Disease," *Annals of Neurosciences* 24, no. 2 (May 12, 2017): 111–22, http://doi.org/10.1159/000475900.
4. Venkata Ramana Vollala, Subramanya Upadhya, and Satheesha Nayak, "Enhancement of Basolateral Amygdaloid Neuronal Dendritic Arborization Following *Bacopa monnieri* Extract Treatment in Adult Rats," *Clinics (Saõ Paulo)* 66, no. 4 (April 2011): 663–71, http://doi.org/10.1590/S1807-59322011000400023.
5. Sangeeta Raghav et al., "Randomized Controlled Trial of Standardized *Bacopa monnieri* Extract in Age-Associated Memory Impairment," *Indian Journal of Psychiatry* 48, no. 4 (2006): 238–42, http://doi.org/10.4103/0019-5545.31555.
6. Carlo Calabrese et al., "Effects of a Standardized *Bacopa monnieri* Extract on Cognitive Performance, Anxiety, and Depression in the Elderly: A Randomized, Double-Blind, Placebo-Controlled Trial," *Journal of Alternative and Complementary Medicine* 14, no. 6 (July 2008): 707–13, https://doi.org/1089/acm.2008.0018.
7. C. Stough et al., "The Chronic Effects of an Extract of *Bacopa monnieri* (Brahmi) on Cognitive Function in Healthy Human Subjects," *Psychopharmacology* 156, no. 4 (August 2001): 481–84, https://doi.org/10.1007/s002130100815. See also Stough et al., "Examining the Nootropic Effects of a Special Extract of *Bacopa monnieri* on Human Cognitive Functioning: 90 Day Double-Blind

Placebo-Controlled Randomized Trial," *Phytotherapy Research* 22, no. 12 (December 2008): 1629–34, http://doi.org/10.1002/ptr.2537.

8. Deepali Mathur et al., "The Molecular Links of Re-Emerging Therapy: A Review of Evidence of Brahmi (Bacopa monniera),"*Frontiers in Pharmacology* 7 (2016): 44, http://doi.org/10.3389/fphar.2016.00044.

9. Aguiar and Borowski, "Neuropharmacological Review," 313–26.

10. Aguiar and Borowski, "Neuropharmacological Review," 313–26.

11. Aguiar and Borowski, "Neuropharmacological Review," 313–26.

12. Aguiar and Borowski, "Neuropharmacological Review," 313–26.

Chapter 33

1. Akito Kato-Kataoka et al., "Soybean-Derived Phosphatidylserine Improves Memory Function of the Elderly Japanese Subjects with Memory Complaints," *Journal of Clinical Biochemical Nutrition* 47, no. 3 (November 2010): 246–55, http://doi.org/10.3164/jcbn.10-62.

2. Elizabeth Somer, *Food & Mood: The Complete Guide to Eating Well and Feeling Your Best*, rev. ed. (New York: Henry Holt, 1999), 211.

3. Dani Veracity, "Essential Fatty Acid Phosphatidylserine (PS) Is Powerful Prevention for Memory Loss, Alzheimer's and Dementia," Natural News, January 9, 2006, https://www.naturalnews.com/016646_Phosphatidylserine_Alzheimers .html. Also see Parris M. Kidd, "Phosphatidylserine; Membrane Nutrient for Memory. A Clinical and Mechanistic Assessment," *Alternative Medicine Review* 1, no. 2 (January 1996): 70–84.

4. Y. Richter et al., "The Effect of Soybean-Derived Phosphatidylserine on Cognitive Performance in Elderly with Subjective Memory Complaints: A Pilot Study," *Clinical Interventions in Aging* 8 (May 21, 2013): 557–63, http://doi.org /10.2147/CIA.S40348.

5. T. H. Crook et al., "Effects of Phosphatidylserine in Age-Associated Memory Impairment," *Neurology* 41, no. 5 (May 4, 1991): 644–49, http://doi.org/10.1212 /wnl.41.5.644.

6. Georges Ramalanjaona, "Effects of Phosphatidylserine on Alzheimer's Disease and Age-Related Memory Loss," Integrative Medicine, *Relias Media*, November 1, 2001, https://www.reliasmedia.com/articles/74302-effects-of-phosphatidylserine -on-alzheimer-8217-s-disease-and-age-related-memory-loss.

7. Crook et al., "Effects of Phosphatidylserine," 644–49. See also Timothy J. Smith, *Renewal: The Anti-Aging Revolution* (Emmaus, PA: Rodale, 1999), 387–88.

8. Kidd, "Phosphatidylserine; Membrane Nutrient," 79–80.

Chapter 34

1. Z. Cai, C. Wang, and W. Yang, "Role of Berberine in Alzheimer's Disease," *Neuropsychiatric Disease and Treatment* 12 (October 3, 2016): 2509–20, http://doi.org/10.2147/NDT.S114846.

2. Jing Gong et al., "Berberine Attenuates Intestinal Mucosal Barrier Dysfunction in Type 2 Diabetic Rats," *Frontiers in Pharmacology* 8 (February 3, 2017), http://doi.org/10.3389/fphar.2017.00042.

3. Yifei Zhang et al., "Treatment of Type 2 Diabetes and Dyslipidemia with the Natural Plant Alkaloid Berberine," *Journal of Clinical Endocrinology & Metabolism* 93, no. 7 (July 1, 2008): 2559–65, http://doi.org/10.1210/jc.2007-2404.

4. Zhang et al., "Treatment of Type 2 Diabetes," 2559–65.

5. Laura M. Koppen et al., "Efficacy of Berberine Alone and in Combination for the Treatment of Hyperlipidemia: A Systematic Review," *Journal of Evidence-Based Complementary & Alternative Medicine* 22, no. 4 (October 2017): 956–68, http://doi.org/10.1177/2156587216687695, https://journals.sagepub.com/doi/full/10.1177/2156587216687695

6. Mahila Lotfi Aski et al., "Neuroprotective Effect of Berberine Chloride on Cognitive Impairment and Hippocampal Damage in Experimental Model of Vascular Dementia," *Iranian Journal of Basic Medical Sciences* 21 no. 1 (January 2018): 53–58, http://doi.org/10.22038/IJBMS.2017.23195.5865.

7. Jun Yin, Huili Xing, and Jianping Ye, "Efficacy of Berberine in Patients with Type 2 Diabetes Mellitus," *Metabolism* 57, no. 5 (May 2008): 712–17, http://doi.org/10.1016/j.metabol.2008.01.013.

8. Guangju Zhou et al., "Ameliorative Effect of Berberine on Neonatally Induced Type 2 Diabetic Neuropathy via Modulation of BDNF, IGF-1, PPAR-γ, and AMPK Expressions," *Dose-Response* 17, no. 3 (July 16, 2019), http://doi.org/10.1177/1559325819862449.

Conclusion

1. Riya R. Kanherkar, Naina Bhatia-Dey, and Antonei B. Csoka, "Epigenetics across the Human Lifespan," *Frontiers in Cell and Developmental Biology* 2 (September 9, 2014): 49, http://doi.org/10.3389/fcell.2014.00049.

2. Jose V. Sanchez-Mut and Johannes Gräff, "Epigenetic Alterations in Alzheimer's Disease," *Frontiers in Behavioral Neuroscience* 9 (December 17, 2015): 347, http://doi.org/10.3389/fnbeh.2015.00347.

3. Samuel A. Lambert et al., "The Human Transcription Factors," *Cell* 172, no. 4 (February 8, 2018): 650–65, http://doi.org/10.1016/j.cell.2018.01.029.

4. Bruce Alberts et al., "Chromosomal DNA and Its Packaging in the Chromatin Fiber," in *Molecular Biology of the Cell*, 4th ed. (New York: Garland Science, 2002), https://www.ncbi.nlm.nih.gov/books/NBK26834/.

5. Shibu M. Poulose et al., "Nutritional Factors Affecting Adult Neurogenesis and Cognitive Function," *Advances in Nutrition* 8, no. 6 (November 15, 2017): 804–11, http://doi.org/10.3945/an.117.016261.

6. Ashley Yeager, "How Exercise Reprograms the Brain," *Scientist* (October 31, 2018), https://www.the-scientist.com/features/this-is-your-brain-on-exercise-64934.

7. Beate Winner and Jürgen Winkler, "Adult Neurogenesis in Neurodegenerative Diseases," *Cold Springs Harbor Perspectives in Biology* 7, no. 4 (April 2015), http://doi.org/10.1101/cshperspect.a021287.

8. Niladri Basu, Jaclyn. M. Goodrich, and Jessica Head, "Ecogenetics of Mercury: From Genetic Polymorphisms and Epigenetics to Risk Assessment and Decision

Making," *Environmental Toxicology and Chemistry* 33, no. 6 (August 27, 2013): 1248–58, http://doi.org/10.1002/etc.2375.

9. Bailey Kirkpatrick, "Epigenetics, Nutrition, and Our Health: How What We Eat Could Affect Tags on Our DNA," *What Is Epigenetics* (May 15, 2018), https://www.whatisepigenetics.com/epigenetics-nutrition-health-eat-affect-tags-dna/.

10. James Greenblatt, "Nutritional Lithium: Orchestrating Our Genes and Optimizing Our Moods," *ZRT Laboratory Blog* (September 8, 2017), https://www.zrtlab.com/blog/archive/nutritional-lithium-deficiency-genes-mental-health/.

11. Jayakumar Preethi, Hemant K. Singh, and Koilmani E. Rajan, "Possible Involvement of Standardized *Bacopa monniera* Extract (CDRI-08) in Epigenetic Regulation of *reelin* and Brain-Derived Neurotrophic Factor to Enhance Memory," *Frontiers in Pharmacology* 27 (June 27, 2016): 166, http://doi.org/10.3389/fphar.2016.00166.

12. Faiz-ul Hassan et al., "Curcumin as an Alternative Epigenetic Modulator: Mechanism of Action and Potential Effects," *Frontiers in Genetics* 10 (June 4, 2019): 514, http://doi.org/10.3389/fgene.2019.00514.

13. Jansen Fernandes, Ricardo M. Arida, and Fernando Gomez-Pinilla, "Physical Exercise as an Epigenetic Modulator of Brain Plasticity and Cognition," *Neuroscience and Biobehavioral Reviews* 80 (September 2017): 443–56, http://doi.org/10.1016/j.neubiorev.2017.06.012.

14. Riya R. Kanherkar et al., "Epigenetic Mechanisms of Integrative Medicine," *Evidence-Based Complementary and Alternative Medicine* 2017 (February 21, 2017): 4365429, http://doi.org/10.1155/2017/4365429.

Acknowledgments

I want to express my deep, heartfelt gratitude to Sharon Goldinger for all the wonderful energy and hard work she contributed to this book. And I forgive her for refusing to let me italicize *anything* and for getting rid of all my exclamation marks. I thank Kristin Loberg for a huge gift: she referred me to Sharon.

My wonderful, awesome wife, Dellie Kohl—supermom, supergrandma, incredible partner, and best friend for fifty years—fed me scrumptious food and came to assist me whenever I needed help—which was often. Dellie had the dedication and confidence to solve problem after problem as the book developed. Her keen insights brought this project to life. Without Dellie's support, not only would this book not have come about, but I would also have starved to death. Thank you so much!

I want my two exceptional daughters, Emma Kohlsmith and Dr. Hana Paterno, to know that over the five years I worked on this book, every time they asked me "How is the book coming along, Dad?" I got a three-day surge of support energy that made me happy and propelled me forward toward completion.

My wonderful mother-in-law, Freeke van Nouhuys Kohl, first introduced me to Dr. Bredesen's work and then kept telling me to write.

I also want to express my deep gratitude to Peter Rowell for being a good and remarkably generous friend who helped me with so many things that I gave up keeping a list a long time ago (San Diego hasn't been—and never will be—the same without him); my wonderful brother-in-law Bob Stupp and my extremely supportive sister Christy Foote-Smith, who gave strong encouragement every step of the way (hearing Christy say she actually enjoyed reading my draft gave me hope); Cynthia Miller, who kept encouraging me and steering me onto the right path, and she knows her paths; my dear friend Kani Comstock, who supported my book from beginning to end, was full of ideas and support, and helped me with all aspects of writing and publishing; Stephen Langer, MD, my Buddha buddy for lots of great ideas and for reminding me that nothing is everything and everything is nothing; Gale Young, PhD, for caring and for great ideas; Bob Frost, who was an endless font of encouragement and made many suggestions that improved the quality of the book; and Karl Smith, PhD, who provided lots of great advice and some help navigating the at-times shark-infested waters of the publishing industry.

Also, much gratitude goes out to Craig Comstock; Tony Paterno; Marguerite Sierra; Wendy Coy and Michael Coy; Cecile Biltekoff; Catherine Conner; Maria Rowell; Janey Paterno; Diane WeberShapiro, PhD; Vu Tran, MD; Jeff Bland, PhD; David Miller; William G. Kraybill, MD; Elaine Chernoff, PhD; Starr Sutherland; Karla Herbold; and last but definitely not least, Jan Winitz.

Great appreciation goes to Kenneth Pelletier, PhD, MD; Rudolph Tanzi, PhD; Ann Louise Gittleman, PhD; Jacob Teitelbaum, MD; Bill Gray, MD; and Ann Hathaway, MD, for their generous words of support and encouragement.

I have personally thanked Dale Bredesen, MD, for his research and teaching contributions and his many great ideas, not the least of which has been bringing functional medicine to the Alzheimer's table. Without his work, this book would not have been possible (and I appreciate his insistence that my discussion of AD-associated infections didn't belong in the microbiome chapter—good call).

And finally, above all, thanks to my entire family—for love, ideas, food, fun, and making space in your lives for my writing. I am so proud—and beyond grateful—to have all of you in my life!

Index

abstract thinking, 9
acetylcholine (ACh), 60, 272–275, 289
acidophilus, 82, 142
adenosine monophosphate-activated protein kinase (AMPK), 291–292
adrenal hormones, 79–80
advanced disease, 17–18
age-related cognitive decline (ARCD), 255, 284–286
aging, 18, 68–69, 147–148, 208, 210
Aguiar, Sebastian, 282
ALA (alpha-linolenic acid), 254
alcohol consumption, 34, 68, 172, 188, 210
allergenic foods, 82, 139, 143
Allergy Research Group, 82, 143
alpha-linolenic acid (ALA), 254
alpha-lipoic acid, 103
ALS, 208–209
alternative, defined, 21
Altman, Joseph, 52
aluminum, 33, 161, 174, 194. See also toxic metals
Alzheimer, Alois, 1, 38–44, 45, 109, 216
Alzheimer's Association, 1, 11
Alzheimer's disease
    autophagy and, 205–212 (see also autophagy)

biomarkers, 75–83 (see also biomarkers)
blueberries as prevention, 224–232
cause, 53–54
chocolate and cocoa as prevention, 233–241
defining, 9–10, 15–16
determining time to test, 18–19
diagnosing, 14–18
diets preventing, 185–196 (see also diets for prevention)
discovery, 38–44
epigenetics and future research, 295–298
multiple systems/causes of, 22–24
nutritional supplements reversing, 243–294 (see also nutritional supplements)
polyphenols as prevention, 218–223
statistics of, 11–13
suspecting, 19–20
terminology, 10
amalgam dental fillings, 83, 165–166
American Academy of Neurology, 91
American Academy of Sleep Medicine, 31
American Association of Clinical Endocrinologists, 149

American College for the
Advancement of Medicine, 170
*American Journal of Respiratory and
Critical Care Medicine,* 31
American Thyroid Association, 32,
148
AMPK (adenosine monophosphate-
activated protein kinase),
291–292
amyloid beta
autophagy and, 208–209
berberine reducing, 102–103
cholesterol and, 106–107
cocoa and, 239
DHA and, 257
discovery, 43
EGCG and, 271
and estradiol, 179–180
vitamin D and, 118
amyloid beta plaque
in advanced disease, 18
cholesterol and, 78
coconut oil preventing/removing,
216
curcumin and, 265–266
and high cholesterol, 106–107
vitamin D and, 30
Annals of Neurosciences, 280
Annweiler, Cédric, 117
anthocyanins, 226–227
antibiotics, 136, 140
antimicrobial peptides, 118
antioxidants, 52, 219–220. *See also*
chocolate and cocoa
antithyroglobulin, 79
antithyroid antibody (ATA) panel,
155
apnea, sleep. *See* sleep apnea
ARCD (age-related cognitive
decline), 255, 284–286

Archives of Neurology, 256
Armour Thyroid, 154–155
arsenic, 33
artificial sweeteners, 195, 201
Aski, Mahila, 291
aspartame, 195, 201
As You Sow, 102, 167, 234–236
ATA (antithyroid antibody) panel,
155
atherosclerosis, 96–97, 112, 157, 201,
230, 292
atherosclerotic plaque, 105
Atkins, Robert, 203
attention, estradiol supporting,
178–179
autoimmune diseases, 81, 137–138,
155–156
autoimmune thyroid disease,
155–156
autophagosomes, 206
autophagy, 205–212
about, 35–36, 185, 206
after, 212
benefits, 206–210
foods boosting, 211
initiating, 206
lowering blood sugar, 98
practicing, 210–211
as prevention, 186–187
avocado oil, 100, 191

Bacopa monnieri, 245, 279–282
bacteria
autophagy removing, 207
and gut microbiome, 30, 47, 131
healthy, 82
in human genome, 134–135
Barnes, Broda O., 149, 158–159
Barnes Basal Metabolic Temperature
Test (BMTT), 158–159

Bartzokis, George, 171–172
baseline testing, 15
B-complex vitamins, 109–114
   for BDNF production, 68
   as brain atrophy protection,
     110–111
   elevated homocysteine and, 29,
     79, 112
   and methyl groups/methylation,
     111–112
   supplemental, 112–114
BDNF. *See* brain-derived
   neurotrophic factor
beer, 193
behavioral symptoms, 14
Ben Cao Jing, 289
berberine, 36, 288–294
   benefits, 245
   drug interactions, 293–294
   lowering blood sugar, 102–103,
     290
   lowering cholesterol, 104, 107
   mechanisms, 291–292
   metformin vs., 292–293
   protective properties, 289–290
   VaD and, 290–291
bergamot, 104, 108
berries, 102. *See also* blueberries
Bifidobacterium, 142, 143
Bifidobiotics, 82
biofilm disruptors, 82–83, 142–143
bioidentical estradiol, 175–182
   as AD prevention, 178
   delivery systems, 180–181
   enhancing brain health, 178–180
   and fear of hormones, 176–178
   and NHRT, 181–182
biology, molecular, 22, 39, 52
biomarkers, 75–83
   about, 24–25

blood pressure, 76–77
blood tests, 77–80
cost of testing, 76
and microbiome, 81–83
obstructive sleep apnea and,
   80–81
testing (*see* molecular biomarker
   testing)
toxic metal hair analysis, 83
Biotagen, 82, 143
bisphenol A (BPA), 193
black tea, 191, 271
Bland, Jeffrey, 48
blood pressure, 84–89
   about, 85
   lowering, 87–88
   monitoring, 86–87
   normal range, 76, 87
   OSA and, 80
   rapid reduction, 88–89
   testing, 76–77, 86–87
   treatment, 27
blood pressure devices, 76
blood sugar, 90–103
   berberine lowering, 290
   and carbohydrate
     overconsumption, 93–96
   damaging effects of high, 90–93
   and insulin resistance, 95–97, 201
   lowering, 98–103
   testing FBS, 97
   treatment, 27–28
blood tests
   ATA panel, 155
   biomarker, 77–80
   iron, 173
   vitamin D, 119
blood vessels
   blueberries and, 230–231
   brain blood vessel disease, 26

blood vessels (*continued*)
    damaged, 84–85
    estradiol benefiting, 180
    homocysteine damaging, 112
blueberries, 224–232
    BDNF and, 66–67, 220
    benefits, 226–231
    products with, 231–232
    pterostilbene in, 226–227
BMTT (Barnes Basal Metabolic
    Temperature Test), 158–159
Borowski, Thomas, 282
Bowtell, Joanna L., 228
BPA (bisphenol A), 193
Brahmi. See *Bacopa monnieri*
brain
    advanced disease, 17
    atrophy, 17, 110–111, 251
    cholesterol in, 105
    gray matter, 150
    hypertension damaging, 85
    nerve cells, 46–47
    and phosphatidylserine, 284
brain blood vessel disease, 26
brain-derived neurotrophic factor
    (BDNF)
    about, 62
    blueberries enhancing, 227–228
    cocoa stimulating production, 239
    DHA increasing, 258
    and epigenetics, 297
    estradiol increasing, 179
    exercise and, 33–34
    increasing, 66–68
    lead blocking, 169
    lithium and, 252
    as neuroprotection, 63
    polyphenols and, 66–68, 220,
        221–222
brain health

estrogen enhancing, 178–180
    foods damaging, 192–196
    and gut microbiome, 137–138
Brain Maker (Perlmutter), 97, 139,
    188
breast-feeding women, 278
breathing techniques, 89
Bredesen, Dale, 2, 46, 48
Brickman, Adam M., 220, 237
Brooks, Fred, 225
Buck Institute for Research on
    Aging, 46
butter, 100

Cache County Study on Memory in
    Aging, 181–182
cadmium, 33, 101, 166–168, 234–
    235
calcium regulation, 119, 169
California poppies, 288
caloric intake, 199
carbohydrates
    about, 200–202
    calories from, 199
    effects, 187
    and gut microbiome, 139
    and high-carbohydrate diets,
        199–200
    overconsumption
        (*see* carbohydrate
        overconsumption)
carbohydrate overconsumption
    effects, 199–200
    epidemic of, 93–95
    inhibiting microbiome, 136
    and insulin resistance, 95–96
Cardiovascular Research, 261
caregivers, 12
causality, 13, 48–49
CDP-choline. *See* citicoline

cell signaling, 252

Centers for Disease Control and Prevention, 162

central nervous system (CNS), 22–23

central sleep apnea, 124

cerebral blood flow, 180

cerebral small vessel disease, 56

cerebrovascular injury, 84

Chaudhari, K. S., 280

cheese, processed, 192

Cherbuin, Nicolas, 91

chocolate and cocoa, 101–102, 191–192, 233–241

  benefits, 236–240

  cadmium in, 83, 167, 234–236

  milk, 237

  types, 240–241

  unsweetened, 101

CholestePure Plus, 108

cholesterol, 28, 78, 104–108, 256

chronic high blood pressure, 16

chronic traumatic encephalopathy, 208–209

cinnamon extract, 103

citicoline, 60–61, 113, 244, 272–278, 286, 297

Clinical Research Center (Massachusetts General Hospital), 92

Clostridium, 143

CNS (central nervous system), 22–23

cocoa. *See* chocolate and cocoa

coconut oil, 67, 100, 191, 203, 213–217

coenzyme Q10 (CoQ10), 88, 108

coenzyme QH (CoQH), 88, 108

coffee, 63, 191, 210. *See also* polyphenols: foods containing

cognitive functioning

  assessing levels, 15

  autophagy reversing decline, 208

  blueberries enhancing, 228–229

  high-carb diets damaging, 199–200

  mild impairment, 18–19

cognitive symptoms, 14

Cole, Greg M., 257

combination products, 103

complementary, defined, 21

Contour, 97

conventional neurologists, 19

conventional treatment, 19

cookware, 194

CoQ10 (coenzyme Q10), 88, 108

CoQH (coenzyme QH), 88, 108

coronary artery disease, 180

Coville, Frederick Vernon, 225–226

CPAP machines, 123, 130

Creutzfeld, Hans-Gerhard, 41

curcumin, 190–191, 244, 263–269

dark chocolate. *See* chocolate and cocoa

Das, Gopal, 52

DaTerra Cucina Vesuvio frying pan, 194

DeCarli, Charles, 106

deep slow breathing, 89

defective methylation, 110

dementia

  defining, 10–11, 14

  elevated blood sugar and, 90–91

  functional medicine treatment, 2–3

  mixed, 16

  prevalence, 1, 11–12

  and sleep apnea, 125–126

  types of, 15–17

  and vitamin D deficiency, 117

dental fillings, amalgam, 83, 165–166
depression, 286, 290
Deter, Auguste, 39–44
DHA. *See* docosahexaenoic acid
DHEA-S, 79–80
diabetes, 293
Diabetes Center (Massachusetts General Hospital), 92
diagnosis, 13–18
  of AD type, 15–17
  advanced disease, 17–18
  assessing levels of cognitive functioning, 15
  biomarkers, 24–25
  dementia, 11
  new ways of, 22
diastolic pressure, 85
diet
  and AD reversal, 53–54
  autophagy, 35–36
  BDNF-generating, 67
  and epigenetics, 297–298
  healthy fats, 99–100
  for healthy gut microbiome, 140–141
  lowering blood pressure, 87–88
  lowering blood sugar, 98–103
  nutritional supplements, 36–37, 102–103
  for prevention (*see* diets for prevention)
  as treatment, 35–37
diets for prevention, 185–196
  about, 185–186
  antidementia superfoods, 190–192
  autophagy, 186–187
  damaging foods, 192–196
  grain-free diet, 185, 187–188
  high fat, 189
  ketogenic (*see* ketogenic diet)
  low carb (*see* low-carb diet)
  low protein, 186, 189–190
digestive enzymes, 82, 141–142
digestive symptoms, 81
Direct Labs, 76, 112, 156, 158
disaccharides, 200
discrimination, 12
DNA, 296
docosahexaenoic acid (DHA), 67, 195, 244, 254–262
Doctor's Data Toxic and Essential Elements Hair Mineral Analysis, 83, 173
Douaud, Gwenaëlle, 110
DreamWear Nasal mask, 123
drinking water, 170, 172–173, 194
drug interactions, berberine, 293
dysbiosis, 81, 138, 141–144

Ecological Formulas' Neuromins, 195
economic impact, 11
EFAs. *See* essential fatty acids
EFT (Emotional Freedom Technique), 89
EGCG (epigallocatechin gallate), 191, 270–271
eggs, 190
Eine eigenartige Erkrankung der Hirnrinde (Alzheimer), 42
Emotional Freedom Technique (EFT), 89
energy, mental, 275–276
enzymes, digestive, 82, 141–142
epigallocatechin gallate (EGCG), 191, 270–271
epigenetics, 295–299
Epstein-Barr virus, 207

Erickson, Kirk, 69
essential fatty acids (EFAs)
    about, 255
    alpha-linolenic acid, 254
    DHA (*see* docosahexaenoic acid
      (DHA))
    importance of, 47
    omega-3s (*see* omega-3 oils)
    phosphatidylserine derived from,
      284
    in seafood, 194
estradiol, bioidentical. *See*
    bioidentical estradiol
estrogen, 80. *See also* bioidentical
    estradiol
exercise, 62–71, 258
    and BDNF, 62–63, 66–68
    benefits, 68–70
    and hippocampus, 63–65
    importance of daily, 70–71
    lowering blood pressure, 87
    lowering blood sugar, 98
    neurogenesis/neurogeneration/
      neuroplasticity, 65–66
    as treatment, 33–34
"Exercise Training Increases Size of
    Hippocampus and Improves
    Memory" (Erickson), 69
"Experiments in Blueberry Culture"
    (Coville), 225

fasting. *See* autophagy
fasting blood sugar (FBS)
    at-home testing, 97
    minimal increases, 27–28
    normal range, 77, 95
    testing, 77–78
fats and oils, 99–100, 202–204,
    213–214
FBS. *See* fasting blood sugar

FDA (US Food and Drug
    Administration), 59, 61
Fels, Anna, 248
ferritin, 79, 173
fish and fish oils, 164–165. *See also*
    seafood
flash-frozen blueberries, 231–232
flaxseed oil, 191, 244, 254–262
Flint, Michigan, 168
Flöel, Anges, 93
Folstein test, 15
food allergens, 143
Food & Mood (Somer), 283
foods
    antidementia superfoods, 190–
      192
    autophagy boosting, 211
    BDNF increasing, 34, 63
    BDNF production blocking, 34,
      68
    blood sugar lowering, 99
    boosting autophagy, 211
    carbohydrates (*see* carbohydrates)
    damaging, 192–196
    grains, 139
    high carbohydrate, 188
    omega-3, 260–261
    polyphenol containing, 28, 88,
      186, 190, 303–306
    processed, 141, 192–193
    starches, 139
    See also diet
Foresterol, 108
Forlenza, Orestes, 250
Framingham Heart Study, 256
Frankfurt, Mya, 179
Frautschy, Sally A., 257
free radicals, 52, 172, 207
free T3, 150–152
free T4, 151–152

Freudianism, 39
Frontiers in Aging Neuroscience,
    136–137
functional, defined, 21
functional medicine, 2, 48–49

GastroThera, 144
Geisenheimer, Cecilia, 39–40
gene expression, 295–299
genetics, 39, 52, 220. *See also*
    epigenetics
Genova Diagnostics GI Effects
    Microbial Ecology Profile,
    81–82
Geophysical Research Letters, 259
glial cells, 118–119
glucose
    and AMPK, 292
    berberine vs. metformin and, 293
    blood (*See* blood sugar)
    citicoline increasing metabolism
        of, 275–276
    as energy source, 94, 202
    from grains, 188
    and hypertension, 107
    See also sugar
glycemic control. *See* blood sugar
glycosylated hemoglobin (HbA1C),
    91
glyphosate, 231
GM. *See* gut microbiome
government recommended daily
    allowances (RDAs), 113
Grain Brain (Perlmutter), 97, 139,
    188
grain-free diet, 185, 187–188
grains, 139, 193
gray matter, 150, 251
green tea, 101, 191, 244, 270–271
gut, leaky, 81, 138

gut microbiome (GM), 131–144
    about, 133–134
    antibiotics damaging, 140
    berberine and, 289
    defined, 133
    and diet, 139–141
    discovery and research, 47
    and DNA, 134–135
    healing, 137–138
    importance of, 131–132
    modern practices damaging,
        135–136
    obtaining medical health for, 144
    pathogenic microbes disrupting,
        136–137
    reestablishing, 141–144
    terminology, 132–133
    testing, 81–82
    treatment, 30–31, 82–83

hair toxic mineral analysis, 33, 83,
    161
*The Handbook of Alzheimer's Disease
    and Other Dementia,* 14
Hashimoto's disease, 79, 81, 138,
    155–156, 158
HbA1C (glycosylated hemoglobin),
    91
HDL cholesterol, 78, 106–107
healthy bacteria, 82
healthy fats, 99–100
heart, hypertension damaging, 85
herpesviruses, 207
high-carbohydrate diets, 199–200,
    214–215. *See also* carbohydrate
    overconsumption
high cholesterol, 105–107
high-dose lithium, 247, 253
"Higher Normal Fasting Plasma
    Glucose Is Associated with

Hippocampal Atrophy"
    (Cherbuin), 91
Hill, James M., 136
hippocampus
    blood sugar affecting, 92–93
    blueberries and, 230–231
    estradiol supporting, 178–179
    exercise and, 69
    lead damaging, 169
    low thyroid hormone slowing,
      150
    polyphenols and, 218
    role, 63–65
    shrinkage, 17, 68–69
    sleep apnea damaging, 125–126
home sleep tests, 129–130
homocysteine, 29, 79, 109, 112
hormone replacement therapy
    (HRT), 176
hormones
    adrenal, 79–80
    BDNF (*see* brain-derived
      neurotrophic factor (BDNF))
    and cholesterol, 105
    estradiol (*see* bioidentical
      estradiol)
    fear of, 176–178
    horse, 176–177
    vitamin D (*see* vitamin D)
horse hormones, 176–177
hot shower or bath, 89
HRT (hormone replacement
    therapy), 176
Human Genome Project, 134
human microbiome, defined, 133
Huntington's disease, 208–209
hyperpermeability, intestinal, 81
hypertension
    blood vessel damage from, 84, 85
    effects, 76–77

high cholesterol and, 107
sleep apnea and, 32
uncontrolled, 16
vitamin D and, 87
hypothyroidism, 145–160
    aging vs., 147–148
    effects, 149–150
    experiential example, 145–146
    hormone levels, 152
    misdiagnosing, 32, 152–153
    prevalence, 148–149
    symptoms, 146–147, 156–157
    testing, 150–152, 158–159
    treatment, 159–160
    and T4-to-T3 peripheral
      conversion problems, 154–155

ICD-10, 76
iHealth Feel wireless blood pressure
    monitor, 76–77, 86
impure water, 194
inflammation
    carbohydrates and, 139, 200
    and cholesterol, 105
    curcumin blocking, 264
    and estradiol, 179
    food allergens and, 143
    foods increasing, 82
    neurodegeneration and, 53
    omega-6 oils and, 99
    omega-3s and, 100, 257
    Teflon and, 194
    thyroid function and, 156
    vitamin D suppressing, 30, 118
Institute of Neuropathology
    (University of Munich), 44
insulin receptors, 94–95, 201
insulin resistance, 77–78, 95–97,
    201–202, 214–215

insurance coverage
   blood tests, 76
   glucose meters, 97
   polysomnogram, 81
   stool testing, 81–82
InterFase, 82, 142
intestinal hyperpermeability, 81
intravenous tPA (tissue plasminogen
   activator), 59–60
iron, 33, 79, 162, 171–173
ischemic damage, 277
ischemic stroke, 276–277

Jakob, Alfons Maria, 41
JAMA Neurology, 106
jogging, 70–71. *See also* exercise
Journal of Alzheimer's Disease, 199,
   239
Journal of Nutrition, 257
Jung, Carl, 38

Kessing, Lars, 249–250
ketogenic diet, 197–204
   about, 185, 188
   for autophagy, 211
   benefits, 198–199
   carbs vs. fat, 199
   fat and oils in, 202–204
   lowering blood sugar, 98
ketone bodies, 100, 215
ketosis, 189
Keys, Ancel, 204
Kidd, Parris, 284
kidney, hypertension damaging, 85
Klaire Labs, 82, 142–144
Kraepelin, Emil, 38–39, 41
Kresser, Chris, 156

LabCorp, 75
laboratory test order form, 301–302

Lactobacillus, 142, 143
lacunar stroke, 16, 26, 55–58
Lancet, 195
language problems, 9
LDL cholesterol, 78, 106–107
lead, 33, 101, 168–170
leaky gut, 81, 138
learning, estradiol supporting,
   178–179
Lewy, Friedrich H., 41
Lewy bodies, 208
lipid hypothesis, 203–204
lipid panel, 78
liposomal delivery systems, 267
lithium, 36, 67, 247, 253. *See also*
   low-dose lithium
Littlejohns, Thomas J., 117
Llewellyn, David, 117
Longvida, 191, 221, 267–268
loss of initiative, 9
low-carb diet
   about, 185, 187–188, 202
   for autophagy, 211
   lowering blood sugar, 98
low-dose lithium, 244, 247–253
low-protein diet, 186, 189–190
low thyroid. *See* hypothyroidism
Luine, Victoria, 179

mad cow disease, 41
Mary S. Easton Center for
   Alzheimer's Disease Research,
   46
Mayo Clinic, 188, 199
MCI. *See* mild cognitive impairment
MCTs (medium chain triglycerides),
   100, 186, 198, 203, 213–217.
   See also coconut oil
meat, 189–190
Medicare, 76, 81, 97

medication
    developing AD, 50–51
    lowering blood pressure, 88
    statin drugs, 108
medium chain triglycerides (MCTs),
    100, 186, 198, 203, 213–217.
    See also coconut oil
Mellanby, Edward, 116
memory
    Bacopa and, 279
    blood sugar affecting, 92
    blueberries enhancing, 229–230
    and B vitamins, 110
    estradiol supporting, 178–179
    foods damaging, 192–196
    and hippocampus, 63–65
    loss, 9
    mental status testing, 15
    navigational, 64, 229–230
    spatial, 229–230
men, soy consumption in, 196
menopause, 181–182
mental energy, 275–276
mental status testing, 15
mercury, 33, 162–166
    in dental fillings, 165–166
    effects, 162–164
    in fish and fish oils, 164–165
    in seafood, 101, 194–195, 259–
        260
    sources, 83, 164
Meridian Valley Lab, 143
Meriva, 191, 221, 267–268
metabolic biomarker testing, 15,
    23–24
metabolic disruptions, 23
metabolic syndrome, 93–94, 96
Metabolism, 293
metals, toxic. *See* toxic metals
metformin, 292–293

methyl groups and methylation,
    111–112
microbiome
    defined, 132
    gut, 30–31, 81–83, 131–144 (*see*
       also gut microbiome (GM))
    human, defined, 133
microbiota, defined, 132
microdose lithium, 247–253
mild cognitive impairment (MCI)
    and B vitamins, 110
    coconut oil for, 100
    and dementia, 10
    DHA and, 255–256
    elevated blood sugar and, 90–91
    reversal, 20
    testing, 18–19
    vitamin D deficiency and, 115
milk chocolate, 237, 240
Mini-Cog, 15
Mini-Mental State Examination
    (MMSE), 15
mitochondria, 207, 266
mixed dementia, 16
mixed sleep apnea, 125
MMSE (Mini-Mental State
    Examination), 15
molecular biology, 22, 39, 52
molecular biomarker testing
    for cause, 23–25
    cost, 76
    and dementia diagnosis/
       treatment, 2
    for diagnosis, 13
    mild cognitive impairment and, 19
    See also blood tests
monosaccharides, 200
monosodium glutamate (MSG), 196
monounsaturated fatty acids
    (MUFAs), 203

mood, 10, 178–179
Morgenthaler, Timothy, 31–32
Mortby, Moyra, 93
Moser, Edvard I., 229
Moser, May-Britt, 229
MSG (monosodium glutamate), 196
MUFAs (monounsaturated fatty
    acids), 203
multi-infarct dementia. *See* vascular
    dementia (VaD)
multiple modality model, 45–49, 53
Municipal Asylum of Frankfurt, 40
musculoskeletal symptoms, 14

Nathan, David, 92
National Institute on Aging, 12, 199
National Testing Laboratories, 170
natural antibiotics, 82, 143
natural hormone replacement
    therapy (NHRT), 181–182
Nature Medicine, 187
Nature Neuroscience, 237
Nature-Throid, 154–155
naturopathic, defined, 21
navigational memory, 64, 229–230
nerve cells, 46–47
nerve growth factor (NGF), 78, 118
neurodegeneration
    allergies and, 139
    as Alzheimer's cause, 23, 53
    autophagy blocking, 209–210
    bioidentical estradiol preventing,
        175, 178–180
    and biomarker testing, 22
    EFAs preventing, 258
    foods preventing (*see* diets for
        prevention)
    OSA and, 80
    polyphenols and, 236
    strokes and, 58

toxic metals causing, 33
neurofibrils, 42
neurogenesis, 65–66
    blueberries enhancing, 227–228
    defined, 34
    discovery, 52
    enhancing, 297
    exercise and, 70
    and vitamin D, 118
neurologists, conventional, 19
Neurology, 59, 91, 92, 117
Neuromins, 195, 261
neurons, 42, 163
neuroplasticity, 3, 23*fig*, 34, 62, 65–
    66, 69, 169, 185, 228, 258, 277
    disrupts neurogenesis, 152
    and epigenetics, 297
    and thyroid, 150
neuroprotection, 62–63
neuroregeneration, 34, 52, 65–66
neurotransmitter systems, 179, 275
New England Journal of Medicine, 92
New York Times, 248
NGF (nerve growth factor), 78, 118
NHRT (natural hormone
    replacement therapy), 181–
    182
Nilsson, Per, 208
Nissl, Franz, 38
Nixon, Ralph, 187
nonstick coatings on cookware, 194
normal range
    blood pressure, 76, 87
    BMTT, 159
    cholesterol, 78, 107
    fasting blood sugar, 77, 95
    ferritin, 79, 173
    homocysteine, 112
    thyroid, 79, 152
    vitamin D, 75, 78, 119, 120

Nunes, M. A., 250
Nunes, Paula, 249
nutrient deficiencies, 68
nutritional medicines, 48, 98,
    107–108
nutritional supplements, 243–294
    Bacopa monnieri, 245, 279–282
    B-complex vitamins, 112–114
    BDNF enhancing, 34, 36–37
    berberine (*see* berberine)
    citicoline (*see* citicoline)
    for cognitive decline, 36–37
    curcumin (*see* curcumin)
    docosahexaenoic acid (*see*
        docosahexaenoic acid (DHA))
    flaxseed oil (*see* flaxseed oil)
    green tea (*see* green tea)
    iron reducing, 173
    low-dose lithium, 244, 247–253
    lowering blood pressure, 87–88
    lowering blood sugar, 102–103
    omega-3, 100
    phosphatidylserine, 245, 283–287

obstructive sleep apnea (OSA),
    31–32, 80–81
oils. *See* fats and oils
O'Keefe, John, 229
olive leaf extract, 87
omega-3 oils, 100, 185, 201–202,
    256–257. *See also* flaxseed oil
omega-6 oils, 99, 186, 203, 255
oolong teas, 271
oral consumption of hormones, 180
orthomolecular treatment, 48
OSA (obstructive sleep apnea),
    31–32, 80–81
oxidative stress, 219, 252–253
oxygen
    deprivation, 31, 80, 122–123

role of, 94
Oz, Mehmet, 279

Palfrey, Sean, 235
Parkinson's disease, 41, 171, 208–209
Pasinetti, Giulio Maria, 239–240
pathogenic microbes, 136–137, 289
"Pathogenic Microbes, the
    Microbiome, and Alzheimer's
    Disease (AD)" (Hill et. al),
    136–137
Pauling, Linus, 48
periventricular white matter
    changes. *See* white matter
    disease (WMD)
Perlmutter, David, 97, 139, 188
pesticides, 33
phagocystosis, 206
Philips Repironics, 123
phosphatidylserine (PS), 245,
    283–287
pituitary gland, 151
plant sterols, 104, 107
policosanol, 104, 108
polyphenols, 218–223
    and BDNF, 66–68, 221–222
    benefits, 218–219
    cocoa, 237–238 (*see also*
        chocolate and cocoa)
    foods containing, 28, 88, 186,
        190, 221–223, 303–306
    function, 219–220
    lowering blood pressure, 88
    lowering blood sugar, 101–102
    most important, 221
polysaccharides, 201
polysomnogram, 81, 122, 129
polytetrafluoroethylene (PTFE), 194
poppies, California, 288
prebiotics, 82, 143

pregnancy, 195, 260, 278
Premarin, 176–177
prevention
    bioidentical estrogen, 178
    biomarker testing, 13–14
    diets for (*see* diets for prevention)
    importance of early, 299
    stroke, 60
prion-like proteins, 207
probiotics, 82, 142
Proceedings of the American Thoracic Society, 122
Proceedings of the National Academy of Sciences of the United States of America, 69, 110
processed cheese, 192
processed foods, 141, 192–193
processed meats, 192
progesterone, 79–80, 177–178
Proposition 65 (California), 234–236
protein aggregates, 208
protein in diet
    and autophagy, 211–212
    from fish and fish oil, 164
    and grains, 139
    low, 186, 189–190
    and low-carb dieting, 202
    to lower blood sugar, 98
    partially digested, 141
    target ratio of, 199
Provera, 177
PS (phosphatidylserine), 245, 283–287
psychological change, 14
pterostilbene, 226–227
PTFE (polytetrafluoroethylene), 194
Puglielli, Luigi, 106
Punjabi, Naresh M., 122

Rajiv Gandhi Institute of Medical Sciences, 280

Ramalanjaona, Georges, 285–286
rapid blood pressure reduction, 88–89
Rasgon, Natalie, 178
RDAs (government recommended daily allowances), 113
red yeast rice extract, 104, 107
Reed, Bruce, 106
Rendeiro, Catarina, 229–230
resveratrol, 34, 68, 221, 227, 263
"Reversal of Cognitive Decline: A Novel Therapeutic Program" (Bredesen), 46
RIKEN Brain Science Institute, 208
Roberts, H. J., 195
Royal Psychiatric Clinic in Munich, 41
Rush University Medical Center, 12

S-adenosyl methionine (SAMe), 113
Safe Drinking Water and Toxic Enforcement Act (California), 234
SAMe (S-adenosyl methionine), 113
saturated fats, 203–204, 213–214
seafood, 101, 194, 254, 259–260
sex steroid, 79–80
"Should We All Take a Bit if Lithium?" (Fels), 248
silent strokes. *See* lacunar stroke
Sleep, 124
sleep apnea, 121–130
    about, 124–125
    central, 124
    diagnosis, 129–130
    and hippocampus damage, 125–126
    lack of diagnosing, 126–129
    obstructive, 31–32, 80–81
    prevalence, 126

sleep apnea (*continued*)
   as risk factor, 124
   testing, 76
Sleep Heart Health Study, 31
sleep quality, 125–126
small vessel disease, 57
small vessel ischemic disease. *See*
     white matter disease (WMD)
Smith, A. David, 110
snoring, 32, 81, 127, 129
Somer, Elizabeth, 283
soy, 196
spatial memory, 229–230
starches, 139, 201
statin drugs, 108
steroid, sex, 79–80
stool testing, 81
stroke, 55–61
   and cholesterol, 105
   and citicoline, 60–61, 276–277
   estrogen and, 180
   experiential example, 55–57, 86
   ischemic, 276–277
   lacunar (*see* lacunar stroke)
   response to, 59–60
   and VaD prevalence, 57–59
Stroke, 59
sucrose, 200–201
sugar, 200–201. *See also* blood sugar;
    carbohydrates
supplementation
   citicoline, 278
   EFA, 261–262
   nutritional (*see* nutritional
    supplements)
   phosphatidylserine, 283–284
sweeteners, 188
sweeteners, artificial, 195, 201
symptoms
   behavioral, 14

categories, 14
cognitive, 14
digestive, 81
gut microbiome imbalance, 137,
   139
hypothyroidism, 32, 146–147,
   153, 157–158
insulin resistance, 214
low thyroid hormone, 149–150
mild cognitive impairment, 18
musculoskeletal, 14
sleep apnea, 31, 129
stroke, 58–59
synapses, 66
synaptoplasticity
   about, 34, 66
   Bacopa and, 279–280
   BDNF enhancing, 62–63
systolic pressure, 85

tap water, lead in, 170
tau protein, 208, 257
tea
   black, 191, 271
   green (*see* green tea)
   oolong, 271
Teflon, 194
testing
   baseline, 15
   blood (*see* blood tests)
   home sleep tests, 129–130
   mental status, 15
   metabolic biomarker, 15, 23–24
   molecular biomarker (*see*
    molecular biomarker testing)
   stool, 81
testosterone, 79–80
"The Epidemiology of Adult
    Obstructive Sleep Apnea"
    (Punjabi), 122

Ther-Biotic Complete, 82, 142
"The Role of Autophagy in
    Neurodegenerative Disease"
    (Nixon), 187
thyroperoxidase antibody (TPO), 79
thyroid function, 145–160
    about, 32, 149
    autoimmune thyroid disease,
        155–156
    hypothyroidism (*see*
        hypothyroidism)
    inflammation disrupting, 156
    low thyroid hormone, 149–150
    normal ranges, 79
    testing, 79, 150–152
    treatment, 159–160
thyroid hormone replacement,
    159–160
TMG (trimethylglycine or betaine
    HCl), 113
TNFα (tumor necrosis factor alpha),
    264
tofu, 196
toxic metals, 161–174
    aluminum, 174
    cadmium (*see* cadmium)
    hair analysis, 33, 83
    iron, 171–173
    lead, 168–170
    mercury, 162–166
    testing risks, 161–162
    treatment, 33
TPO (thyroperoxidase antibody), 79
Tran, Vu, 123
transdermal estradiol, 180–181
traumatic brain injury, 252
traumatic encephalopathy, chronic,
    208
treatment, 26–37
    blood pressure, 27

blood sugar, 27–28
    causality and, 13, 24
    cholesterol, 28
    conventional, 19
    diet, 35–37
    exercise and BDNF, 33–34
    gut microbiome, 30–31
    homocysteine, 29
    low thyroid, 32–33
    pillars of, 141–144
    research for, 45–46
    sleep apnea, 31–32
    toxic metals, 33
    vitamin D, 29–30
Tricycline, 82, 143
triglycerides, 78, 186
trimethylglycine or betaine HCl
    (TMG), 113
TSH, 150–152
T4-to-T3 peripheral conversion
    problems, 154–155
Tübinger Chronik, 43
tubulin, 163
tumor necrosis factor alpha (TNFα),
    264
turmeric, 221, 263, 266–267

University of Calgary, 163
University of California, 46, 90, 106,
    171
University of Exeter, 228
University of Munich, 44
University of Oxford, 110, 117
University of Pittsburgh, 69
University of Wisconsin, 124
unsaturated fats, 213
unsweetened chocolate, 101
US Department of Agriculture
    (USDA), 197, 225

US Environmental Protection Agency, 162
US Food and Drug Administration (FDA), 59, 61

van Leeuwenhoek, Antön, 131–132
vascular blockages, 58, 291
vascular dementia (VaD)
    and AD, 26–27
    blueberries and, 230
    defining, 16
    elevated cholesterol and, 78
    and high blood pressure, 84–89
    prevalence of, 57–59
    and stroke, 55–61
    and white matter disease, 57
vitamins
    B-complex (*see* B-complex vitamins)
    hormones vs., 116
    quality, 36–37
    vitamin C, 114
    vitamin D (*see* vitamin D)
    vitamin E, 114
vitamin C, 114
vitamin D, 115–120
    achieving optimum levels, 119–120
    deficiency, 29, 115–116, 117
    as dementia protection, 117–119
    importance of, 30, 116
    lowering blood pressure, 87
    normal range, 75, 78, 119, 120
    receptors, 117–118
    and sunlight, 120

supplementing, 88
testing, 78
vitamin E, 114
Vollala, Venkata Ramana, 280

walking, 70–71, 96
walnuts and walnut oil, 191
water, impure, 194
Weuve, Jennifer, 12
White, Elizabeth Coleman, 224–226
white foods, 193
white matter disease (WMD), 57–58
white matter hyperintensities, 26, 56
white sugar, 188
WHI (Women's Health Initiative), 175–176
women
    and bioidentical estradiol, 175–182
    breast-feeding, 278
    elevated HbA1C in, 91
    hypothyroidism in, 32, 148
    pregnancy, 195, 260, 278
Women's Health Initiative (WHI), 175–176
World Health Organization, 12, 234, 249
Wu, Aiguo, 258

zinc, 114
zonulin, 139

About the Author

Timothy J. Smith, MD, wandered aimlessly through his undergraduate years, attending the University of Wisconsin, the University of Illinois, Harvard University, and Northwestern University before deciding on a career in medicine. He graduated from the University of Cincinnati College of Medicine in 1970, completing his internship at Presbyterian Hospital at Pacific Medical Center in San Francisco and residency in psychiatry, specializing in brain biochemistry, at the University of California, San Francisco, and San Francisco General Hospital. He then trained to become a doctor of traditional Chinese medicine (TCM) in San Francisco, Japan, and China. In addition to his busy clinical family medicine practice, Dr. Smith taught TCM to thousands of physicians at the University of California, Los Angeles. He designed and administered the first TCM certifying examinations for the states of California and Florida and joined the team that created the first national acupuncture certifying examination for physicians, served as president of the American Acupuncture Association, was a founding member of the American Academy of Medical Acupuncture, and was honored to be selected as a delegate member of the first group of American doctors practicing traditional Chinese medicine to travel to China as guests of the government in 1979. In the 1980s and '90s, he turned his attention to integrative, functional, nutritional, and anti-aging medicine, publishing his bestseller *Renewal: The Anti-Aging Revolution* (Rodale, Saint Martin's) in 2000. Since then, Dr. Smith has continued his focus on finding and addressing the molecular causes of disease. Now in his fiftieth year of practicing medicine, he continues to apply the latest research developments in molecular and nutritional medicine, as well as epigenetics, to the prevention and treatment of Alzheimer's and all disease.

Dr. Smith invites you to stay in touch with him:

Email: drsmith@renewalresearch.com
Website: www.timsmithmd.com
Twitter: @TimothyJSmithMD
LinkedIn: https://bit.ly/33fbXIU